Coronary Restenosis

GENERAL SERIES EDITOR
Ronald E. Vlietstra, MD
Department of Medicine (Cardiology)
The Watson Clinic
Lakeland, Florida

OTHER VOLUMES IN THE SERIES
Frank Litvack, *Coronary Laser Angioplasty*
David R. Holmes, Jr. and Kirk N. Garratt, *Atherectomy*

FORTHCOMING VOLUMES
Gerald V. Naccarelli and Enrico P. Veltri, *Implantable Cardioverter Defibrillators*
Steven E. Nissen, *Intracoronary Imaging Techniques*

SERIES IN INTERVENTIONAL CARDIOLOGY

· ·

Coronary Restenosis

EDITED BY

ROBERT S. SCHWARTZ, M.D.

Assistant Professor of Medicine
Consultant, Division of Cardiovascular Diseases
Department of Medicine
Mayo Clinic
Rochester, Minnesota

BOSTON

Blackwell Scientific Publications
Oxford   London   Edinburgh
Melbourne   Paris   Berlin   Vienna

Blackwell Scientific Publications

EDITORIAL OFFICES:
238 Main Street, Cambridge, Massachusetts 02142, USA
Osney Mead, Oxford OX2 0EL, England
25 John Street, London WC1N 2BL, England
23 Ainslie Place, Edinburgh EH3 6AJ, Scotland
4 University Street, Carlton, Victoria 3053, Australia
Arnette SA, 2 rue Casimir-Delavigne, 75006 Paris, France
Blackwell-Wissenschaft, Meinekestrasse 4, D-1000 Berlin 15, Germany
Blackwell MZV, Feldgasse 13, A-1238 Vienna, Austria

DISTRIBUTORS:
USA
Blackwell Scientific Publications
238 Main Street
Cambridge, MA 02142
(Telephone orders: 800-759-6102 or 617-876-7000)

Canada
Times Mirror Professional Publishing
130 Flaska Drive
Markham, Ontario L6G 1B8
(Telephone orders: 800-268-4178 or 416-470-6739)

Australia
Blackwell Scientific Publications (Australia) Pty Ltd
54 University Street
Carlton, Victoria 3053
(Telephone orders: 03-347-0300)

Outside North America and Australia
Blackwell Scientific Publications, Ltd.
c/o Marston Book Services, Ltd.
P.O. Box 87, Oxford OX2 0DT, England
(Telephone orders: 44-865-791155)

Typeset by Pine Tree Composition
Printed and bound by The Maple-Vail Book Manufacturing Group
Designed by Joyce C. Weston

© 1993 by Blackwell Scientific Publications
Printed in the United States of America
92 93 94 95 5 4 3 2 1

Library of Congress Cataloging in Publication Data
Coronary restenosis / edited by Robert S. Schwartz.
　　　p.　cm. — (Series in interventional cardiology)
　　Includes bibliographical references and index.
　　ISBN 0–86542–222–2
　　1. Coronary artery stenosis.　2. Transluminal angioplasty–
–Complications and sequelae.　I. Schwartz, Robert S. (Robert
Stockton), 1951– .　II. Series.
　　[DNLM: 1. Angioplasty, Transluminal, Percutaneous Coronary.
2. Coronary Disease—therapy.　3. Recurrence.　WG 300C8256]
RC685.C58C67　1992
616.1'23—dc20
DNLM/DLC
for Library of Congress　　　　　　　　　　　　　　92–13565
　　　　　　　　　　　　　　　　　　　　　　　　　　　　　CIP

Contents

Contributors

J. J. Badimon
Associate Professor of Medicine
Harvard Medical School
Massachusetts General Hospital
Boston, Massachusetts

L. Badimon
Assistant Professor of Medicine
Harvard Medical School
Massachusetts General Hospital
Boston, Massachusetts

Peter Barath, MD, PhD
Research Scientist
Department of Cardiology
Cedars-Sinai Medical Center
Los Angeles, California

Malcolm R. Bell, MBBS, FRACP
Cardiovascular Division
Mayo Clinic
Rochester, Minnesota

Bojan Cercek, MD
Associate Cardiologist
Cedars-Sinai Medical Center
Los Angeles, California

James H. Chesebro, MD
Division of Cardiovascular
    Diseases and Internal Medicine
Mayo Clinic
Rochester, Minnesota

Jesse W. Currier, MD
Assistant Professor of Medicine
Boston University School of
    Medicine
Evans Memorial Department
    of Clinical Research and
    Department of Medicine
Boston University Medical
    Center
Boston, Massachusetts

William D. Edwards, MD
Professor of Pathology
Mayo Medical School
    and Mayo Graduate School
    of Medicine;
Consultant, Division of Pathology
Mayo Clinic Foundation
Rochester, Minnesota

James A. Fagin, MD
Director, Vascular Biology
    Program
Cedars Sinai Medical Center
Assistant Professor of Medicine
UCLA School of Medicine
Los Angeles, California

David P. Faxon, MD
Professor of Medicine
Boston University School
of Medicine
Director, Interventional
Cardiology
The University Hospital
Boston, Massachusetts

James J. Ferguson, III, MD
Cardiology Research
Texas Heart Institute
Houston, Texas

David P. Foley
Thoraxcenter, Erasmus
University
Rotterdam, The Netherlands

James S. Forrester, MD
Director, Division of Cardiology
George Burns and Gracie Allen
Professor
Cedars Sinai Medical Center
Professor of Medicine
UCLA School of Medicine
Los Angeles, California

George I. Frank, MD, FACP
Associate Clinical Professor
of Medicine
University of Washington
Seattle, Washington

Robert Leo Frye, MD
Past President, American College
of Cardiology
Chairman, Department
of Medicine
Mayo Clinic
Rochester, Minnesota

V. Fuster, MD
Chief, Cardiac Unit
Mallinkrodt Professor of Medicine
Harvard Medical School
Massachusetts General Hospital
Boston, Massachusetts

Kirk N. Garratt, MD
Consultant, Division
of Cardiovascular Diseases
and Department
of Internal Medicine
Mayo Clinic;
Instructor in Medicine
Mayo Medical School
Rochester, Minnesota

Bernard J. Gersh, MB, ChB, DPhil, FRCP
Consultant in Cardiovascular
Diseases
Mayo Clinic
Professor of Medicine
Mayo Medical School
Rochester, Minnesota

Geoffrey O. Hartzler, MD, FACC
Consulting Cardiologist
Mid America Heart Institute
St. Luke's Hospital;
Clinical Professor of Medicine
University of Missouri at Kansas
City
Kansas City, Missouri

James Hearn, MD
Division of Cardiovascular Diseases
University of Alabama at
Birmingham
Birmingham, Alabama

Walter R. M. Hermans
Thoraxcenter, Erasmus
  University
Rotterdam, The Netherlands

David R. Holmes, Jr., MD
Director, Adult Cardiac
  Catheterization Laboratory
Division of Cardiovascular
  Diseases
Mayo Clinic
Rochester, Minnesota

Kenneth C. Huber, MD
Senior Interventional Fellow
Division of Cardiovascular
  Diseases
Mayo Clinic
Rochester, Minnesota

Spencer B. King, III, MD
Professor of Medicine
Director, Andreas Gruentzig
  Cardiovascular Center
Emory University School
  of Medicine
Atlanta, Georgia

**David William Marshall Muller,
  MBBS, FRACP**
Director, Experimental
  Angioplasty Program
University of Michigan Medical
  Center
Ann Arbor, Michigan

Elizabeth G. Nabel, MD
Associate Professor of Medicine
Attending Physician, University
  Hospital
University of Michigan Medical
  Center

Ann Arbor, Michigan

Gary J. Nabel
Associate Professor of Medicine
  and Biological Chemistry
Associate Investigator, Howard
  Hughes Medical Institute
University of Michigan Medical
  Center
Ann Arbor, Michigan

James H. O'Keefe, Jr, MD, FACC
Assistant Professor of Medicine,
  Cardiology
University of Missouri at Kansas
  City
Kansas City, Missouri

Gregory Plautz, MD
Post Doctoral Fellow
Departments of Internal
  Medicine and Biological
  Chemistry
University of Michigan Medical
  Center
Ann Arbor, Michigan

Benno J. Rensing, MD
Thoaxcenter, Erasmus University
Rotterdam, The Netherlands

Gary S. Roubin, MD, PhD, FACC
Associate Professor of Medicine
Director of Interventional
  Cardiology and Cardiac
  Catherization Laboratory
Division of Cardiovascular
  Diseases
University of Alabama
  at Birmingham
Birmingham, Alabama

Robert S. Schwartz, MD
Assistant Professor of Medicine
Consultant, Division of
    Cardiovascular Diseases
Department of Medicine
Mayo Clinic
Rochester, Minnesota

P. W. Serruys, MD, PhD
Professor of Interventional
    Cardiology
Erasmus University
Rotterdam, The Netherlands

**Professor Ulrich Sigwart, MD,
    FACC, FESC**
Professor of Medicine
Department of Invasive
    Cardiology
Royal Brompton National Heart
    & Lung Hospital
London, England

Eric J. Topol, MD
Chairman, Department of
    Cardiology

The Cleveland Clinic Foundation
Cleveland, Ohio

Willem J. van der Giessen, MD
Department of Cardiology
Thoraxcenter, Academic Hospital
Laboratory for Experimental
    Cardiology
Erasmus University
Rotterdam, The Netherlands

James T. Willerson, MD
Professor and Chairman
Department of Internal Medicine
University of Texas Medical
    School; Director, Cardiology
    Research
Texas Heart Institute
Houston, Texas

P. Zoldhelyi, MD
Cardiology Fellow
Division of Cardiovascular
    Diseases and Internal Medicine
Mayo Clinic
Rochester, Minnesota

Foreword

UTILIZATION of percutaneous transluminal coronary angioplasty (PTCA) in the management of patients with coronary artery disease has expanded dramatically during the decade of the 1980s. It is estimated that well over 200,000 PTCAs were performed in 1989. The dramatic increase in frequency of PTCA has occurred in spite of the persisting problem of restenosis. However, from a clinician's point of view, restenosis remains as a major flaw in the overall expectations associated with PTCA. While those performing PTCA point to the ease with which repeat PTCA can be performed, the costs and utilization of resources to accomplish repeated dilatations in a given patient cannot easily be ignored. Fortunately, as reflected in the work of the contributors to this volume, those engaged in performance of PTCA and others are committed to a careful study of the perplexing problem of restenosis.

Restenosis has forced a review of the most fundamental, biologic responses to injury, as well as the development of the atherosclerotic plaque and its instability. Von Rokitansky was the first to suggest recurrent thrombosis as an important factor in the development of atheroma and Duguid provided graphic support for this concept in 1946 with simple but elegant descriptive studies of human coronary atheroma. The essential components of a rational approach to thrombus formation can be focused in Virchow's triad which includes changes in the vessel wall, coagulation, and blood flow. This triad seems an essential framework for approaching the biology of restenosis and the current monograph reflects such a consideration of all components of the triad.

The intensity of the local response to angioplasty contributes to the resistance for any easy solution to the problem of restenosis. I suspect we will not solve the problem of restenosis without the ability to modify not only thrombotic propensities, but the stimulating effects of growth factors, all of which is addressed in the current volume.

Can we identify why specific patients or specific lesions do not develop restenosis? While there is a great deal of pessimism with such high restenosis rates noted currently, it is remarkable that in fact restenosis is not even higher given the trauma within the artery at the site of dilatation. What are the instrinsic patient or lesion features that resist restenosis? Efforts to characterize noninvasively the composition and characteristics of targeted lesions seems an attractive approach for further investigation. Hopefully with the new knowledge derived from carefully planned experiments, it will be possible to reduce the restenosis rate from the 30% to 40% range to more acceptable levels. I applaud the efforts of those contributing to this important monograph and their efforts to deal with a pressing clinical problem in the management of patients with coronary artery disease.

ROBERT L. FRYE, M.D.
Mayo Clinic
Rochester, Minnesota

Preface

CORONARY angioplasty has become an integral and important part of the practice of cardiology since its beginnings in the late 1970s. Tremendous technical advances have enabled the percutaneous approach to combat complex coronary disease virtually anywhere in the coronary tree. Newer interventional technologies are undergoing evaluation, many of which will add even more to our technical prowess. Despite these advances in an explosive field, there has been virtually no progress made in solving the "Achilles' Heel" of angioplasty: coronary restenosis. The restenosis problem remains perplexing and recalcitrant. Many ideas for effective treatments and subsequent trials have been shown to be clinical failures.

Indeed, we may be more confused than ever about this problem, as evidenced by the disparity of markedly different approaches ranging from smooth muscle cell toxins to arterial gene therapy and advanced molecular biology. In many ways, our view of restenosis resembles that of the six blind men feeling different parts of the elephant, each relating to only a single aspect of the problem.

This book was thus difficult to plan, since it was important to not only cover the basic hypotheses regarding restenosis, but also to gain perspective on our current failure in many expensive and time-consuming clinical trials. Needless to say, in this first edition there are no solutions to the problem, only material that when taken as a whole may permit a better overall perspective on the problems and potential solutions.

With research into restenosis moving so rapidly, it was critical to plan and execute the book in as short a time as possible. Planned obsolescence is thus inherent in this undertaking, so that future editions may be able to track the research and clinical trials to the point where a totally effective therapy has been found. If an effective therapy is to be found, it now seems that it will result only from calculated and methodical research into fundamental cellular mechanisms and processes. The time and money spent on negative clinical trials should serve as a note of caution to avoid planning additional trials based on scant data or unsupported hypotheses. Future editions of the book will track the exciting stories which are no doubt currently unfolding, one or more of which may lead to the solution.

I must give enormous credit in the production of this book to Ron Vlietstra for his guidance, vision, and persistence. Vicky Reeders of Blackwell Scientific Publications also deserves much credit for her patience and technical direction. I am also especially grateful to Mr. John DeHaan of the DeHaan Foundation for his ongoing support. Finally, I want to thank my wife Beth and my children Jonathan, Andrew, and Elise for their patience and understanding during all the lonely evenings spent while manuscripts were being prepared.

ROBERT S. SCHWARTZ, M.D.

Series Preface

T H I S is the third book in a series dedicated to bringing the clinician authoritative up-to-the-minute information on new interventional cardiology issues. Interestingly, this particular volume posed some conceptual problems in planning. At first one might consider the issue of restenosis to be out of place in a series dealing with techniques. However, restenosis complicates and frustrates every coronary interventional technique. Indeed many of the newer approaches have been developed with the primary objective of lessening the luminal obstruction that this healing process causes.

The expert contributors summarize the diverse and determined efforts that are being brough to bear on the issue. At a time when there are real financial and regulatory disincentives to clinical research, an impressive body of data has been accumulated. It is pleasing that there is now a growing involvement of basic scientists as well as clinicians. The contributions of both blend especially well in this book.

The finished product is also a tribute to Dr. Schwartz. His pleasant, but persistent, manner has led to the prompt development of a most comprehensive manuscript. To his accomplishments as an engineer and a clinician/investigator, he demonstrates that he is also a most competent book editor.

Vicky Reeders, Kathleen McCormack and Katie Grimes continue to steer the project from Blackwell Scientific Publications. Their astute, accelerated processing of this and other manuscripts in the series has been accomplished with a calm, lucid handling of the diverse challenges posed by sometimes demanding physician contributors (and editors!).

We often hear rather confident predictions that the clinical problem of restenosis will soon be solved. I hope so, but is is not outside the bounds of possibility that the problem of restenosis will outlive each of the current devices that provoke it. Whatever the outcome, this book will stand as an accurate and current statement of the issues.

RONALD E. VLIETSTRA
Series Editor

Coronary Restenosis

CHAPTER **1**

· ·

Restenosis: Historical Perspectives

——

GARY S. ROUBIN

——

Early Concepts and Confusion

EARLY in the application of percutaneous transluminal coronary angioplasty (PTCA)—the late 1970s and early 1980s—fascination with the initial angiographic and clinical results and efforts to master the various technical problems dominated the practice of PTCA. Andreas Gruentzig saw little restenosis in his first 30 patients, but as his experience increased he noted between 25% and 30% of patients in his carefully studied initial series returned with angiographic evidence of lesion recurrence (1,2). Because the long-term consequences of coronary dilatation were still unknown and all of the initial patients were surgical candidates, many were referred for bypass surgery. Realization that the vast majority of patients with restenosis could be managed with repeat dilatation had to wait another 5 years. Gruentzig made another initial observation that continues to complicate the study of coronary intervention and restenosis. In some patients, initial suboptimal results (usually luminal haziness) improved over time as the balloon injury healed. He also noted that a simple 20% reduction in luminal diameter narrowing produced salutary clinical results in the majority of patients. Into the early 1980s there was still confusion and debate concerning the mechanism of balloon dilatation. Gruentzig's early "compression and remodelling" concepts were probably partly true for his early patients with "young" lesions consisting of ulcerated plaque and organized thrombus. However, the importance of stretching and splitting of the vessel wall soon became apparent (3). Patients returned then, as they do now, from weeks to many months after PTCA with recurrent narrowing at the PTCA site. Debate focused on the contribution of thrombus versus neointimal proliferation. Some even suggested an inflammatory response. However, there were very few deaths and a paucity of material for direct pathologic examination. A number of early clinical observations and reports added to the confusion and were responsible for the direction of early pharmacologic intervention studies. Patients with coronary spasm had an increased risk of restenosis, a finding later confirmed by French investigators (4). More importantly, young patients with early symptoms, unstable ischemic syndromes, severe symptoms, soft lesions, and evidence of thrombus seemed to present more frequently with lesion recurrence (5,6).

Early Randomized Trials and Observational Studies

The value of antiplatelet therapy with aspirin and anticoagulant therapy with heparin in preventing acute thrombosis during or soon after PTCA was recognized from the outset. Based on early clinical observations, it seemed reasonable to assume that accumulation of clot at the dilatation site after heparin withdrawal might cause or predispose to restenosis. Gruentzig instigated the first randomized trial in interventional cardiology. This trial compared aspirin therapy alone to periprocedural aspirin followed by coumadin therapy alone at the time of hospital discharge (7). Always cautious of complications and searching for practical therapies, Gruentzig's first trial was flawed in that therapeutic levels of anticoagulation were not achieved for some days after vessel wall injury. Thrombus was probably not prevented in this trial and the negative results did not dispel the thrombus theory of restenosis. A later trial examined the effect of 12 to 18 hours of heparin but not the effect of longer term anticoagulation (8). The issue is now being reexamined with more effective antithrombin and antiplatelet agents. It is of some historical interest that one German group reported restenosis of only 15% in a carefully followed group of patients treated with up to 1 gram aspirin daily (9).

With the contribution of arterial spasm in mind, another early randomized trial examined the effect of the calcium antagonist nifedipine on restenosis, again with a negative result (10). Other calcium channel blockers also failed to prevent restenosis (11). These studies were the forerunners of numerous randomized trials of systemic therapies, all of which have failed to have a clinically significant impact on restenosis rates. The instigation of randomized trials and the accumulation of observational data raised the question of definitions of restenosis, and much intellectual effort was wasted in debating these issues rather than devoting energies toward understanding the underlying mechanism. From a practical standpoint, all three commonly used definitions were of value: (1) loss of 50% of the original gain, (2) increase by 30% of the luminal diameter stenosis, and (3) return of the lumen to 50% diameter narrowing. Each emphasized a binary outcome of late angiographic success versus late angiographic "failure." Although these were not as sensitive a measure for detecting a difference in outcome as analysis using the follow-up angiographic stenoses as continuous variables, they had practical advantages. Any therapy likely to have an important beneficial clinical impact on patients after PTCA would have been detected by any of these definitions.

Regardless of definition, observational studies provided some well-established patterns in the occurrence of restenosis after PTCA. The most consistent finding was the relationship between inadequate initial results and the recurrence of an angiographically and clinically significant lesion (5,6,12–14). This observation became the primary impetus for the development of techniques that would optimize initial angiographic results. A number of studies also confirmed the difference between coronary vessels. Restenosis occurred more frequently in the left anterior descending artery than in the right coronary and left circumflex arteries (6). Proximal lesions had more restenosis than distal lesions, as did ostial lesions, branch point stenoses, and lesions in tortuous segments (14). The unifying but unrecognized relationships were probably related to increased arterial medial damage and inadequate initial results. One interesting observation that could not be explained at the time was the presence of localized intimal flaps and tears having a positive effect in decreasing the restenosis rate (15). After a decade of hindsight and the benefit of contemporary imaging technology such as intraarterial ultrasound, it appears the presence of an intimal tear reflected adequate dilatation and less frequent vessel wall recoil, a mechanism now recognized as important in restenosis for some patients (J.M. Tobis, personal communication).

Unstable ischemic syndromes and unstable coronary lesions were recognized as descriptors for restenosis. Risk factors for coronary atherosclerosis also emerged in some studies. The most important of these was insulin-dependent diabetes mellitus (5). Cigarette smoking (16) and hyperlipidemia (16–18) were also noted in some studies.

About the same time, Waller and colleagues published the first pathologic studies in patients dying from cardiac and noncardiac causes from weeks to many months after PTCA (19). They reported a proliferative lesion in some patients, but lesions indistinguishable from native atherosclerosis in others. They were criticized for the latter finding and their methodology was questioned. Most recently, these findings have been vindicated by atherectomy specimens from some restenotic lesions, showing a predominance of mature atherosclerotic plaque. Similarly, recent angiographic and ultrasound studies have documented early "recoil" of the vessel wall and residual plaque early after balloon dilatation (20,21). In one study, 73% of the available cross-sectional area was taken up by plaque after PTCA (21). It is now recognized that residual mature plaque is an important component of the restenotic lesion in many patients. At the same time, however, Waller's pathologic observations and the emergence of some atherosclerotic risk factors as descriptors for restenosis led some groups to pursue atherosclerosis risk modification as a potential method for reducing restenosis. In general, these efforts have been ineffective. Most recently, however, an aggressive pharmacologic approach to reducing serum lipids has produced some encouraging results.

Understanding the Time Course and Clinical Consequences of Restenosis

As the late clinical and angiographic outcome after PTCA became better understood, clearer concepts of restenosis emerged. It became apparent that restenosis could occur from days to months after PTCA with the peak occurring at about 4 months (22,23). Early restenosis was associated with residual atherosclerotic plaque and severe intimal dissection and the probable accumulation of thrombus at the dilatation site.

Later restenosis usually represented the accumulation of significant neoproliferative tissue or small amounts of contracted healed proliferative tissue in combination with large amounts of residual atherosclerotic tissue (24–26). These processes probably represented a continuum. Early restenosis was frequently associated with unstable ischemic syndromes and myocardial infarction; later restenosis was frequently manifested by return of exertional angina or recurrence of a positive exercise stress study. Late myocardial infarction was rare, a finding consistent with the understanding of underlying pathology. It also became apparent that symptom status late after PTCA had only a modest correlation with angiographic restenosis.

Predischarge exercise scintigraphy was not particularly helpful in predicting late outcome. Although a negative predischarge exercise thallium scan was somewhat predictive of less restenosis, a positive scan was a poor predictor of restenosis. These findings suggested that both "beneficial healing" and "detrimental changes," possibly elastic or plastic recoil, may occur in the days and weeks after PTCA.

By the mid 1980s, repeat PTCA had been performed on many thousands of patients and was recognized as a safe and effective procedure. Success rates of approximately 98% were reported and complications were rare. A difference of opinion emerged concerning the incidence of subsequent restenosis in these patients. In at least one large follow-up study, the restenosis rates after a second PTCA were approximately 30% and not different from initial de novo PTCA (27). Other studies reported higher restenosis rates, especially in patients with two or more previous dilatations to the same site (28).

An important and interesting observation over time has been that many lesions respond to repeated dilatations and that lesion recurrence is not an inevitable event. It also raised mechanistic questions concerning the ability to achieve more optimal results in restenotic lesions and the "limited proliferative potential" of neointimal smooth muscle cells.

Also by the mid 1980s sufficiently large numbers of patients with multilesion and multivessel PTCA had undergone angiographic restudy to allow some assessment of restenosis rates in these circumstances. In multilesion PTCA where the lesions were in the same vessel, restenosis rates per patient were increased, but lesion-specific factors appeared to predispose to restenosis in one lesion and not in another (29). Curiously, a consistent observation was that multivessel PTCA was associated only with modest increases in restenosis rates compared to single vessel

PTCA (29–31). Speculation about this phenomenon continues to center on the increased proliferative potential of unstable, culprit lesions whether they occur in a single or multivessel environment.

Attention to Optimizing Initial Geometry with Balloon Dilatation

As repeated observational studies confirmed a lower incidence of restenosis in lesions with optimal initial results, attention in the mid 1980s turned to how this might be achieved with balloon dilatation. Until this time most experienced operators had chosen balloon sizes equal to or slightly smaller than the diameter of the artery to avoid severe dissection or even rupture of the vessel. If suboptimal results were obtained with initial inflations, balloon size could be increased by 0.5 mm with slightly higher pressures. Two European groups published compelling retrospective observational data showing that dilatation in which the balloon-to-artery diameter ratio was greater than 1:1 had less restenosis (32,33). One study showed that optimal diameter stenosis results were obtained with a balloon-artery diameter ratio of 1.1:1.3 and that arterial dissection was primarily related to lesion morphology. The other group reported restenosis rates as low as 5% in concentric stenoses where the balloon-artery ratio was greater than 1:1. A prospective randomized trial designed to test this hypothesis was undertaken in a larger group of patients with more complex lesion morphology. This study was halted prematurely because of the increased incidence of complications, particularly dissection and coronary artery bypass grafting (CABG) in the oversized balloon group (34). Final analysis of restenosis rates in the prospectively randomized group showed no trend toward lower restenosis in the oversized balloon group. Because of the unreliable immediate effect of oversized balloon dilatation and the disappointing late results, this approach has been largely abandoned.

Over the years attention has also been directed toward inflation pressures, rate of inflation, the number of balloon inflations, and total inflation time (35,36). Higher balloon pressures have been associated with better initial results but higher restenosis rates (37). However, these studies did not account for the important confounding effect of inflation pressure on balloon size and the influence of different balloon materials that determine the inflation pressure–balloon diameter relationship. Controlled studies examining these factors have not been done.

The number and duration of balloon inflations have also been associated with increased restenosis rates, but it has been difficult to separate these factors from lesion response to repeated balloon inflations. Prolonged balloon inflations have been recognized for many years as being associated with more optimal initial results, but prospective randomized studies have had to await the development of balloon technology, particularly autoperfusion balloons. To date, however, no convincing evidence has emerged to show that restenosis can be reduced by prolonged balloon inflations.

Understanding and Controlling the Reparative Response to Endoluminal Injury

By the late 1980s, interventional cardiologists began to focus attention on the biology of vascular healing after endoluminal injury (38). They appreciated the importance of a process that had for more than two decades been the research focus of vascular surgeons and vascular biologists. Interestingly, this coincided with the growth of molecular biology and a growing interest in molecular cardiology. Also, several good pathologic studies confirmed (24,25,39) the importance of smooth muscle cell proliferation in the restenotic process and the types of balloon injury that might predispose to an "exuberant overgrowth" response. In particular, multiple anatomic specimens, carefully examined, have shown the apparent migration of cells specifically from deep fissures in the media into the neoproliferative lesion (25).

Over the last 5 years our understanding of smooth muscle cell biology has grown exponentially (40). Initial emphasis on modulating single "growth factors" (e.g., platelet-derived growth factor) has shifted to understanding the complex and large array of extracellular and intracellular factors that modulate protein synthesis smooth muscle cell migration, replication, and hypertrophy. There has been an increasing understanding of the importance of extracellular, proteoglycan matrix secretion in the genesis of the neointimal lesion after PTCA.

We now recognize that smooth muscle cells undergo transformation from the dormant contractile phenotype to the migratory, proliferative, or secretory phenotype as new genes are expressed. These changes are reflected by a marked increase in certain types of receptors on the smooth muscle cell membrane. By linking certain naturally occurring toxins to proteins recognized by these receptors, the potential exists for targeting and disabling only actively proliferating cells. Other investigators have linked specific ribosomal toxins to monoclonal antibodies that have a high specificity for medial and subintimal smooth muscle cells (41). It seems inevitable that advancing biotechnology will allow us to control the proliferation and secretion of the smooth muscle cell, but local delivery of these agents to the offending arterial wall segment still seems crucial (42). One current challenge is the development of catheters capable of placing drugs at the potentially restenotic site without causing additional vascular injury.

Molecular studies have also opened the way for more innovative medical therapies. Based on our understanding of the expression of angiotensin mRNA in the arterial wall and the promotion of platelet derived growth factor-like substances by angiotensin, investigators have been able to show that high doses of angiotensin-converting enzyme inhibitors could prevent smooth muscle cell proliferation in the rat model (43). Administered in clinically tolerable doses, however, these agents have failed to provide any salutary effect in man. Whether this represents species differences in response or dosage effects or other factors has not been determined. Other studies are now focusing on the relationship between smooth muscle cell injury, O_2 free radical generation, and the effect of this process on smooth muscle cell protein synthesis. Further studies are unraveling the importance of the fibrinolytic system on directing smooth muscle cell migration. The complex relationships among the endothelium, platelets, procoagulant proteins, and endoluminal injury are increasingly better understood.

Optimizing Luminal Geometry with New Interventional Devices

The late 1980s also saw the introduction of a plethora of new interventional devices, all conceived to address the shortcomings of balloon dilatation. Restenosis after balloon angioplasty was a dominant concern, but reducing acute closure (acute restenosis) and procedural complications were also important objectives. It is increasingly clear that these processes are related. The principle behind the development of new devices was the need to optimize the initial luminal result while limiting the amount of smooth muscle cell damage. It has also been thought for many years that both the stretching of smooth muscle cells and fissuring of the medial layer by the balloon were primary stimulants to smooth muscle cell overgrowth. Blood flow characteristics, which may be important to smooth muscle cell proliferation, were also thought to be suboptimal after balloon dilatation.

Two approaches were adopted—plaque ablation and intraluminal stenting. The first plaque ablation device to be used clinically was directional atherectomy (44). Despite producing optimal angiographic results, restenosis rates have been disappointing (45). This may be related to the "Dotter" and stretching effect of this device in addition to its cutting or ablating effect. The other ablation devices now in use (i.e., excimer laser and rotablator probes) do not stretch the medial layers, but are limited in the amount of plaque they ablate. They deliver their own form of "traumatic" energy to the vessel wall. Because adjunctive balloon dilatation is frequently necessary, the perceived possible benefit on restenosis now seems ill conceived and this has been borne out in clinical studies. Only stenting with the tubular slotted (Palmaz–Schatz) stent has been shown in observational studies to possibly reduce restenosis (46). Randomized trials are pending. Since the cost of using this device is significantly more than stand-alone balloon therapy and there are potential risks of acute problems, any reduction in restenosis rates will need to be substantial. It is now clear that neither the quantity nor nature of smooth muscle cell proliferation is reduced by any of the new devices (47,48). In the case of stenting, the reliable and optimal initial result seems to mitigate against clinically relevant luminal renarrowing despite a given amount of proliferative response (49).

The availability of new devices has accelerated efforts of interventional cardiologists to approach a large number of stenotic lesions not previously thought appropriate for balloon dilatations. Diffuse and long lesions, tortuous anatomy, and severely diseased saphenous bypass grafts have now become treatable. Importantly, it has been known for many years that the opportunity for restenosis is increased in such lesions. Thus, although these devices had the potential for reducing restenosis, they have paradoxically highlighted the problem.

Restenosis—A Heterogeneous Entity

To the seasoned observer of clinical and angiographic restenosis after PTCA, it is apparent that we are dealing with a heterogeneous entity. Following balloon dilatation, vessel wall recoil, residual plaque burden, thrombus formation, and smooth muscle cell proliferation must all contribute to luminal narrowing to varying degrees (50).

The relative importance of each of these factors varies according to the lesion morphology, procoagulant factors in the blood and vessel wall, and proliferative potential of the vessel wall, the nature of which is still poorly understood. Accordingly, single therapies targeting only one of the contributing causal mechanisms should be expected to have only a modest effect on restenosis. Thus, a stent that addresses only the initial geometric result might be expected to reduce the restenosis rate by only one third (assuming in this proportion of patients, vessel recoil and residual plaque play an important role). Similarly, an overwhelmingly effective antiproliferative agent (and none is yet available) might be expected to reduce the restenosis rate only in that subpopulation of patients who have initially optimal results with little recoil and residual plaque burden. Clearly, overlap between mechanisms occurs and combination therapy may be necessary in certain patients. If we have learned from our past experiences in restenosis research, we should now understand that effective therapies must be based on a clear understanding of the relevant mechanisms in humans and that no single therapy is likely to be effective in all patients.

References

1. Gruentzig AR, Senning A, Siegenthaler WE. Non-operative dilatation of coronary artery stenosis: percutaneous transluminal coronary angioplasty. N Engl J Med 1979;301:61–68.
2. Gruentzig A. Results from coronary angioplasty and implications for the future. Am Heart J 1982;103:779–782.
3. Faxon DP, Sanborn TA, Weber VJ, et al. Restenosis following transluminal angioplasty in experimental atherosclerosis. Arteriosclerosis 1984;4:189–195.
4. Bertrand ME, LaBlanche JM, Fourrier JL, Traisnel G. Percutaneous transluminal coronary angioplasty in patients with spasm superimposed on atherosclerotic narrowing. Br Heart J 1987;58:469–472.
5. Holmes DR Jr, Vlietstra RE, Smith HC, et al. Restenosis after percutaneous transluminal coronary angioplasty (PTCA): a report from the PTCA Registry of the National Heart, Lung, and Blood Institute. Am J Cardiol 1984;53:77C–81C.
6. Leimgruber PP, Roubin GS, Hollman J, et al. Restenosis after successful coronary angioplasty in patients with single-vessel disease. Circulation 1986;73,74:710–717.

7. Thornton MA, Gruentzig AR, Hollman J, King SB, Douglas JS. Coumadin and aspirin in prevention of recurrence after transluminal coronary angioplasty: a randomized study. Circulation 1984;69:721–727.

8. Ellis SG, Roubin GS, Wilentz J, et al. Effect of 18- to 24-hour heparin administration for prevention of restenosis after uncomplicated coronary angioplasty. Am Heart J 1989;117:777–782.

9. Kaltenbach M, Kober G, Scherer D, Vallbracht C. Recurrence rate after successful coronary angioplasty. Eur Heart J 1985;6:276–281.

10. Whitworth HB, Pilcher GS, Roubin GS, et al. Do proximal lesions involving the origin of the left anterior descending artery (LAD) have a higher restenosis rate after coronary angioplasty (PTCA)? Circulation 1985;72:398.

11. Corcos T, David PR, Val PG, et al. Failure of diltiazem to prevent restenosis after percutaneous transluminal coronary angioplasty. Am Heart J 1985;109:926–931.

12. Mata LA, Bosch X, David PR, Rapold HJ, Corcos T, Bourassa MG. Clinical and angiographic assessment 6 months after double vessel percutaneous coronary angioplasty. J Am Coll Cardiol 1985;6:1239–1244.

13. Myler RK, Topol EJ, Shaw RE, et al. Multiple vessel coronary angioplasty: classification, results, and patterns of restenosis in 494 consecutive patients. Cathet Cardiovasc Diagn 1987;13:1–15.

14. Ellis SG, Roubin GS, King SB III, Douglas JS Jr, Cox WR. Importance of stenosis morphology in the estimation of restenosis risk after elective percutaneous transluminal coronary angioplasty. Am J Cardiol 1989;63:30–34.

15. Leimgruber PP, Roubin GS, Anderson HV, et al. Influence of intimal dissection on restenosis after successful coronary angioplasty. Circulation 1985;72:530–535.

16. Galan KM, Hollman JL. Recurrence of stenoses after coronary angioplasty. Heart Lung 1986;15:585–587.

17. Austin GE, Lynn M, Hollman J. Laboratory test results as predictors of recurrent coronary artery stenosis following angioplasty. Arch Pathol Lab Med 1987;111:1158–1162.

18. Jacobs AK, Folan DJ, McSweeney SM, et al. Effect of plasma lipids on restenosis following coronary angioplasty (abstr). J Am Coll Cardiol 1987;9:183A.

19. Waller BF, McManus BM, Gorfinkel J, et al. Status of major epicardial coronary arteries 80 to 150 days after percutaneous transluminal coronary angioplasty. Analysis of 3 necropsy patients. Am J Cardiol 1983;51:81–84.

20. Lehmann KG, Feuer JM, Kumamoto KS, Le HM. Elastic recoil following

coronary angioplasty: magnitude and contributory factors. Circulation 1990;82(suppl III):313.

21. Tobis JM, Mahon D, Lehmann K, Moriuchi M, Honye J, Henry WL. Intracoronary ultrasound imaging after balloon angioplasty 1990;82(suppl III):676.

22. Serruys PW, Luijiten HE, Beatt KJ, et al. Incidence of restenosis after successful coronary angioplasty: a time-related phenomenon. A quantitative angiographic study in 342 consecutive patients at 1, 2, 3, and 4 months. Circulation 1988;77:361–371.

23. Nobuyoshi M, Kimura T, Nosaka H, et al. Restenosis after successful percutaneous transluminal coronary angioplasty: serial angiographic follow-up of 229 patients. J Am Coll Cardiol 1988;12:616–623.

24. Essed CE, Van den Brand M, Becker AE. Transluminal coronary angioplasty and early restenosis: fibrocellular occlusion after wall laceration. Br Heart J 1983;49:393–396.

25. Gravanis MB, Roubin GS. Histopathologic phenomena at the site of percutaneous transluminal coronary angioplasty: the problem of restenosis. Human Pathol 1989;20:477–485.

26. Kimura T, Ohishi H, Horiuchi H, Nosaka H, Nobuyoshi K. Temporal histologic changes of coronary arteries after coronary angioplasty (abstr). Circulation 1990;82(suppl III):616.

27. Black AJ, Anderson HV, Roubin GS. Repeat coronary angioplasty: correlates of a second restenosis. J Am Coll Cardiol 1988;11:714–718.

28. Teirstein PS, Hoover C, Ligon B, et al. Repeat restenosis: efficacy of the third and fourth coronary angioplasty (abstr). J Am Coll Cardiol 1987;9:63A.

29. Roubin GS, Redd D, Leimgruber P, et al. Restenosis after multilesion and multivessel coronary angioplasty (PTCA) (abstr). J Am Coll Cardiol 1986;7:22.

30. Vandormael MG, Deligonul U, Kern MJ, Kennedy H, Galan K, Chaitman B. Restenosis after multilesion percutaneous transluminal coronary angioplasty. Am J Cardiol 1987;60:44B–47B.

31. Lambert M, Bonan R, Cote G, et al. Early results, complications and restenosis rates after multilesion and multivessel percutaneous transluminal coronary angioplasty. Am J Cardiol 1987;60:788–791.

32. Schmitz HJ V, Essen R, Meyer J, Effert S. The role of balloon size for acute and late angiographic results in coronary angioplasty (abstr). Circulation 1984;70(suppl II):295.

33. Hamm C, Kupper W, Thier W, Mathey DG, Bleifeld W. Factors predicting recurrent stenosis in patients with successful coronary angioplasty (abstr). J Am Coll Cardiol 1985;5:518.

34. Roubin GS, Douglas JS Jr, King SB III, et al. Influence of balloon size on initial success, acute complications, and restenosis after percutaneous transluminal coronary angioplasty—A prospective randomized study. Circulation 1988;78:557–565.

35. Sarembock IJ, LaVeau PJ, Sigal SL, et al. The influence of inflation pressure and balloon size on the development of intimal hyperplasia following balloon angioplasty. A study in the atherosclerotic rabbit. Circulation 1989;80:1029–1040.

36. Quigley PJ, Perez J, Mikat E, et al. Effective prolonged balloon inflation on arterial hyperplasia in rabbits. Circulation 1986;4:184.

37. Marantz T, Williams DO, Reinert S, Gewirtz H, Most AS. Predictors of restenosis after successful coronary angioplasty (abstr). Circulation 1984;70(suppl II):176.

38. Liu MW, Roubin GS, King SB III. Restenosis after coronary angioplasty: potential biologic determinants and role of intimal hyperplasia. Circulation 1989;79:1374–1387.

39. Austin GE, Ratliff NB, Hollman J, Tabei S, Phillips DF. Intimal proliferation of smooth muscle cells as an explanation for recurrent coronary artery stenosis after percutaneous transluminal coronary angioplasty. J Am Coll Cardiol 1985;6:369–375.

40. Clowes AW, Schwartz SM. Significance of quiescent smooth muscle migration in the injured rat carotid artery. Circ Res 1985;56:139–145.

41. Casscells W, Wai C, Shrivastav S, et al. Smooth muscle proliferation in vessel injury is characterized by expression of fibroblast growth factor receptors and is inhibited by a toxin-fibroblast growth factor conjugate (abstr). Circulation 1990;82(suppl III):201.

42. Naftilan AJ. Chemical atherectomy: a novel approach to restenosis. Circulation 1991;84:945–947.

43. Powell JS, Clozel JP, Muller RKM, et al. Inhibitors of angiotensin-converting enzyme prevent myointimal proliferation after vascular injury. Science 1989;245:I86–I88.

44. Simpson J, Rowe M, Robertson G, et al. Directional coronary atherectomy: success and complication rates and outcome predictors (abstr). J Am Coll Cardiol 1990;15:196.

45. Hinohara T, Rowe M, Sipperly ME, et al. Restenosis following directional coronary atherectomy of native coronary arteries (abstr). J Am Coll Cardiol 1990;15:196.

46. Schatz RA, Leon M, Baim D, et al. Short-term results and complications with the Palmaz–Schatz coronary stent (abstr). J Am Coll Cardiol 1990;15:117.

47. Hanke H, Haase KK, Hanke S, et al. Excimer laser angioplasty in rabbit

carotid arteries: proliferative response of smooth muscle cells (abstr). Circulation 1990;82(suppl III):494.

48. Kuntz RE, Schmidt DA, Levine MJ, Reis GJ, Safian RD, Baim DS. Importance of post-procedure luminal diameter on restenosis following new coronary interventions (abstr). Circulation 1990;82(suppl III):314.

49. Strauss BH, de Scheerder IK, Beatt KJ, Tijssen J, Serruys PW. Angiographic predictors of restenosis in the coronary wall stent (abstr). Circulation 1990;82(suppl III):540.

50. Waller BF, Pinkerton CA, Orr CM, Slack JD, VanTassel JW. Two distinct types of restenosis lesions after coronary balloon angioplasty: intimal proliferation and atherosclerotic plaques only. An analysis of 20 necropsy patients (abstr). Circulation 1990;82(suppl III):314.

. . . .

CHAPTER 2

Restenosis: A Clinician's Perspective

—

MALCOLM R. BELL
BERNARD J. GERSH

—

Magnitude of the Problem

SINCE the introduction of percutaneous transluminal coronary angioplasty (PTCA) into clinical cardiology practice in 1977 (1), interventional cardiology has developed into a large field that has continued to grow each year. In 1990, approximately 300,000 patients underwent PTCA in the United States alone (data from National Center for Health Statistics) and industry estimates of the number of patients who underwent PTCA in 1991 was approximately 335,000 (Figure 2.1). The introduction of steerable guidewire systems in the early 1980s, increased operator experience, and further refinements in balloon technology have all helped broaden the clinical and anatomic indications for PTCA. More complex lesions (e.g., eccentric, long, or total occlusions) as well as more high-risk patients (e.g., with multivessel disease, unstable angina, acute myocardial infarction, or poor left ventricular function) are being approached with PTCA today. Despite the wider application of PTCA, primary success rates have continued to increase; success rates of over 90% can generally be anticipated with PTCA of nonoccluded vessels in the modern era. Although the risk of abrupt total occlusion

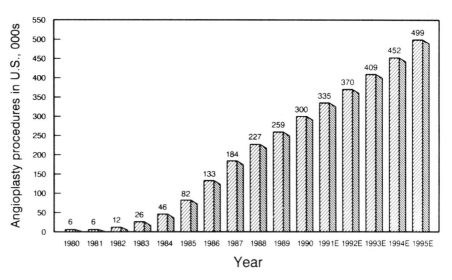

Figure 2.1. Number of coronary angioplasty procedures performed in the United States since 1980. Data from 1980–1990 obtained from the National Center for Health Statistics; estimates (E) for 1991–1995 obtained courtesy of Christopher G. Sassouni, D.M.D. of Raymond James and Associates, Inc., St. Petersburg, Fla.

has decreased since the advent of PTCA (about 5% of procedures at the present time), it is the single most important acute complication of this procedure, often leading to myocardial infarction, emergency surgery, or death.

From the clinician's perspective, the major limitation of PTCA is the high incidence of *restenosis*—emphasized by the realization that after more than a decade of experience, no effective prevention of this problem has been developed. The reported frequency of restenosis varies considerably depending on the definition used and completeness of angiographic follow-up in each series. The overall incidence of restenosis is generally considered to be approximately 35%, although it is considerably higher for some lesions (Figure 2.2; 2). The clinical, social, and economic impact of restenosis may be better appreciated when one considers the absolute number of PTCA failures that currently occur in the United States. Assuming that 335,000 patients in this country underwent PTCA in 1991 and that 301,500 (90%) had an initially successful procedure, at least 106,000 (approximately 35% of 301,500) developed restenosis. Therefore, little more than 50% of the original total treat-

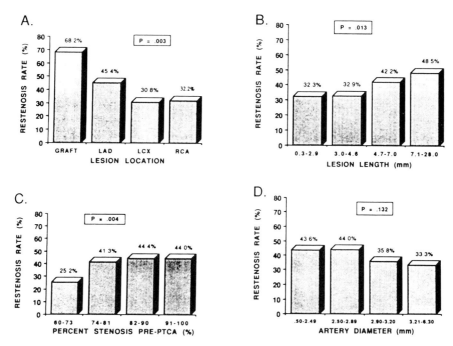

Figure 2.2. Relation of selected preangioplasty variables to coronary restenosis rates among 510 patients (598 successfully dilated lesions) undergoing follow-up coronary angiography. Restenosis rates are divided according to: (*A*) lesion location. LAD = left anterior descending coronary artery; LCX = left circumflex coronary artery; RCA = right coronary artery. (*B*) lesion length (mm) with the lesions segregated by quartiles of length. (*C*) percent stenosis before PTCA with the lesions segregated by quartiles of percent stenosis. (*D*) diameter of the arterial segment (mm) immediately adjacent to the dilated lesion with the lesions segregated by arterial diameter. (Reprinted with permission of the American College of Cardiology from Hirshfeld et al. Restenosis after coronary angioplasty: a multivariate statistical model to relate lesion and procedure variables to restenosis. J Am Coll Cardiol 1991; 18:647–656.)

ment population should be finally considered as having had a completely successful initial procedure.

Since the late 1980s a number of new coronary catheter-based devices have been evaluated and introduced into the interventional cardiology practice. Included among these are various laser angioplasty systems, coronary atherectomy devices, and intracoronary stents. Although these devices have undoubtedly expanded the indications for coronary intervention, a major hope attached to these technologies was that they would significantly affect a reduction of restenosis. Perhaps related to the fact that these devices have simultaneously broadened the indications for coronary intervention with more complex cases being attempted (e.g., long diffuse stenoses, chronic total occlusions, highly eccentric stenoses, ostial locations, vein graft stenoses), restenosis appears to have increased rather than decreased in frequency. For example, the overall frequency of restenosis among patients after excimer laser angioplasty appears to be about 50% (3,4), after directional coronary atherectomy the rate ranges from 26% in de novo native vessel lesions (5) to 50% for all lesions (6), and after rotational atherectomy it has been reported to be 54% for de novo lesions (7). These recent data, some of which are preliminary, support the notion that the new devices have clearly not reduced the incidence of restenosis, and at first glance they appear to be spawning more restenosis; an alternative explanation is that the "true" restenosis rate associated with PTCA may have been underestimated, as suggested by the elegant study of Nobuyoshi and colleagues documenting a restenosis rate after PTCA of almost 50% at 6 months (8).

What impact does restenosis have on event-free outcome following PTCA? The 1-year follow-up findings of the 1985–1986 National Heart, Lung, and Blood Institute (NHLBI) PTCA Registry demonstrated reductions in all major untoward cardiac events compared to the earlier 1977–1981 data, but the use of repeated angioplasty for restenosis had increased by 50% (9). Among all patients in this registry study, 21% required repeat angioplasty by 1 year with similar rates among patients with single and multivessel disease. Only 74% of all successfully treated patients were free of death, myocardial infarction, bypass surgery, or PTCA after 1 year and only 58% were free of these events and asymptomatic—a sobering finding when one recalls that half these patients had single vessel disease. Although restenosis cannot be blamed for all these events, a major reduction in the frequency of restenosis will have an enormous impact on the number of follow-up events occurring after PTCA, particularly with respect to repeat procedures and bypass surgery.

The risk of restenosis increases in patients who have multilesion or multivessel PTCA, although fortunately it does not appear to be arithmetically linear. Two recent reports of patients with multivessel disease undergoing PTCA documented that 50% to 54% of patients returning for catheterization had restenosis in at least one dilated segment and 14% had multiple restenoses (10,11). Restenosis is a time-related phenomenon, tending to occur within the first few months following

PTCA (8,12), and if initially avoided or successfully treated with repeat PTCA or bypass surgery within this first year, the incidence subsequently declines. Although incomplete revascularization and progression of native coronary disease are important factors affecting long-term outcome after PTCA, they play a much smaller role in the first year (Figure 2.3; 10).

Restenosis Definitions: Clinical Interpretation

There is currently no consensus regarding the optimal angiographic definition of restenosis. Quantitative coronary angiographic analysis is now considered by some to be essential to the reporting of restenosis. It avoids the pitfalls of visual diameter stenosis estimation before and

Figure 2.3.   Pie diagrams show angiographic follow-up results within 6 months of multivessel angioplasty. Multilesion restenosis was significantly more frequent in patients with three versus two vessel disease ($p < 0.01$). Progression of native disease was uncommon in both groups. (Reprinted by permission of the American College of Cardiology from Deligonul et al. Coronary angioplasty: a therapeutic option for symptomatic patients with two and three vessel coronary disease. J Am Coll Cardiol 1988; 11:1173–1179.)

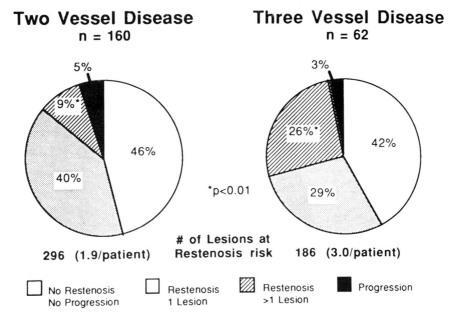

after coronary angioplasty but has limitations in routine clinical practice. It presently remains an investigative tool. Using these methods, the absolute change in minimum luminal diameter can be measured and when used as a continuous variable, these absolute measurements may be useful to those interested in the biologic aspects of the restenosis process. Restenosis viewed as a binary event has been defined by relative changes of vessel diameter (the four NHLBI definitions) (13). These were conceived when visual estimations of lesion severity were common. The definition proposed by Serruys and colleagues (12) entailed a decrease from the post-PTCA luminal diameter of 0.72 mm or greater. This latter criterion may be especially useful for quantitatively defining the degree of restenosis, although it is limited somewhat by not relating the extent of restenosis to the size of the vessel. For instance, a diameter decrease of 1 mm (thus qualifying as restenosis) in a 3- to 4-mm vessel may be of no functional significance. Other definitions using the various NHLBI definitions have been helpful when using visual estimates of coronary stenoses but become more problematic when quantitative angiographic analysis is attempted. The lack of agreement between different definitions of restenosis and the potential confusion that this may produce are illustrated in Figure 2.4.

Although the presence of restenosis defined anatomically is relevant, the major interest for the clinician is whether the lesion results in ischemia or symptoms. Restenosis by some definitions cannot necessarily be extrapolated to imply the presence of a functionally significant coronary obstruction and if, in addition, the patient is asymptomatic, no further mechanical or surgical intervention may be necessary. Therefore, although restenosis may represent a natural response to injury inflicted at the time of angioplasty and should probably be viewed as a continuum, the implications of this process vary for each patient depending on the severity of the resulting luminal obstruction.

Patient Demographic Risk Factors of Restenosis

Methodological Aspects of Restenosis Trials

A multitude of studies report the association of restenosis with specific patient, lesion, and procedural characteristics. The majority, however, have not had the benefit of complete angiographic follow-up. In any re-

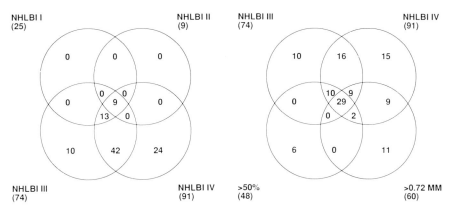

Figure 2.4. The relationships among different restenosis criteria are illustrated with two Venn diagrams. On the left, the relationships among the four NHLBI restenosis criteria are shown while on the right the relationships among the NHLBI III and IV criteria and two additional criteria are shown. The total number of lesions fulfilling each of these criteria are shown in parentheses. (Redrawn by permission of the American Heart Association, Inc. from Serruys et al: Incidence of restenosis after successful coronary angioplasty: a time-related phenomenon. A quantitative angiographic study in 342 consecutive patients at 1, 2, 3, and 4 months. Circulation 1988; 77:361–371.)

view of the incidence and predictors of restenosis, conclusions must be tempered by the fact that symptomatic patients are more likely to undergo repeat coronary angiography than those who remain asymptomatic. This will skew the results toward higher frequencies of restenosis among those patients if only those with follow-up angiography are included in the denominator. The opposite will occur if *all* patients undergoing the procedure are included, not just those undergoing angiography. Symptoms by themselves are not reliable because not all recurrent chest pain can be attributed to restenosis since incomplete revascularization and progression of native coronary disease may also contribute. The sample sizes chosen for these studies have also not always had adequate power to detect patient characteristics that portend a high risk of restenosis (i.e., there is potential for a type II statistical error).

Predictors of Restenosis: Patient Related

Notwithstanding these important limitations, a number of patient-related predictors of restenosis have been documented (Table 2.1). These clinical predictors should be distinguished from lesion- or procedural-

Table 2.1. Patient-Related Potential Restenosis Risk Factors

Strongly Associated

Diabetes mellitus
Continued smoking
Unstable angina pectoris
Variant angina

Less Strongly Associated

Male gender
Hypercholesterolemia
No history of previous myocardial infarction

related predictors, which are discussed in subsequent chapters. Unfortunately, there does not appear to be a consensus regarding the correlation and importance of patient-related risk factors for restenosis, which may be explained in part by the fact that lesion or procedural variables have not always been simultaneously examined in detail. The importance of lesion and procedural variables as predictors of restenosis has been emphasized (14–16). Once these variables have been accounted for, clinical predictors of restenosis are scarce—for example, diabetes mellitus was the only clinical variable independently predictive of restenosis in a model developed by Lambert and colleagues to discriminate clinical and procedural factors in 119 patients undergoing coronary angiography 6 months after PTCA (14).

Diabetes Mellitus: Diabetes mellitus is positively associated with restenosis in many studies (14,17,18) and after multivariate analysis appears to be an important independent risk factor (14,18). However, the lack of consensus in the literature is underlined by the failure of four recently published studies to identify diabetes as a significant risk factor for restenosis (19–22). The M-HEART Group study (22) reported their observations of patient-related variables and risk of restenosis in 722 patients who had successful PTCA, 71% of whom had repeat angiography at a mean of 6 months later. Neither diabetes nor other patient characteristics such as age, sex, cigarette smoking history, history of previous myocardial infarction, or anginal duration and severity were found to be associated with increased frequency of restenosis. Guiteras Val and colleagues, in a study involving 178 patients with a follow-up angiography rate of 98%, also found no association between diabetes and restenosis (20).

Cigarette Smoking: A history of cigarette smoking prior to and up to the time of PTCA has not been correlated with increased risk of restenosis. In contrast, restenosis occurs more frequently among patients who continue to smoke compared to those who do not (19,23,24). Galan and coworkers (24) retrospectively reviewed the frequency of restenosis among 160 patients who underwent follow-up coronary angiography after PTCA, 84 of whom continued to smoke and 76 of whom ceased smoking after the initial PTCA. Continued smoking was associated with a significantly higher risk of restenosis compared with cessation of smoking (55% versus 38%) and was identified as an independent predictor of restenosis.

Unstable and Variant Angina: Follow-up studies of patients with unstable angina who underwent PTCA have documented an overall restenosis rate of 30% to 35%, similar to that anticipated in patients with stable angina (25–35). However, angiographic follow-up rates were not consistently high in these studies and in the majority there were no direct comparisons to patients with stable angina; in addition, widely varied definitions of unstable angina and restenosis were used.

In contrast, several direct comparisons of patients with unstable versus stable angina suggest an increase in incidence of restenosis among patients with unstable angina (21,27,36–38). Bentivoglio and colleagues (36) studied the initial NHLBI PTCA Registry patients and reported that restenosis occurred in 30% of patients with stable compared to 36% of patients with unstable angina; the severity of angina as an independent risk factor for restenosis was confirmed in another NHLBI PTCA Registry study in the same year (13). Leimgruber and coworkers (37) also found that unstable angina was a significant risk factor for restenosis in a study of 998 patients with single vessel disease who underwent PTCA. These findings have been confirmed recently in a study by Johansson and colleagues (38) who found a significantly higher restenosis rate in unstable angina versus stable angina patients (46% versus 29%). In contrast, Luitjen and colleagues (39) examined coronary angiograms from 339 consecutive patients with a quantitative automated edge-detection technique and found no differences in restenosis rates between patients with unstable angina and stable angina, regardless of the restenosis definition used.

The apparent higher frequency of restenosis in unstable angina patients compared to those with stable symptoms may reflect the presence of a more active lesion at the time of dilatation. These lesions are often more complex and more likely to contain thrombus than those not producing unstable symptoms. This might contribute to a more active healing phase with more cellular proliferation leading to more restenosis. Restenosis has also recently been reported to occur much more quickly in patients with unstable angina than in patients with stable symptoms (40). Other factors that may increase the risk of restenosis in patients with unstable angina include the location of lesions in the left anterior descending coronary artery, presence of collateral vessels, ST segment depression, multivessel disease, recent onset of chest pain, multiple luminal irregularities, and poor distal flow (30,41).

An interesting and consistent finding has been the strong association of variant angina with restenosis (20,42–44). Restenosis occurred in 45% of patients with variant angina compared to only 21% of those with stable symptoms in the aforementioned study reported by Guiteras Val and colleagues (20). Recently, abnormal coronary vasoconstriction induced by hyperventilation at the lesion site prior to PTCA has been associated with a greater frequency of restenosis compared to no response to this stimulus (44).

Male Gender: In some studies men have been reported to have a slightly higher restenosis rate than women. Data from the initial NHLBI PTCA Registry revealed that restenosis (an increase of $\geq$ 30% from the immediate post-PTCA stenosis or a loss of $\geq$ 50% of the initial gain) occurred in 187 of 557 patients who had follow-up angiography (33.6%) (13). These data were obtained from 27 clinical centers representing a total of 665 patients who underwent successful angioplasty. Using these criteria ($p < 0.01$), 36% of men and 22% of women developed restenosis. This gender difference persisted even after multivariate analysis was performed. Vandormael and colleagues (45) also showed that male gender was associated with an increased frequency of restenosis among 209 patients undergoing multilesion PTCA. However, recent studies have failed to find significant association between male gender and restenosis (18,19). In summary, the association between gender and restenosis has not been consistent, but a slight preponderance seems to occur in men (16,37,46,47).

Hypercholesterolemia: Hypercholesterolemia as a risk factor for restenosis has not been well characterized. Whereas some studies have suggested that hypercholesterolemia may increase the risk of restenosis

(23,48), others have shown no association (19,49). It is possible that, although hypercholesterolemia is important in atherogenesis, it plays less of a role in the fibroproliferative response that constitutes restenosis. However, methodological issues should also be addressed; for example, many other investigators have studied hypercholesterolemia as a categorical variable that may have less power in detecting an association with restenosis than if serum cholesterol were studied as a continuous variable. Few data are available regarding the association between restenosis and the various apolipoproteins, although in a preliminary study by Hearn and coworkers (50) higher serum levels of lipoprotein-a (Lp[a]) and apolipoprotein B were associated with restenosis. A recent study has described an apparent reduction in restenosis rates with the use of lovastatin after PTCA (51). Problems with interpretation of this study, however, include the relatively small number of patients, the lack of complete follow-up angiography (as well as a significantly lower rate of angiography in the control group), and the fact that some patients did not have elevated lipids at baseline. Further research in this area may be particularly rewarding in view of the recently reported studies describing the regression of coronary atherosclerosis with lipid-lowering agents (52).

History of Prior Myocardial Infarction and Emergency PTCA: The absence of prior myocardial infarction appears to have some protective effect against restenosis after PTCA, although the reasons for this are not clear. Restenosis rates following direct PTCA (primary or adjunctive) for acute myocardial infarction may be associated with a lower risk of restenosis compared to elective PTCA, but the evidence is conflicting. This is particularly interesting since PTCA is often used in some centers as primary therapy for acute infarction, particularly when contraindications for thrombolytic therapy exist. PTCA is also used acutely in cases of apparent thrombolytic failure (adjunctive PTCA). Simonton and colleagues (53) found the restenosis rate among 79 consecutive patients after successful emergency PTCA for acute infarction (90% of whom received high-dose intravenous streptokinase therapy in conjunction with their PTCA) was 19% compared to a restenosis rate of 35% among a contemporary group of consecutive patients who had elective PTCA performed. However, the rate of acute reocclusion was higher in the emergency group than in the elective group (13% versus 2%) and when both the early closure and late restenosis events are summed, no major difference in lesion recurrence is apparent between the two groups.

Direct PTCA without thrombolytic therapy in one large study of 151 patients was associated with a restenosis rate of 31% (54). Recent data from France showed no difference in restenosis rates according to the use of thrombolytic agents in conjunction with PTCA (55). In this study, with 100% angiographic follow-up, the low restenosis rate of 16% in those with thrombolytic therapy was similar to the restenosis rate of 20% in those not receiving thrombolytic therapy. Again, many patients in both groups suffered early reocclusion resulting in combined reocclusion/restenosis rates for each of the two groups of 44% and 47%, respectively. Therefore, interpretation of apparently low restenosis rates after acute PTCA should consider the significant number of vessels that reocclude during hospitalization. A recent analysis of overall restenosis rates following PTCA alone, combined with streptokinase, and PTCA after delayed presentation showed no decrease compared to restenosis following elective procedures (56).

Conclusions

Our ability to predict which patients will experience restenosis based on identification of baseline patient characteristics is poor. This is exemplified by the confusion and the many inconsistencies in the literature in the reporting of patient-related predictive factors. Although methodological problems of such studies may partly explain these inconsistencies, it is becoming increasingly apparent that lesion and procedural variables assume far more importance in the prediction of restenosis. Further support for this is provided by a recently reported statistical model for predicting restenosis based on lesion and procedural variables from the M-HEART study group (2). Although these have not been discussed in detail here, they are discussed at length in the following chapter. From the clinician's standpoint, however, it seems appropriate to pursue the following objectives:

1. Obtain good control of daily serum glucose levels in diabetic patients undergoing PTCA.
2. Counsel smokers to cease smoking after PTCA.
3. Carefully follow patients who have PTCA in the setting of unstable angina to detect early signs of restenosis.
4. Attempt to lower lipid levels in those with elevated levels.

Strategies of Revascularization

How can a clinician choose the most appropriate revascularization strategy, taking into account the risk of future restenosis yet being unable to predict this event with any degree of certainty for an individual patient? This is a difficult question to address and will naturally depend on the specific situation of each patient. As will be discussed in a subsequent chapter, certain lesion characteristics predict an increased risk of restenosis and so these should also be considered when assessing alternative revascularization strategies.

Single and Multivessel Disease

Assuming that the risk of restenosis and repeat intervention are "acceptable" to the patient and physician, PTCA still is a reasonable first approach in the patient with single vessel disease who is refractory to medical therapy. However, since the risk of restenosis is increased in patients with multivessel disease (10), the likelihood of returning for repeat PTCA will be high in this situation. In addition, incomplete revascularization, which occurs in more than 50% of patients with multivessel disease undergoing PTCA, is usually predictable prior to the procedure (10,11). It should also be considered because the combination of both this and restenosis will adversely affect outcome. Nevertheless, PTCA can be effective treatment for many patients with multivessel disease who might otherwise require bypass surgery or for those who have already had surgery and are unsuitable for further surgery. PTCA of vein grafts is generally successful but the high rates of restenosis (> 50%) should be considered when planning a PTCA strategy that includes dilating one or more vein grafts.

Repeat PTCA for Restenosis

Once restenosis occurs, repeat PTCA usually has a high chance of success. An 85% success rate with redilatation of restenotic lesions was reported for the 203 patients who underwent repeat PTCA in the initial NHLBI PTCA Registry (57), with very few major complications. More recent data confirm these findings although the success rates have improved to 92%–98% (58–60). In the study of Black and coworkers (58), a second restenosis occurred in 31% of 151 patients having angiographic follow-up. Correlates were: an interval less than 5 months between the first and second angioplasties, male gender, lesion length of 15 mm or more, and dilatation of an additional site at the time of the second angioplasty.

An intriguing question about the risk of restenosis, relating to the importance of constitutional factors, is whether the risk of restenosis after a second PTCA is higher in patients with a history of restenosis at another site. Berger and coworkers (61) recently reported data from Mayo Clinic comparing 54 patients with no history of restenosis to 67 patients with a history of restenosis at another site—all patients underwent a second PTCA of a de novo lesion. Following the second PTCA, subsequent restenosis rates were 25% and 30%, respectively. This difference was not statistically significant although the small number of patients may have introduced a type II statistical error. However, these preliminary results suggest that there is no substantial increase in restenosis rates for patients with previous restenosis and support the concept that constitutional factors are less important than local anatomic and procedural factors for the development of restenosis.

The Clinical Presentation of Restenosis

Acute closure after successful PTCA occurs in up to 5% of patients during the initial hospitalization phase but probably relates more to the presence of thrombus, intimal dissection, or inadequate dilatation than the primary process of restenosis. Intriguing evidence that "silent" restenosis, or evidence of future restenosis, may be present in some patients within a day or so of PTCA has recently been reported and will be discussed later in this chapter.

Recurrent Angina

The temporal sequence of follow-up angiography, recurrent symptoms, and restenosis was first analyzed in a cohort of patients from the initial NHLBI PTCA Registry by Holmes and coworkers in 1984 (13). In this study, 557 patients who underwent a first angioplasty and had follow-up coronary angiography were evaluated, representing 84% of the total number of eligible patients. The overall restenosis rate in this population was 34%, diagnosed at a median of approximately 6 months following PTCA. The distribution in time to follow-up angiography and com-

RELATIONSHIP BETWEEN TIMING OF FOLLOW-UP
ANGIOGRAPHY AND RESTENOSIS

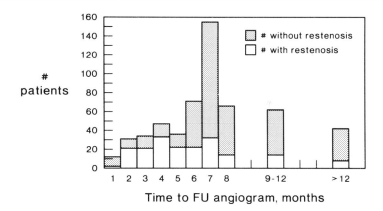

Figure 2.5. Distribution of 557 patients with and without restenosis after PTCA according to time to follow-up (FU) angiography. Restenosis was defined as an increase in stenosis of 30% or greater at follow-up compared to immediately after PTCA. Reprinted by permission of the publisher from Holmes et al. Restenosis after percutaneous transluminal coronary angioplasty (PTCA): a report from the PTCA Registry of the National Heart, Lung and Blood Institute. American Journal of Cardiology, 1984 (13).

parison of patients with and without restenosis is shown in Figure 2.5. It is evident from this figure that the probability of restenosis at angiography was higher in the first 5 months, whereas angiography performed after this time was less likely to reveal restenosis. Of the asymptomatic patients, representing almost half of the total number of patients, only 14% had restenosis confirmed by angiography (Figure 2.6). In contrast, patients with definite or probable angina had a restenosis rate of 56%.

Subsequent reports have confirmed these early findings. An angiographic follow-up study from Emory University of 998 patients with single vessel disease confirmed that the highest rate of restenosis (53%) was observed within the first 4 months after PTCA and that restenosis was an uncommon finding if angiography was performed after 1 year (37). The corresponding percentage of patients with symptoms of chest pain during each of these two periods was 84% and 44%, respectively. The Montreal Heart Institute experience has been similar: in a study

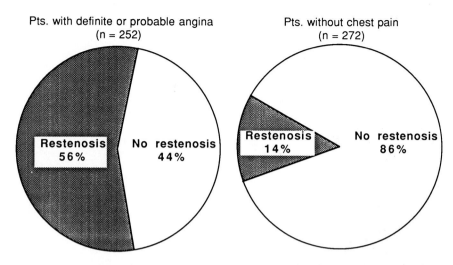

Figure 2.6. Relationship between symptoms and frequency of restenosis in 524 patients returning for follow-up angiography after PTCA. Redrawn by permission of the publisher from Holmes et al: Restenosis after percutaneous transluminal coronary angioplasty (PTCA): a report from the PTCA Registry of the National Heart, Lung and Blood Institute. American Journal of Cardiology, 1984 (13).

where the repeat angiography rate was 98%, restenosis was documented at a median of 4.7 months after PTCA and 92% of patients had restenosis documented within 6 months (20).

In 1988, however, the relationship between the angiographic appearance of restenosis and its clinical consequences was challenged by two elegant and important angiographic studies showing the incidence of restenosis was progressive up to the third month, after which the plateau was reached (8,12). At the time of angiography only 23% of the total population in Serruys' study was symptomatic (12). In contrast, 76% of patients with restenosis in the initial NHLBI PTCA Registry had definite or probable angina at the time of angiography (13). Repeat catheterization in the study of Serruys and colleagues was predetermined per protocol, whereas it was performed voluntarily at the various NHLBI registry sites at intervals determined by patient symptoms or physician preference. Therefore, although many patients with restenosis will present to their physician with anginal symptoms, these more recent data emphasize that restenosis is primarily an angiographic diagnosis and thus its true incidence can be determined only by routine angiography.

The discrepancy between the incidence of angiographic restenosis and the relative lack of symptom recurrence in some patients raises several issues. First, although the "gold" standard is an angiographic definition, from the perspective of the clinician and patient, the presence of symptoms or ischemia on functional testing may be the most important end point. Second, although a 70% lesion may indicate restenosis, it may not be as significant as the original 95% stenosis that was the target of the initial PTCA. Finally, in patients with multivessel disease, is the lack of symptoms following restenosis a function of misidentification of the "culprit lesion" or is it a reflection of concomitant medical therapy?

Myocardial Infarction and Death

Clinical experience and the paucity of myocardial infarction or death secondary to restenosis suggest that these untoward cardiac events rarely result from restenosis. In view of the high incidence of restenosis, this indeed is fortunate. The findings of two studies with a combined population of 457 patients indicate that the risk of myocardial infarction or death as a direct result of restenosis is less than 2% (62,63).

Noninvasive Detection of Restenosis

Restenosis is generally considered an angiographic definition and therefore coronary angiography is currently considered to be the "gold" standard for defining its presence or absence. Numerous reports in the literature over the last decade describe the value of various noninvasive techniques for detecting restenosis compared to coronary angiography. Moreover, functional testing identifies the contribution of restenosis to ischemia. For the clinician and patient, this may be the most relevant end point. However, any comparisons between noninvasive techniques and coronary angiography should consider a number of important caveats.

In the early era of PTCA in this country, follow-up angiography was commonly performed. This has become far less common in the last 5 years. Instead, patients are generally sent for angiography because of symptoms or findings on functional testing. The timing of angiography also varies considerably from patient to patient, and many studies have not included consecutive series of patients who have all had noninvasive testing and catheterization. In addition, not all patients with symptoms or with objective evidence of ischemia will have restenosis since progression of native disease and residual ischemia from incomplete revascularization may also contribute to these events. With the introduction over the last few years of new coronary intervention devices, many investigators at various testing sites have insisted on more complete angiographic follow-up, which may provide the opportunity for evaluation of newer noninvasive techniques to detect restenosis.

Exercise Electrocardiography Testing

Bicycle exercise tests proved to be valuable in the documentation of restenosis among the initial patients treated by Gruentzig (64). However, although treadmill or bicycle exercise electrocardiography (ECG) may be useful for follow-up after PTCA for single vessel disease (65), it is less likely to be useful for multivessel disease (66). Although a positive exercise test may identify patients with restenosis after PTCA, up to 20% of patients with restenosis will be missed by using this method alone (67). The predictive value of ST segment depression alone is low (68), but in patients who are asymptomatic and have a negative exercise test, the risk of missing restenosis is quite low (68,69). Little information about exercise ECG testing to detect restenosis after emergency PTCA for acute myocardial infarction is available, but the observations of Honan and colleagues (70) suggest it is of limited value.

A divergence of opinion remains as to the real utility of exercise ECG testing after PTCA to detect restenosis. When used alone it probably has limited value when performed routinely after PTCA, particularly in patients with multivessel disease. In patients with multivessel disease restenosis will undoubtedly involve more complex physiologic responses compared to single vessel disease. For example, whether patients with multivessel disease are symptomatic or not, a positive test generally cannot distinguish restenosis and ischemia from incomplete revascularization or identify the number or location of restenosis sites. Laarman and colleagues (69) have emphasized that low sensitivity of the exercise ECG for detecting restenosis in asymptomatic patients mitigates against the value of routine stress testing. It is also uncertain whether subsequent intervention in patients with single vessel disease and silent restenosis will improve long-term prognosis.

Exercise Thallium 201 Scintigraphy

In contrast to the limited value of exercise ECG testing to detect restenosis, thallium 201 perfusion imaging considerably improves the value of treadmill testing. The superiority of perfusion imaging over exercise ECG testing has been clearly demonstrated in a number of studies (71–75). Wijns and coworkers (74) reported the results of exercise thallium scintigraphy performed in 89 patients within 4 weeks after PTCA and compared them to follow-up coronary angiography performed at approximately 6 months. An abnormal test (reversible defect) predicted the recurrence of angina in 66% of patients in whom it occurred versus 38% with an abnormal exercise ECG (ST segment depression or angina at peak exercise) and predicted restenosis in 74% in whom it occurred versus 50% of patients with an abnormal exercise ECG (Figures 2.7 and 2.8).

The usefulness of exercise thallium imaging in predicting recurrent chest pain and restenosis was also evaluated by Breisblatt and coworkers (71) in a study involving the performance of sequential thallium studies. Patients undergoing successful PTCA were studied with thallium imaging early after PTCA (4–6 weeks) and on two later occasions (3–6 months and 11–13 months). At the initial evaluation, 25% of the 104 asymptomatic patients (from a total of 121 patients) had positive thallium scans (reversible ischemia); by 6 months 86% of this subgroup had developed restenosis and by 1 year 96% had restenosis. Similarly, 9 of the 17 patients with chest pain had positive thallium scans, correlating perfectly with the presence of restenosis. Thus, both low- and high-risk subgroups for restenosis were identified at this early evaluation. Of the symptomatic patients studied at 3 to 6 months, 60% had a positive thallium scan; of these, 93% had restenosis at catheterization. At this stage the majority of patients (35 of 40) who would develop restenosis at 1 year were identified by thallium imaging. Eighty-four patients were followed for up to 13 months and of the 24 who were symptomatic, 5 had positive thallium scans with all but 1 showing angiographic evidence of restenosis. Although only symptomatic patients underwent catheterization in this study, thallium imaging appeared useful for predicting restenosis. Therefore, at 4 to 6 weeks after PTCA, a positive scan in a symptomatic patient was highly predictive of restenosis, whereas in an asymptomatic patient a positive scan was predictive of future symptoms and restenosis.

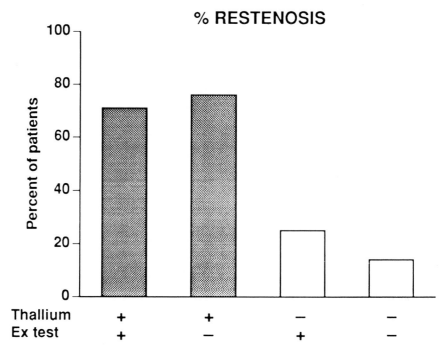

Figure 2.7. Predictive value for angiographic restenosis (defined as an increase of the stenosis to more than 50% luminal diameter) for the possible combinations of noninvasive test results performed 4 weeks after PTCA: (+) = abnormal test and (−) = normal test; EX TEST = exercise ECG. All 89 patients studied underwent coronary angiography within 6 months of PTCA. The shaded columns represent the patients with abnormal thallium tests. Redrawn by permission of the publisher from Wijns et al: Early detection of restenosis after successful percutaneous transluminal coronary angioplasty by exercise-redistribution thallium scintigraphy. American Journal of Cardiology, 1985 (74).

In 1990, Hecht and coworkers (76) reported the results of single photon emission computed tomographic (SPECT) thallium imaging in 116 patients (185 vessels) who underwent PTCA (47% of whom had multivessel disease). Angiographic restenosis was documented in 60% of patients (46% of vessels) at a mean of 6.4 months following PTCA. SPECT thallium imaging was 93% sensitive and 77% specific in detecting restenosis with comparable findings in both completely and partially revascularized patients (Figure 2.9) and had a high accuracy for localizing restenosis to specific vessels in patients with both single and multivessel disease.

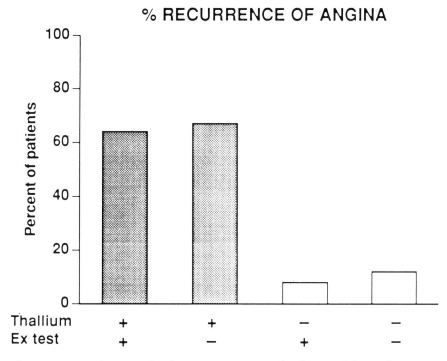

Figure 2.8. Predictive value for recurrent angina for the possible combinations of noninvasive test results performed 4 weeks after PTCA (abbreviations and legend as in Figure 2.7). Redrawn by permission of the publisher from Wijns et al: Early detection of restenosis after successful percutaneous transluminal coronary angioplasty by exercise-redistribution thallium scintigraphy. American Journal of Cardiology, 1985 (74).

This same group of patients was further evaluated to determine the usefulness of SPECT thallium imaging in the prediction of restenosis among symptomatic versus asymptomatic patients (77). The important finding in this study was that the accuracy of SPECT thallium imaging in detecting restenosis was similar for both groups of patients (Table 2.2) and considerably more sensitive and accurate than exercise ECG alone. Additionally, the overall accuracy of detection of restenosis in individual vessels was similar in those with and without symptoms (Table 2.3). The restenosis rate of 59% in the asymptomatic group, much higher than rates reported from other studies, suggests some bias in patient selection in this nonconsecutive series of patients and

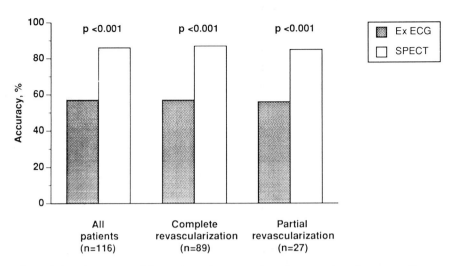

Figure 2.9. Accuracy of detection of restenosis using exercise electrocardiography (Ex ECG) and single photon emission computed tomographic (SPECT) thallium 201 imaging in patients after coronary angiography. Comparison between the two modalities are shown for all patients as well as for those in whom revascularization was considered complete and in those it was considered partial. The number of patients in each group is shown in parentheses. Adapted by permission of the publisher from Hecht et al: Usefulness of tomographic thallium-201 imaging for detection of restenosis after percutaneous transluminal coronary angioplasty. American Journal of Cardiology, 1990 (76).

should be taken into account when interpreting the results of these two studies. Therefore, SPECT thallium imaging appears to be a particularly useful approach to the noninvasive assessment of restenosis and is ideally suited to the assessment of patients with multivessel disease.

Radionuclide Angiography

DePuey and coworkers (78) demonstrated that exercise-gated radionuclide ventriculography also is useful for predicting the severity of coronary restenosis after PTCA. In their study, radionuclide ventriculography performed 4 to 12 months after PTCA distinguished those patients with mild, moderate, and severe degrees of restenosis (based on percent change in luminal stenosis at repeat angiography) by using the magnitude of the change in ejection fraction and presence of exercise-induced

Table 2.2. Detection of Restenosis after Angioplasty by SPECT Thallium Imaging and Exercise ECG: Silent versus Symptomatic Ischemia

	SENSITIVITY (%)	SPECIFICITY (%)	ACCURACY (%)
Silent Ischemia			
SPECT	96*	75	88*
Exercise ECG	40	50	44[†]
Symptomatic Ischemia			
SPECT	91*	77	85*
Exercise ECG	59	71	64

(Reprinted by permission of the American College of Cardiology from Hecht et al. Silent ischemia after coronary angioplasty: evaluation of restenosis and extent of ischemia in asymptomatic patients by tomographic thallium-201 exercise imaging and comparison with symptomatic patients. J Am Coll Cardiol 1991; 17:670–677.)
$p < 0.001$ vs exercise ECG; [†]$p < 0.05$ vs symptomatic ischemia. SPECT = single photon emission computed tomography; ECG = electrocardiography.

Table 2.3. Detection of Restenosis in Individual Vessels by SPECT Thallium Imaging: Silent versus Symptomatic Ischemia

	SENSITIVITY (%)	SPECIFICITY (%)	ACCURACY (%)
Silent Ischemia			
All vessels	90	89	89
Left anterior descending	93	89	91
Right coronary	90	100	95
Left circumflex	83	75	79
Symptomatic Ischemia			
All vessels	84	77	84
Left anterior descending	87	100	92
Right coronary	86	72	77
Left circumflex	83	75	81

(Reprinted by permission of the American College of Cardiology from Hecht et al. Silent ischemia after coronary angioplasty: evaluation of restenosis and extent of ischemia in asymptomatic patients by tomographic thallium-201 exercise imaging and comparison with symptomatic patients. J Am Coll Cardiol 1991; 17:670–677.)
Abbreviations as for Table 2.2.

Table 2.4. Results of Exercise-Gated Radionuclide Ventriculography at Time of 4–12-Month Postangioplasty Follow-up Angiography

	GROUP I (≤20% RESTENOSIS) n = 23	GROUP II (>20% <50% RESTENOSIS) n = 10	GROUP III (≥50% RESTENOSIS) n = 8	p VALUE (I vs III)
Duration, sec	764 ± 303	695 ± 486	614 ± 430	NS
RPP (× 10²)	267 ± 93	243 ± 91	268 ± 61	NS
Angina	0	45%	13%	NS
≥ 2 mm ST depression	5%	36%	25%	NS
Abnormal ΔEF	23%	64%	88%	<0.005
Abnormal wall motion	14%	45%	50%	<0.10
Abnormal GRNV*	27%	73%	88%	<0.01

Reprinted by permission of the American College of Cardiology from DePuey et al: Restenosis after transluminal coronary angioplasty detected with exercise-gated radionuclide ventriculography. J Am Coll Cardiol 1984; 4:1103–1113.

*Abnormal gated radionuclide ventriculography (GRNV) defined by either a failure to increase ejection fraction (EF) by 5 percentage points or an exercise-induced wall motion abnormality, or both.

Duration = duration of bicycle exercise; RPP = maximal heart rate–systolic blood pressure product.

regional wall motion abnormalities (Table 2.4). Twenty-seven percent of those without significant restenosis had abnormal radionuclide ventriculograms compared to 78% with restenosis. Restenosis occurred in 70% of those patients with an abnormal ejection fraction response or an exercise-induced regional wall motion abnormality compared to only 20% of those with normal responses.

Similar results were found in a retrospective study from Mayo Clinic reported by O'Keefe and colleagues (79) who evaluated the usefulness of radionuclide ventriculography performed within 1 month of PTCA. All patients had follow-up angiography at a mean of 8 months following PTCA. None of the 35% of patients who had normal or negative radionuclide tests developed restenosis. In contrast, 42% of the remaining patients with abnormal tests developed restenosis. The negative predictive value of the test was 100% (lower confidence limit, 81%) and the positive predictive value was 42%, leading the authors to conclude that exercise radionuclide ventriculography is useful in separating low- and high-risk groups for restenosis.

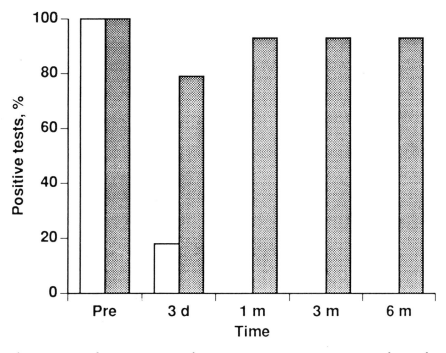

Figure 2.10. The percentages of positive ECG exercise tests are shown for patients before PTCA and at 3 days (d), 1, 3, and 6 months (m) following PTCA. The 17 patients without angiographically documented restenosis are represented by the open bars and the 14 patients with subsequent restenosis are represented by the shaded bars. (Adapted by permission of the American College of Cardiology from el-Tamimi et al. Very early prediction of restenosis after successful coronary angioplasty: anatomic and functional assessment. J Am Coll Cardiol 1990; 15:259–264.)

Early Stress Testing after PTCA and Possible Implications for Early Prediction of Late Restenosis

Recent data suggest that prediction of subsequent restenosis in patients with single vessel disease and stable chronic angina may be possible as early as 3 days after angioplasty with exercise ECG testing (80). In this study, 3 of 17 patients with no documented restenosis had a positive exercise ECG test 3 days after PTCA compared to 11 of 14 patients who did develop restenosis. After 1 month all exercise tests were negative in the patients without restenosis and positive in all but 1 with restenosis with similar findings at 3 and 6 months (Figure 2.10). No differences in

Table 2.5. Results of Exercise-Gated Radionuclide Ventriculography Within 4 Days of Coronary Angioplasty in Patients Divided into Groups According to Subsequent Angiographic Findings at Follow-up Angiography 4–12 Months Later

	GROUP I (≤20% RESTENOSIS) n = 23	GROUP II (>20% <50% RESTENOSIS) n = 10	GROUP III (≥50% RESTENOSIS) n = 8	p VALUE (I vs III)
Duration, sec	656 ± 242	684 ± 239	745 ± 400	NS
RPP ($\times 10^2$)	276 ± 63	275 ± 85	264 ± 38	NS
Angina	0	0%	0%	NS
≥ 2 mm ST depression	0	9%	0%	NS
Abnormal ΔEF	13%	27%	50%	< 0.05
Abnormal wall motion	5%	27%	50%	< 0.05
Abnormal GRNV	18%	36%	75	< 0.01

Reprinted by permission of the American College of Cardiology from DePuey et al: Restenosis after transluminal coronary angioplasty detected with exercise-gated radionuclide ventriculography. J Am Coll Cardiol 1984; 4:1103–1113.
Abbreviations and definitions as for Table 2.4.

the percentage narrowing of the immediate post-PTCA lesion were found between the two groups of patients as measured by an automated edge-detection technique. Although these results may stimulate debate about the possible mechanisms of late restenosis and the intriguing possibility that this may be detected within a few days of PTCA, or certainly within a month, they apply only to patients with single vessel disease and probably should not be extrapolated to patients with multivessel disease for whom more sophisticated functional testing should be considered.

In this regard, dipyridamole SPECT thallium imaging offers a potentially convenient and early physiologic assessment of the future risk of restenosis as early as 3 days after PTCA as suggested by the study of Jain and colleagues (81). Following PTCA, 65% of the patients in this study had no reversible tomographic defects, whereas 35% had reversible defects in the territory of the successfully dilated vessel: 71% of those with reversible defects developed restenosis compared to only 12% of those without reversible defects. The study reported by DePuey and colleagues (78) some years earlier also suggested that restenosis might be predictable from the results of radionuclide ventriculography performed within 4 days of PTCA (Table 2.5).

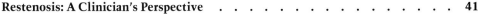

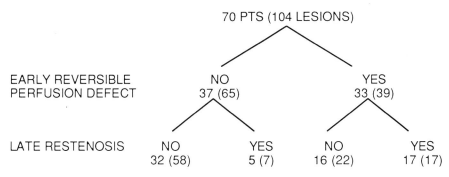

Figure 2.11. Relationship between the results of thallium 201 scintigraphy performed at rest and during atrial pacing on day 1 after PTCA and late angiographic restenosis. Numbers in parentheses represent lesions; PTS = patients. Redrawn by permission of the American College of Cardiology from Hardoff et al: Predicting late restenosis after coronary angioplasty by very early (12 to 24 h) thallium-201 scintigraphy: implications with regard to mechanisms of late coronary restenosis. J Am Coll Cardiol 1990; 15:1486–1492.

The earliest time noninvasive functional testing has been performed after PTCA was described in a recently reported Israeli study aimed at the early stratification of patients into low- and high-risk groups for restenosis (82). Ninety consecutive patients who underwent successful PTCA were studied with thallium scintigraphy at rest and during atrial pacing, 12 to 24 hours after PTCA. Reversible perfusion defects during atrial pacing were demonstrated in 33 patients of whom 52% developed late restenosis compared to 14% of the 37 patients in whom no thallium abnormalities were documented (Figure 2.11). One limitation to this study was that thallium data for the 19 patients who did not undergo catheterization were not presented—even if it could be assumed that the majority of these did not have restenosis, it would be important to know whether their initial thallium scans were normal.

In contrast to these studies, some investigators have cautioned against the use and interpretation of stress imaging so soon after PTCA (83–85). For example, in the study by Manyari and colleagues (83), the use of sequential exercise thallium perfusion imaging at a mean of 9 days following PTCA in patients without documented recurrence resulted in abnormal results in 28% of patients; all showed progressive improvement in perfusion over the next few months. The authors concluded that an abnormal myocardial perfusion scan soon after PTCA does not necessarily imply that there is residual stenosis or restenosis but might reflect hibernating or stunned myocardium secondary to repeated episodes of myocardial ischemia or acute ischemia during balloon inflation. The discordance between thallium scintigraphy and angiographic findings immediately after angioplasty (84), suggesting that coronary flow reserve is abnormal at this stage, is supported by the results of intracoronary Doppler flow studies demonstrating that coronary flow reserve may not return to normal immediately after PTCA, despite an adequate angiographic PTCA result (86).

Possible causes for conflicting findings in these studies include different patient populations, the use of exercise versus dipyridamole as the cardiac stressor, the type of radionuclide imaging (planar versus SPECT thallium imaging or radionuclide ventriculography), and the small but significant differences in the timing of the scans relative to PTCA. It is also conceivable that abnormalities in coronary flow reserve early after PTCA may not be as marked when dipyridamole or atrial pacing (vide infra) are used for cardiac stress as during exercise. In this regard, exercise can cause coronary spasm at the site of obstructive coronary disease, whereas dipyridamole acts as a powerful coronary vasodilator and the stress of pacing may be less than that induced by exercise—both nonexercise approaches could therefore conceivably be associated with fewer false positive predictions of restenosis compared to exercise.

The results of these studies suggest that the mechanisms of restenosis may be operative within the first day or so after PTCA. From the available evidence, the postprocedural residual stenosis does not seem to be well correlated with the physiologic abnormalities of perfusion at this time although the limitations of coronary angiography in this regard should be recognized. The potentially important roles for such early phenomena as platelet and thrombus deposition and the dynamic vasoactive behavior of the vascular endothelium in the later development of restenosis will require further examination (87). The implications of these findings include the need to focus research onto the prevention of restenosis during this critical time during and immediately after PTCA, the potential implementation and timing of therapy to prevent restenosis, and the in-hospital identification of high-risk patients who will require intensive "anti-restenosis" therapy (although currently not available) and careful follow-up.

Stress Echocardiography

Recently, stress echocardiography using exercise or pharmacologic agents (e.g., dipyridamole or dobutamine) has been introduced into clinical practice for assessment of patients with coronary artery disease. A recent study by Pirelli and colleagues (88) found that dipyridamole echocardiography early after PTCA appeared to be useful in predicting recurrence of angina as an alternative to exercise ECG. However, these results should be considered preliminary since more than half of the eligible patient population were excluded from the study for various clinical or technical reasons, and the results were correlated to recurrence of angina as the standard rather than to angiographic restenosis. Direct comparisons with radionuclide techniques will better determine the usefulness of stress echocardiography in the prediction of restenosis than comparisons to exercise ECG testing alone. The relative merits of dobutamine compared to dipyridamole as the more appropriate stressor agent for echocardiographic studies are currently being debated. Results of further studies in this area as well as other imaging modalities such as ultrafast computed tomography or positron emission tomography are likely to be reported in the future.

The Cost of Restenosis

In view of the enormous impact that coronary restenosis currently has on the practice of PTCA in North America and abroad, it is surprising that so little documentation of the resulting monetary costs has appeared in the literature. Although the costs of PTCA are appropriately compared to those associated with coronary artery bypass surgery, comparison to costs of medical treatment of ischemic heart disease are lacking.

The best analysis comparing the cost of PTCA with bypass surgery was performed by Reeder and colleagues in 1984 (89). These investigators studied the 1-year monetary outlay for unselected patients with single vessel disease who underwent either elective bypass surgery (89 patients) or elective PTCA (79 patients) at Mayo Clinic between 1979 and 1981. The mean initial hospitalization charge (adjusted for patient baseline differences between the different groups) for PTCA patients was $7571, which was 38% lower than the mean charge for surgical patients. Adding the 1-year follow-up costs yielded a total average charge to the PTCA patients of $11,384 compared to $13,387 for the surgical patients. Eighteen patients who underwent PTCA developed restenosis, which was treated by surgery in 9 patients, repeat PTCA in 6 patients, and medically in 3 patients. The adjusted mean follow-up charge was $10,641 for patients with restenosis, which was substantially higher than the adjusted follow-up charges of $2123 for patients without restenosis and the $1422 for surgical patients. The overall charges for restenosis patients (initial plus follow-up) were more than double those for patients without restenosis.

Therefore, during the first year after PTCA, restenosis was responsible for a major loss of the initial monetary saving by performing PTCA instead of bypass surgery. The primary success rate in this study was only 70% (before 1982) compared to current success rates of about 90%. Although medical and hospital charges have both increased since this study was performed, initial hospitalization charges may be lower now for PTCA patients relative to surgical patients. On the other hand, the cost differential could also be in the opposite direction as the spectrum of patients treated today includes patients who are much sicker and have more advanced coronary disease than their predecessors. Recently, a comparison of costs between patients with multivessel disease undergoing PTCA and patients undergoing bilateral mammary artery bypass surgery showed that PTCA could still be performed at considerable cost saving, but that after approximately 2 years this was almost neutralized by the added cost of continuing antianginal medication and repeat procedures (90).

The economic consequences of restenosis were recently described in a preliminary report by Brush and colleagues (91) using cost estimates based on a contemporary series of patients undergoing PTCA. By using the average charge for each PTCA in this consecutive series of patients ($11,727 per patient) and assuming an initial restenosis rate of 28%, these investigators constructed a model to compare the costs of performing one to five PTCA procedures for restenosis before finally resorting to bypass surgery. For example, the average charge for all patients was $18,727 if bypass surgery was performed for all cases of restenosis after the initial PTCA, but the average charge fell to $15,986 if patients underwent a strategy of up to two further PTCAs in the event of restenosis. The authors concluded that the added cost of performing the extra PTCAs was offset by the diminishing number of patients returning for repeat procedures (PTCA or surgery) although the total cost of PTCA increased by approximately 60% because of restenosis.

Three important caveats to cost analysis studies should be mentioned. First, cost analysis studies that examine only hospital charges may be misleading in terms of assigning costs to a procedure or in defining the relative monetary savings between two different treatments. Alternative cost accounting models that do not simply use the hospital charge may result in different conclusions, as illustrated recently by Hlatky and colleagues who demonstrated that the actual economic cost savings of PTCA over bypass surgery may be significantly overestimated using hospital charge data alone (92). Also, the cost of providing back-up cardiac surgical services, even if not used, should be considered. Second, cost analysis studies do not necessarily take into account the cost-benefit or risk-benefit of particular procedures such as PTCA and bypass surgery. Finally, none of these studies has been randomized, although in the study of Reeder and coworkers (89), adjustment of baseline differences between different patient populations was performed. Nevertheless, to put the issue of restenosis into financial perspective, it has been proposed that a reduction in the restenosis rate from 33% to 25% would result in an annual saving of $300 million in the United States as a result of the reduced need for treatment for the consequences of restenosis (93).

Restenosis and Ongoing Randomized Revascularization Trials

A number of major randomized studies are now under way comparing PTCA and coronary bypass surgery as revascularization strategies for patients with coronary artery disease. These include the Bypass Angioplasty Revascularization Investigation (BARI, supported by the NHLBI), Coronary Artery Bypass/Revascularization Investigation (CABRI, in Europe), the Emory Angioplasty/Surgery Trial (EAST, Emory University in the United States), the German Angioplasty Bypass Investigation (GABI), and the Randomized Intervention Treatment of Angina (RITA, in the United Kingdom). The results of the Veterans Administration trial of PTCA compared to medical therapy for single vessel disease (ACME) show PTCA is an effective, practical alternative to medical therapy alone.

These trials occur at a time when restenosis remains nonpreventable. Whether or not an approach to the successful prevention of restenosis will be developed within the next few years is still uncertain. Although there has been some debate as to whether these costly studies are being conducted prematurely, their results will undoubtedly be important and highly relevant to our current choices of revascularization strategies for hundreds of thousands of patients worldwide per year. These trials are subject to the limitations of all studies carried out during the "learning phase" or changing "state of the art." They do, therefore, run the risk of obsolescence, but this is outweighed by the potential benefits of directly comparing the outcomes of two widely used strategies. The sudden appearance of an effective means of preventing restenosis, however, will demand a retrospective and complex adjustment of the long-term follow-up results in all these trials. Data regarding the comparative monetary costs of these treatment modalities, particularly with respect to the impact of restenosis, should also be forthcoming as these studies are completed.

Conclusion

Restenosis remains a formidable clinical issue and is the major limitation to the long-term efficacy of PTCA, particularly in patients with multivessel disease. The search for prevention is now widespread and has appropriately focused on the biologic phenomena underlying the problem. A solution is not yet apparent, but if found, could radically alter current expectations of the results of PTCA.

References

1. Gruentzig A. Transluminal dilatation of coronary artery stenosis (letter). Lancet 1978;1:263.
2. Hirshfeld JW Jr, Schwartz JS, Jugo R, et al. Restenosis after coronary angioplasty: a multivariate statistical model to relate lesion and procedure variables to restenosis. J Am Coll Cardiol 1991;18:647–656.
3. Margolis JR, Litvack F, Krauthamer D, Trautwein R, Goldenberg T, Grundfest W. Excimer laser coronary angioplasty: American multicenter experience. Herz 1990;15:223–232.
4. Rothbaum D, Linnemeier T, Landin R, et al. Excimer laser coronary angioplasty: angiographic restenosis rate at six month follow-up (abstr). J Am Coll Cardiol 1991;17:205A.
5. Simpson JB, Baim DS, Hinohara T, et al. Restenosis of de novo lesions in native coronary arteries following directional coronary atherectomy: multicenter experience (abstr). J Am Coll Cardiol 1991;17:364A.
6. Garratt KN, Holmes DR Jr, Bell MR, et al. Restenosis after directional

coronary atherectomy: differences between primary atheromatous and restenosis lesions and influence of subintimal tissue resection. J Am Coll Cardiol 1990;16:1665–1671.

7. Niazi K, Cragg DR, Strzelecki M, Friedman HZ, Gangadharan V, O'Neill W. Angiographic risk factors for coronary restenosis following mechanical rotational atherectomy (abstr). J Am Coll Cardiol 1991; 17:218A.

8. Nobuyoshi M, Kimura T, Nosaka H, et al. Restenosis after successful percutaneous transluminal coronary angioplasty: serial angiographic follow-up of 229 patients. J Am Coll Cardiol 1988;12:616–623.

9. Detre K, Holubkov R, Kelsey S, et al. One-year follow-up results of the 1985–1986 National Heart, Lung, and Blood Institute's Percutaneous Transluminal Coronary Angioplasty Registry. Circulation 1989;80:421–428.

10. Deligonul U, Vandormael MG, Kern MJ, Zelman R, Galan K, Chaitman BR. Coronary angioplasty: a therapeutic option for symptomatic patients with two and three vessel coronary disease. J Am Coll Cardiol 1988;11:1173–1179.

11. Bell MR, Bailey KR, Reeder GS, Lapeyre AC III, Holmes DR Jr. Percutaneous transluminal coronary angioplasty in patients with multivessel disease: how important is complete revascularization for cardiac event-free survival? J Am Coll Cardiol 1990;16:553–562.

12. Serruys PW, Luijten HE, Beatt KJ, et al. Incidence of restenosis after successful coronary angioplasty: a time-related phenomenon. A quantitative angiographic study in 342 consecutive patients at 1, 2, 3, and 4 months. Circulation 1988;77:361–371.

13. Holmes DR Jr, Vlietstra RE, Smith HC, et al. Restenosis after percutaneous transluminal coronary angioplasty (PTCA): a report from the PTCA Registry of the National Heart, Lung and Blood Institute. Am J Cardiol 1984;53:77C–81C.

14. Lambert M, Bonan R, Cote G, et al. Multiple coronary angioplasty: a model to discriminate systemic and procedural factors related to restenosis. J Am Coll Cardiol 1988;12:310–314.

15. Vallbracht C, Klepzig HJ, Giesecke A, Kaltenbach M, Kober G. Transluminal coronary angioplasty: parameters of increased risk of recurrence. Z Kardiol 1987;76:727–732.

16. Ellis SG, Roubin GS, King SB III, Doublas JS Jr, Cox WR. Importance of stenosis morphology in the estimation of restenosis risk after elective percutaneous transluminal coronary angioplasty. Am J Cardiol 1989; 63:30–34.

17. Lambert M, Bonan R, Cote G, et al. Early results, complications and

restenosis rates after multilesion and multivessel percutaneous transluminal coronary angioplasty. Am J Cardiol 1987;60:788–791.

18. Hollman J, Badhwar K, Beck GJ, Franco I, Simpfendorfer C. Risk factors for recurrent stenosis following successful coronary angioplasty. Cleve Clin J Med 1989;56:517–523.

19. Arora RR, Konrad K, Badhwar K, Hollman J. Restenosis after transluminal coronary angioplasty: a risk factor analysis. Cathet Cardiovasc Diagn 1990;19:17–22.

20. Guiteras Val P, Bourassa MG, David PR, et al. Restenosis after successful percutaneous transluminal coronary angioplasty: the Montreal Heart Institute experience. Am J Cardiol 1987;60:50B–55B.

21. Rupprecht HJ, Brennecke R, Bernhard G, Erbel R, Pop T, Meyer J. Analysis of risk factors for restenosis after PTCA. Cathet Cardiovasc Diagn 1990;19:151–159.

22. Macdonald RG, Henderson MA, Hirshfeld JW Jr, et al. Patient-related variables and restenosis after percutaneous transluminal coronary angioplasty—a report from the M-HEART Group. Am J Cardiol 1990;66:926–931.

23. Myler RK, Topol ET, Shaw RE, et al. Multiple vessel coronary angioplasty: classification, results, and patterns of restenosis in 494 consecutive patients. Cathet Cardiovasc Diagn 1987;13:1–15.

24. Galan KM, Deligonul U, Kern MJ, Chaitman BR, Vandormael MG. Increased frequency of restenosis in patients continuing to smoke cigarettes after percutaneous transluminal coronary angioplasty. Am J Cardiol 1988;61:260–263.

25. Williams DO, Riley RS, Singh AK, Gewirtz H, Most AS. Evaluation of the role of coronary angioplasty in patients with unstable angina pectoris. Am Heart J 1981;102:1–9.

26. Meyer J, Schmitz H, Erbel R, et al. Treatment of unstable angina pectoris with percutaneous transluminal coronary angioplasty (PTCA). Cathet Cardiovasc Diagn 1981;7:361–371.

27. Meyer J, Schmitz H, Kiesslich T, et al. Percutaneous transluminal coronary angioplasty in patients with stable and unstable angina pectoris: analysis of early and late results. Am Heart J 1983;106:973–980.

28. de Feyter P, Serruys P, van den Brand M, et al. Emergency coronary angioplasty in refractory unstable angina. N Engl J Med 1985;313:342.

29. de Feyter PJ, Serruys PW, Suryapranata H, Beatt K, van den Brand M. Coronary angioplasty early after diagnosis of unstable angina. Am Heart J 1987;114:48–54.

30. de Feyter PJ, Suryapranata H, Serruys PW, et al. Coronary angioplasty for unstable angina: immediate and late results in 200 consecutive patients

with identification of risk factors for unfavorable early and late outcome. J Am Coll Cardiol 1988;12:324–333.

31. Quigley PJ, Erwin J, Maurer BJ, Walsh MJ, Gearty GF. Percutaneous transluminal coronary angioplasty in unstable angina: comparison with stable angina. Br Heart J 1986;55:227–230.

32. Steffenino G, Meier B, Finci L, Rutishauser W. Follow up results of treatment of unstable angina by coronary angioplasty. Br Heart J 1987; 57:416–419.

33. Timmis AD, Griffin B, Crick JC, Sowton E. Early percutaneous transluminal coronary angioplasty in the management of unstable angina. Int J Cardiol 1987;14:25–31.

34. Plokker THW, Ernst SM, Bal ET, et al. Percutaneous transluminal coronary angioplasty in patients with unstable angina pectoris refractory to medical therapy: long-term clinical and angiographic results. Cathet Cardiovasc Diagn 1988;14:15–18.

35. Sharma B, Wyeth RP, Kolath GS, Gimenez HJ, Franciosa JA. Percutaneous transluminal coronary angioplasty of one vessel for refractory unstable angina pectoris: efficacy in single and multivessel disease. Br Heart J 1988;59:280–286.

36. Bentivoglio LG, van Raden J, Kelsey SF, Detre KM. Percutaneous transluminal coronary angioplasty (PTCA) in patients with relative contraindications: results of the National Heart, Lung, and Blood Institute PTCA Registry. Am J Cardiol 1984;53:82C–88C.

37. Leimgruber P, Roubin G, Hollman J, et al. Restenosis after successful coronary angioplasty in patients with single vessel disease. Circulation 1986;73:710–717.

38. Johansson SR, Ekstrom L, Emanuelsson H. Higher recurrence rate after coronary angioplasty in unstable angina pectoris. Angiology 1991; 42:273–280.

39. Luijten HE, Beatt KJ, de Feyter PJ, van den Brand M, Reiber JH, Serruys PW. Angioplasty for stable versus unstable angina pectoris: are unstable patients more likely to get restenosis? A quantitative angiographic study in 339 consecutive patients. Int J Card Imaging 1988;3:87–97.

40. Foley JB, Chisolm RJ, Armstrong PW. Restenosis after PTCA for unstable angina has a different natural history (abstr). Circulation 1990;82(suppl III):338.

41. Halon DA, Merdler A, Shefer A, Flugelman MY, Lewis BS. Identifying patients at high risk for restenosis after percutaneous transluminal coronary angioplasty for unstable angina pectoris. Am J Cardiol 1989;64:289–293.

42. Bertrand ME, LaBlanche JM, Thieuleux FA, Fourrier JL, Traisnel G, Asseman P. Comparative results of percutaneous transluminal coronary angioplasty in patients with dynamic versus fixed coronary stenosis. J Am Coll Cardiol 1986;8:504–508.

43. Leisch F, Schützenberger W, Kerschner K, Herbinger W. Influence of variant angina on the results of percutaneous transluminal coronary angioplasty. Br Heart J 1986;56:341–345.

44. Ardissino D, Barberis P, de Servi S, et al. Abnormal coronary vasoconstriction as a predictor of restenosis after successful angioplasty in patients with unstable angina pectoris. N Engl J Med 1991;325:1053–1057.

45. Vandormael MG, Deligonul U, Kern MJ, Kennedy H, Galan K, Chaitman B. Restenosis after multilesion percutaneous transluminal coronary angioplasty. Am J Cardiol 1987;60:44B–47B.

46. Renkin J, Melin J, Robert A, et al. Detection of restenosis after successful coronary angioplasty: improved clinical decision making with use of a logistic model combining procedural and follow-up variables. J Am Coll Cardiol 1990;16:1333–1340.

47. Glazier JJ, Varricchione TR, Ryan TJ, Ruocco NA, Jacobs AK, Faxon DP. Factors predicting recurrent restenosis after percutaneous transluminal coronary balloon angioplasty. Am J Cardiol 1989;63:902–905.

48. Austin GE, Lynn M, Hollman J. Laboratory test results as predictors of recurrent coronary artery stenosis following angioplasty. Arch Pathol Lab Med 1987;111:1158–1162.

49. Austin GE, Hollman J, Lynn MJ, Meier B. Serum lipoprotein levels fail to predict postangioplasty recurrent coronary artery stenosis. Cleve Clin J Med 1989;56:509–514.

50. Hearn JA, Donohue BC, King SB III, et al. Does serum LP(a) predict restenosis after PTCA? (abstr). J Am Coll Cardiol 1990;15:205A.

51. Sahni R, Maniet AR, Voci G, Banka VS. Prevention of restenosis by lovastatin after successful coronary angioplasty. Am Heart J 1991; 121:1600–1608.

52. Brown G, Albers JJ, Fisher LD, et al. Regression of coronary artery disease as a result of intensive lipid-lowering therapy in men with high levels of apolipoprotein B. N Engl J Med 1990;323:1289–1298.

53. Simonton CA, Mark DB, Hinohara T, et al. Late restenosis after emergent coronary angioplasty for acute myocardial infarction: comparison with elective coronary angioplasty. J Am Coll Cardiol 1988;11:698–705.

54. Rothbaum DA, Linnemeier TJ, Landin RJ, et al. Emergency percutaneous transluminal coronary angioplasty in acute myocardial infarction: a 3 year experience. J Am Coll Cardiol 1987;10:264–272.

55. Tison E, Gommeaux A, LaBlanche JM, Bauters C. Long term risk/benefit

of PTCA of infarct related vessel (abstr). J Am Coll Cardiol 1991; 17:266A.

56. Almany SL, Meany BE, Cragg DR, Grines CL, O'Neill WW. Long term patency and incidence of restenosis after primary angioplasty therapy of acute myocardial infarction (abstr). J Am Coll Cardiol 1991;17:336A.

57. Williams DO, Gruentzig AR, Kent KM, Detre KM, Kelsey SF, To T. Efficacy of repeat percutaneous transluminal coronary angioplasty for coronary restenosis. Am J Cardiol 1984;53:32C–35C.

58. Black AJ, Anderson HV, Roubin GS, Powelson SW, Douglas JS Jr, King SB III. Repeat coronary angioplasty: correlates of a second restenosis. J Am Coll Cardiol 1988;11:714–718.

59. Deligonul U, Vandormael M, Kern MJ, Galan K. Repeat coronary angioplasty for restenosis: results and predictors of follow-up clinical events. Am Heart J 1989;117:997–1002.

60. Steffenino G, Meier B, Finci L, Rutishauser W. Recurrence of stenosis after first and repeat coronary angioplasty. Clinical and angiographic follow-up. G Ital Cardiol 1987;17:473–478.

61. Berger PB, Bell MR, Bresee SJ, Hammes L, Holmes DR Jr. Is the risk of restenosis after a second PTCA higher among patients with a history of prior restenosis at another site? (abstr). J Am Coll Cardiol 1991; 17:267A.

62. Levine S, Ewels CJ, Rosing DR, Kent KM. Coronary angioplasty: clinical and angiographic follow-up. Am J Cardiol 1985;55:673–676.

63. Piovaccari G, Fattori R, Marzocchi Z, Marrozzini C, Prati F, Magnani B. Percutaneous transluminal coronary angioplasty of the very proximal left anterior descending artery lesions: immediate results and follow-up. Int J Cardiol 1991;30:151–155.

64. Meier B, Gruentzig AR, Siegenthaler WE, Schlumpf M. Long-term exercise performance after percutaneous transluminal coronary angioplasty and coronary artery bypass grafting. Circulation 1983;68:796–802.

65. Schroeder E, Marchandise B, De-Coster P, et al. Detection of restenosis after coronary angioplasty for single-vessel disease: how reliable are exercise electrocardiography and scintigraphy in asymptomatic patients? Eur Heart J 1989;10(suppl G):18–21.

66. Weiner DA, Chaitman BR. Role of exercise testing in relationship to coronary artery bypass surgery and percutaneous transluminal coronary angioplasty. Cardiology 1986;73:242–258.

67. Bengtson JR, Mark DB, Honan MB, et al. Detection of restenosis after elective percutaneous transluminal coronary angioplasty using the exercise treadmill test. Am J Cardiol 1990;65:28–34.

68. LaBlanche JM, Magy JM, Pruvost P, Fourrier JL, Gommeaux A, Bertrand

ME. Valeur prédictive du sous-décalge de ST à l'effort dans le diagnostic de la resteenose après angioplastie coronaire. Arch Mal Coeur 1989; 82:871–875.

69. Laarman G, Luijten HE, van Zeyl LGPM, et al. Assessment of "silent" restenosis and long-term follow-up after successful angioplasty in single vessel coronary artery disease: the value of quantitative exercise electro-cardiography and quantitative coronary angiography. J Am Coll Cardiol 1990;16:578–585.

70. Honan MB, Bengtson JR, Pryor DB, et al. Exercise treadmill testing is a poor predictor of anatomic restenosis after angioplasty for acute myocar-dial infarction. Circulation 1989;80:1585–1594.

71. Breisblatt WM, Weiland FL, Spaccavento LJ. Stress thallium-201 imag-ing after coronary angioplasty predicts restenosis and recurrent symp-toms. J Am Coll Cardiol 1988;12:1199–1204.

72. Shiba N, Nishimura T, Uehara T, et al. Detection of restenosis after suc-cessful percutaneous transluminal coronary angioplasty (PTCA)—use-fulness of exercise thallium scintigraphy. Kaku Igaku 1990;27:693–701.

73. Lusson JR, Citron B, Peycelon P, et al. Détection de la resténose coronarienne par la tomoscintigraphie myocardique au thallium 201. Série de 85 observations. Arch Mal Coeur 1989;82:1679–1683.

74. Wijns W, Serruys PW, Reiber JHC, et al. Early detection of restenosis after successful percutaneous transluminal coronary angioplasty by exercise-redistribution thallium scintigraphy. Am J Cardiol 1985;55: 357–361.

75. Wijns W, Serruys PW, Simoons ML, et al. Predictive value of early maximal exercise test and thallium scintigraphy after successful percutaneous transluminal coronary angioplasty. Br Heart J 1985; 53:194–200.

76. Hecht HS, Shaw RE, Bruce TR, Ryan C, Stertzer SH, Myler RK. Useful-ness of tomographic thallim-201 imaging for detection of restenosis after percutaneous transluminal coronary angioplasty. Am J Cardiol 1990;66:1314–1318.

77. Hecht HS, Shaw RE, Chin HL, Ryan C, Stertzer SH, Myler RK. Silent ischemia after coronary angioplasty: evaluation of restenosis and extent of ischemia in asymptomatic patients by tomographic thallium-201 ex-ercise imaging and comparison with symptomatic patients. J Am Coll Cardiol 1991;17:670–677.

78. DePuey EG, Leatherman LL, Leachman RD, et al. Restenosis after trans-luminal coronary angioplasty detected with exercise-gated radionuclide ventriculography. J Am Coll Cardiol 1984;4:1103–1113.

79. O'Keefe JH Jr, Lapeyre AC III, Holmes DR Jr, Gibbons RJ. Usefulness of

early radionuclide angiography for identifying low-risk patients for late restenosis after percutaneous transluminal coronary angioplasty. Am J Cardiol 1988;61:51–54.

80. el-Tamimi H, Davies GJ, Hackett D, Fragasso G, Crea F, Maseri A. Very early prediction of restenosis after successful coronary angioplasty: anatomic and functional assessment. J Am Coll Cardiol 1990;15:259–264.

81. Jain A, Mahmarian JJ, Borges NS, et al. Clinical significance of perfusion defects by thallium-201 single photon emission tomography following oral dipyridamole early after coronary angioplasty. J Am Coll Cardiol 1988;11:970–976.

82. Hardoff R, Shefer A, Gips S, et al. Predicting late restenosis after coronary angioplasty by very early (12 to 24 h) thallium-201 scintigraphy: implications with regard to mechanisms of late coronary restenosis. J Am Coll Cardiol 1990;15:1486–1492.

83. Manyari DE, Knudtson M, Kloiber R, Roth D. Sequential thallium-201 myocardial perfusion studies after successful percutaneous transluminal coronary artery angioplasty: delayed resolution of exercise-induced scintigraphic abnormalities. Circulation 1988;77:86–95.

84. DePuey EG, Roubin GS, Cloninger KG, et al. Correlation of transluminal coronary angioplasty parameters and quantitative thallium-201 tomography. J Invasive Cardiol 1988;1:40–50.

85. DePuey EG, Roubin GS, Depasquale EE, et al. Sequential multivessel coronary angioplasty assessed by thallium-201 tomography. Cathet Cardiovasc Diagn 1989;18:213–221.

86. Wilson RF, Johnson MR, Marcus ML, et al. The effect of coronary angioplasty on coronary flow reserve. Circulation 1988;77:873–885.

87. Ip JH, Fuster V, Israel D, Badimon L, Badimon J, Chesebro JH. The role of platelets, thrombin and hyperplasia in restenosis after coronary angioplasty. J Am Coll Cardiol 1991;17(6 Suppl B):77B–88B.

88. Pirelli S, Massa D, Faletra F, et al. Exercise electrocardiography versus dipyridamole echocardiography testing in coronary angioplasty: early functional evaluation and prediction of angina recurrence. Circulation 1991;83(suppl III):38–42.

89. Reeder GS, Krishan I, Nobrega FT, et al. Is percutaneous coronary angioplasty less expensive than bypass surgery? N Engl J Med 1984; 311:1157–1162.

90. Berreklouw E, Hoogsten J, van Wandelen R, et al. Bilateral mammary artery surgery or percutaneous transluminal coronary angioplasty for multivessel coronary artery disease? An analysis of effects and costs. Eur Heart J 1989;10(suppl H):61–70.

91. Brush JE, Erario M, McGovern W, Jacobs AK, Faxon DP, Ryan TJ. Eco-

nomic consequences of restenosis: a model to compare relative costs of revascularization strategies (abstr). J Am Coll Cardiol 1990;15:59A.

92. Hlatky MA, Lipscomb J, Nelson C, et al. Resource use and cost of initial coronary revascularization. Coronary angioplasty versus coronary bypass surgery. Circulation 1990;82(suppl IV):208–213.

93. Califf RM, Ohman EM, Frid DJ, et al. Restenosis: the clinical issues. In: Topol EJ, ed. Textbook of interventional cardiology. Philadelphia: WB Saunders, 1990: 363–394.

· ·

CHAPTER 3

Restenosis: An Interventionalist's Perspective

———

KIRK N. GARRATT
DAVID R. HOLMES, JR.

INTERVENTIONAL techniques have had a profound impact on the practice of cardiology (1). More than 300,000 balloon dilatations were performed in 1989 (2), and it is estimated that 500,000 procedures may be performed in 1992, exceeding the number of coronary artery bypass operations (1). Restenosis after balloon dilatation, however, remains the principal drawback of the procedure (3). This condition results in additional health care costs for a substantial portion of treated patients and has a demonstrable impact on clinical outcome in at least some patient subsets (4). Indeed, the cost of evaluation and treatment of restenosis obviates the cost savings of the procedure vis à vis the initially more expensive coronary bypass surgery (5). The issue of recurring stenoses after catheter intervention in the coronary arteries troubles the increasingly sophisticated patient who must face the prospect of further coronary symptoms and treatments, the physician who must address complex management issues associated with an iatrogenic disorder with no effective preventive medical therapy, and the cardiac surgeon who must integrate the potential role of less invasive revascularization techniques when rendering a judgment concerning the suitability of coronary bypass surgery for individual patients. However, it is the interventional cardiologist who creates the condition and, therefore, bears the greatest responsibility for its consequences and appropriate management. For each patient undergoing coronary treatment, the interventionalist must directly address the potential for restenosis and try to individualize therapy for each patient in an effort to limit the development of recurrent stenoses. Despite restenosis, the majority of patients in whom balloon angioplasty is selected as a therapeutic option enjoy marked symptomatic improvement.

In assessing restenosis, clinical, angiographic, and pathophysiologic mechanism issues must be considered. The outcome of the procedure may vary profoundly, depending on the aspect studied. Asymptomatic angiographic restenosis in a patient with no demonstrable ischemia is quite different from return of a severe stenosis resulting in unstable angina or myocardial infarction. Although most restenosis lesions can be easily retreated, the development of measures successful in preventing the problem will rest on a more complete understanding of the underlying pathophysiology.

Recently, study of the cellular biology of restenosis has yielded some important findings. Several medical therapies were expected (on the basis of sound biologic and pharmacologic principles) to reduce restenosis but have had a disappointingly meager impact on the disease. This may be the result of errors in the postulated mechanism of angioplasty and restenosis development. The extent to which the interventionalist may alter the potential for restenosis in an individual patient is still not clear, although some technical and clinical variables appear to be related to the development of restenosis in certain patient subgroups. In this chapter, the clinical features and technical factors that may influence the recurrence of coronary stenoses after intervention will be integrated with the current understanding of restenosis biology, principles of restenosis management, and the impact of alternative coronary intervention devices currently available or under investigation.

Cellular Biology of Restenosis

The cellular basis of restenosis is discussed extensively elsewhere in this book. Because healing of vascular injury underlies the development of atherosclerotic lesions (6), some early writers suggested that restenosis may be considered an accelerated form of atherosclerosis (7–9). The precise cellular nature of restenosis is still debated, but an increasing body of data suggests that intimal fibroplasia is the principal mediator of subsequent luminal encroachment (2,3,10–23). The distinct cellular composition of restenosis lesions suggests that effective treatments for this disorder will be different from those used to manage typical, spontaneous atherosclerosis. In this regard, the response to catheter-based intervention may differ for restenosis lesions and primary atheromatous lesions.

Animal Models of Restenosis

From animal studies, the mechanism of successful percutaneous transluminal coronary angioplasty (PTCA) (8), the role of thrombosis in restenotic lesions (21), and the response of developing intimal fibroplasia to a variety of pharmacologic agents (3) are becoming more clear. Evaluation in animal models may also permit an improved understanding of the nature of restenotic lesions.

Endothelial denudation in hypercholesterolemic rabbit iliac arteries stimulates the development of atheromatous lesions, and balloon dilatation of these lesions results in fibrointimal hyperplasia (8). These findings are consistent with theories of atherogenesis and restenosis in patients, and work with this model has served as one of the standards for modern investigation of catheter-based intervention. However, differences in vessel caliber and compliance, requirements for excessively high lipid diets, and differences between human and rabbit hemorrheology call into question the applicability of rabbit iliac study results to human coronary artery disease (2).

Another model involves barotrauma to rat carotid arteries. Results from such a model formed the basis of two multicenter studies in patients. Differences in vessel size and composition (e.g., smooth muscle content and elastic properties) may have a significant impact on the relevance of these studies.

Although no ideal animal model exists, some animals may be better suited than others for studies of atherosclerosis and restenosis. The hemorrheologic systems of nonhuman primates probably resemble human systems most closely, but these animals are difficult to manage and expensive to study. Porcine blood and vascular responses appear to closely resemble human beings (21,24), and pigs are more manageable and affordable. Hypercholesterolemic pig models, such as the Yucatan miniature swine (25), can develop lesions histologically similar to human atherosclerotic plaques, and it is possible that restenotic lesions produced in these animals will more closely resemble human restenotic lesions. A recent model for coronary artery restenosis research involves normocholesterolemic mixed breed swine. These pigs develop robust neointimal fibroplasia histologically identical to human restenosis material following coronary artery instrumentation with either oversized metallic coil implantation or oversized balloon inflation (see Chapter 6). Results from this model indicate that the degree of intimal fibroplasia after coronary trauma is proportional to the vascular wall injury induced. These findings are in agreement with pathologic studies of patients after coronary intervention, indicating that fibrointimal hyperplasia is greatest in areas of the most vascular disruption after intervention (11,20,26).

Biochemical Mediators of Cellular Hyperplasia

The biologic mediators (Figure 3.1) involved in stimulating myofibroblasts and differentiated smooth muscle cells to migrate and proliferate are described in detail elsewhere in this book. In brief, the luminal surface of normal vessels consists of a monolayer of endothelial cells that constitute the least thrombogenic surface known (27,28). This confluent endothelial layer maintains a thromboresistant surface through active and passive mechanisms (29). When the endothelium is disrupted without deep vascular injury, platelets deposit over the exposed subintimal tissues. They generally do not progress to macroscopic thrombus (21). However, deeper vascular injury exposes collagen (particularly type I), elastic tissue, smooth muscle cells, and fat, all of which activate circulating platelets and the intrinsic coagulation pathway (30). Tissue thromboplastin activates the extrinsic coagulation pathway and is released with deep arterial injury (30).

Platelet adherence to exposed subintimal tissues is mediated through von Willebrand's factor (required at high shear stresses) and platelet collagen receptors (29,31). A variety of mitogens and growth factors are released by aggregated platelets (29) that may be important in local intimal hyperplasia. Platelet-derived growth factor (PDGF) is released. Also, a PDGF-like molecule is released by stimulated endothelial cells and monocytes (29). This molecule may be produced by atherosclerotic plaques (32). PDGF appears to be involved in the development of early atherosclerotic lesions. The exact role of PDGF in restenosis is uncertain, but it is likely to be involved in smooth muscle cell recruitment and hyperplasia.

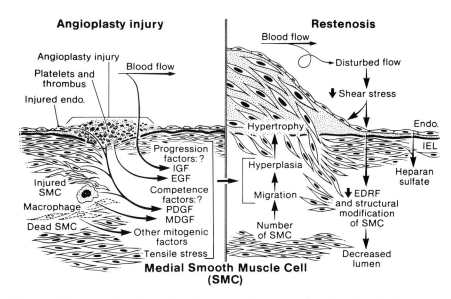

Figure 3.1. Postulated mechanisms mediating restenosis after balloon angioplasty injury. Platelet-derived growth factor (PDGF) or PDGF-like molecules are released by adherent platelets, disrupted endothelial cells, smooth muscle cells, and macrophages. PDGF enables cells to enter the cell replication cycle. Insulin-like growth factor (IGF), epidermal growth factor (EGF), macrophage-derived growth factor (MDGF), and others may facilitate smooth muscle cell migration and proliferation. If sufficient smooth muscle cell replication occurs, the vessel lumen is narrowed; a fall in focal shear stress related to disturbed blood flow over the lesion may cause a reduction in endothelial-derived relaxation factor (EDRF) resulting in structural modifications of the vessel wall that narrow the lumen further. (Adapted by permission of the American Heart Association from Liu et al. Restenosis after coronary angioplasty: potential biologic determinants and role of intimal hyperplasia. Circulation 1989;79:1374–1387.)

Thrombosis occurs when platelet aggregation results in activation of elements of the coagulation pathways; a prothrombinase complex is formed at the platelet surface that is capable of activating thrombin 280,000 times faster than soluble factor Xa alone (30,33). Fibrinogen cleavage by thrombin provides the fibrin monomers that eventually polymerize to stabilize the growing thrombus. Thrombin also provides a positive feedback stimulus that promotes further platelet activation.

One of the prevailing theories of restenosis suggests that two principal mechanisms are operative: intimal hyperplasia, driven by platelet-derived factors, and organization of thrombus, mediated chiefly by activated thrombin (34). The two are interrelated because macroscopic thrombus may be a potent stimulus to release of growth factors participating in smooth muscle cell replication and perhaps vasoconstriction, and may also organize to cause lumen narrowing (Figure 3.2). If these theories are applicable to human beings, restenosis therapies must seek to limit the activation of platelets and thrombin and must blunt the physiologic response to these blood elements once they are activated.

The degree to which the unique pathophysiology of the unstable atheromatous plaque contributes to local cellular hyperplasia is unknown, but since many of the same processes (thrombosis and platelet deposition) are present in unstable lesions before angioplasty is performed, it seems reasonable to conclude that balloon inflations and tissue disrup-

Figure 3.2. Restenosis and extent of arterial injury. Any arterial injury will result in platelet deposition, but deep arterial injury is associated with unlimited platelet deposition and the development of macroscopic thrombus. Growth factor-mediated stimulation of smooth muscle cell replication, organization of macroscopic thrombus, and vasospasm contribute to restenosis. Development of macroscopic thrombus and severe vasoconstriction proximal and especially distal to the dilated vascular segment (*) have been reduced with platelet inhibitor therapy in the porcine carotid artery model of balloon angioplasty injury. (Adapted by permission from Chesebro et al. Restenosis after arterial injury: a hemorrheologic response to injury. Am J Cardiol 1987;10B–16B.)

RESTENOSIS AFTER ARTERIAL ANGIOPLASTY

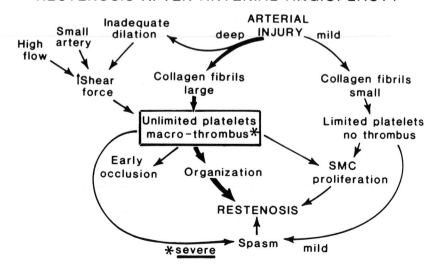

tions in this setting may cause even greater local thrombotic stimulation. This may, in part, explain the observation that restenosis is more common when balloon dilatation is undertaken in patients with acute ischemic syndromes (35–37).

With these facts in mind, it is clear that some form of antithrombin and antiplatelet therapies are mandatory when balloon angioplasty is performed. Theoretically, a drug such as heparin, which has both antithrombin and antimitogenic effects (38,39), should be useful in reducing both the stimuli and the effectors of restenosis. Despite this, limited clinical trials have not demonstrated a beneficial effect of heparin therapy against restenosis (40). Because heparin appears to limit smooth muscle cell growth by regulating entry into the S phase of mitosis (a late phase of mitosis), the short time course and possibly the dosing of heparin may account for this disappointing finding. Aspirin is the most widely used antiplatelet drug; unfortunately, clinical trials with aspirin have also failed to show that it reduces restenosis (41,42). More specific and potent antithrombin, antiplatelet, and antiproliferative agents are under study that may be effective in containing postangioplasty intimal hyperplasia.

Incidence and Time Course of Restenosis

Gruentzig reported that 25% of the first 134 patients to undergo balloon angioplasty developed recurrent stenoses within 1 year (43). Restenosis rates varied widely in subsequent reports, due in part to widely varying definitions of restenosis and to variability in the follow-up time period.

Of the many definitions used, all have some justification, and some have great merit. Angiographic definitions are generally considered the most reliable, although with significant inter- and intra-observer variability in the interpretation of coronary angiograms (44), this may be called into question. Further, clinical definitions address the issue of angioplasty efficacy (i.e., whether the patient derived a benefit from the procedure) rather than angioplasty activity (i.e., the anatomic/physiologic response to angioplasty). However, clinical definitions are less reliable because they rely on patients' perception of symptoms, which may be influenced by many factors; studies indicate that angiographic restenosis will be present in up to 17% of patients who would be considered non-restenosers on the basis of clinical assessment alone (45–47). There is no consensus yet regarding the most appropriate definition, and consequently reports on restenosis must still be interpreted without the benefit of standardized definitions.

Controversy also exists as to whether restenosis follows a Gaussian or bimodal distribution (48). This has important pathophysiologic implications. At present, most investigators believe that restenosis follows a Gaussian distribution. Therefore, quantitative angiography, which allows vessel diameter to be studied as a continuous rather than a discrete variable, is preferred to assess restenosis. Treating angiographic measurements as continuous variables may be especially important when the residual stenosis after PTCA is large (e.g., 45%), and may not need to worsen much to become a clinically important lesion, or when the residual stenosis is small (e.g., 5%), and may have to change greatly before symptoms occur. However, it must be recognized that significant problems exist in quantitative angiographic assessment of results, especially immediately after balloon angioplasty when fresh dissections and thrombus may create indistinct borders.

In studies of restenosis, varying results may be claimed depending on whether restenosis is defined as loss of some percentage of the initial gain in vessel diameter or area, some absolute reduction in vessel dimension, or narrowing that has exceeded some arbitrary threshold value. Some investigators have addressed this problem by reporting restenosis rates for a given study group using multiple definitions. Data from the first NHLBI PTCA Registry were analyzed according to four different, justifiable, and utilized definitions (47). All patients with restenosis according to any of the four definitions tested were accounted for when a combination of two definitions was used (a decrease in lumen dimension of $\geq$ 30% or loss of 50% of the initial gain; Figure 3.3). Using this conservative approach, a restenosis rate of 33.6% over 6 months' follow-up was obtained. This figure has been and continues to be quoted widely as the "standard" risk of restenosis. Although the first NHLBI PTCA Registry focused on patients treated before 1982, it excluded patients with acute myocardial infarction and those who received streptokinase, and it considered the restenosis rates of only the first dilated lesion in cases where multiple lesions were dilated. This figure is generally in keeping with the pooled values obtained from the large number of studies involving a variety of patient subsets that have subsequently been published (42,47,49–57; Table 3.1).

The impact of the definition was nicely illustrated in a study by Serruys and coworkers, who analyzed their experience in 342 patients and found that the incidence of restenosis at 4 months (cumulative)

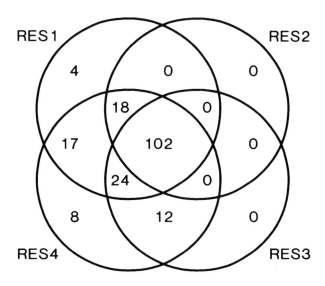

Figure 3.3. Restenosis in the first NHLBI PTCA Registry. When four angiographic definitions of restenosis (RES 1 = increase of ≥ 30% in stenosis severity; RES 2 = post-PTCA lesion < 50% progressing to ≥ 70%; RES 3 = stenosis that is 10% below pre-PTCA severity or higher; RES 4 = loss of 50% of initial gain) were tested in the 557 patients of the first NHLBI PTCA Registry, restenosis was found in 187 (33.6%) patients. Definitions RES 1 and RES 4 identified all patients having restenosis by any tested criteria. (Adapted by permission from Holmes et al. Restenosis after percutaneous transluminal coronary angioplasty (PTCA): a report from the PTCA Registry of the National Heart, Lung and Blood Institute. Am J Cardiol 1984;53:77C–81C.)

varied from 2.3% to 22.9% using the four NHLBI definitions and two other definitions used at the Thoraxcenter at Erasmus University in Rotterdam (58).

An excellent study by Nobuyoshi and colleagues (49) demonstrated that angiographic restenosis developed almost entirely over the first 3 months following angioplasty; thereafter, the risk of restenosis fell dramatically. In this study, 229 patients underwent serial angiography at regular intervals for 1 year after angioplasty. The cumulative prevalence of restenosis in these patients was 12.7% at 1 month, 43% at 3 months, 49.4% at 6 months, and 52.5% at 12 months (Figure 3.4). Analysis of paired angiograms demonstrated that lesion progression (lumen nar

Table 3.1. Restenosis Rates Reported for Balloon Angioplasty

INVESTIGATOR	YEAR	PATIENTS (NO.)	ANGIOGRAPHIC FOLLOW-UP (%)	FOLLOW-UP (MO.)	RESTENOSIS RATE (%)	RESTENOSIS DEFINITION
Gruentzig (43)	1982	184	100	18	25	Unk
Meyer (51)	1983	70	90	6	20	1
Levine (179)	1983	251	92	6	40	2
Holmes (47)	1984	557	74	6	34	3–6
Thornton (42)	1984	248	72	6–9	31	3
Kaltenbach (50)	1985	356	94	6	12	7
Mabin (56)	1985	84	55	18	33	4
Levine (57)	1985	100	92	6	40	3
Leimgruber (53)	1986	998	57	7	33	2–4
Guiteras (55)	1987	181	98	6	28	4
Ernst (54)	1987	1352	62	6	24	3
Serruys (58)	1988	342	100	4	18	8
Nobuyoshi (49)	1988	229	100	1	13	3
"		"	"	3	43	"
"		"	"	6	49	"
"		"	"	12	53	"

Restenosis definition:
1. *> 85% area stenosis at follow-up*
2. *> 50% diameter stenosis at follow-up [NHLBI definition I (47)]*
3. *Loss of ≥ 50 % initial gain in lumen diameter [NHLBI definition II (47)]*
4. *Diameter ≥ 30% narrower than immediate post-PTCA result [NHLBI definition III (47)]*
5. *< 50% stenosis immediate post-PTCA result and > 70% diameter stenosis at follow-up [NHLBI definition IV (47)]*
6. *Increase in stenosis to within 90% of original severity*
7. *Increase in stenosis to within 80% of original severity*
8. *Decrease of ≥ 0.72 mm in minimal lumen diameter*
Unk = unknown

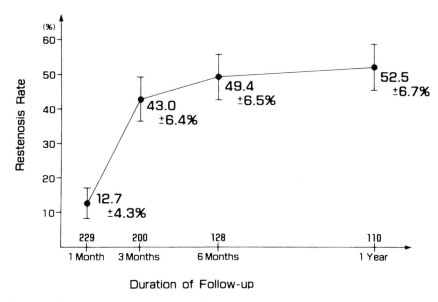

Figure 3.4. Incidence of angiographic restenosis. Actuarial restenosis in 229 patients undergoing serial angiograms after balloon angioplasty. The numbers above the horizontal axis represent the number of patients at risk at the end of each interval. (Adapted by permission from Nobuyoshi et al. Restenosis after successful percutaneous transluminal coronary angioplasty: serial angiographic follow-up of 229 patients. J Am Coll Cardiol 1988; 12:616–623.)

rowing by > 0.5 mm) was most prevalent between 1 and 3 months; earlier progression was highly predictive of eventual restenosis ($> 50\%$ loss of gain, absolute stenotic vessel diameter). This study suggests that restenosis occurs early in most patients and that the incidence of restenosis in a mixed patient population (with regard to clinical presentation and variables) may be high.

Empiric Predictors of Restenosis

Basic and animal research have revealed factors that may impact on restenosis in human beings. Patient and procedural characteristics influencing the incidence of restenosis may be identifiable from clinical investigations, despite the definition problems discussed previously.

Patient Characteristics

Multiple clinical factors associated with restenosis have been identified (Table 3.2), although controversy exists over some of them. The first NHLBI PTCA Registry data indicated that men were at increased risk of restenosis compared with women (59); other investigators have not found this to be the case (55,57,60). One interesting study identified male gender as a risk factor for restenosis after repeat PTCA but not after the first PTCA (61). Age does not appear to be a risk factor for restenosis (47,62,63). Conflicting data exist pertaining to the risk of hypertension (64,65) and diabetes mellitus (47,53,60,61,65–68), but smoking (61, 64,65,67,68) and hyperlipidemia (61,64,65,67) do not appear to be significant risk factors for restenosis. The failure of gender, hypertension, smoking, diabetes, and hyperlipidemia to predict an increase in restenosis has led some investigators to conclude that the pathophysiologic mechanisms of restenosis may have a set of clinical risk factors different from those associated with the progression of atherosclerosis (61).

The clinical setting may influence restenosis rates. Balloon angioplasty undertaken in the setting of acute ischemic syndromes, such as unstable angina or acute myocardial infarction (36,37), may be associated with an increased restenosis risk. However, these observations have not been uniform. Some of the discrepancies may relate to differences in culprit lesion morphology or environment rather than overt clinical syndrome. In particular, a strong theoretical basis exists to support the argument that local thrombus and platelet aggregation contribute to subsequent neointimal proliferation. Therefore, patients with lesions rich in thrombus and platelet aggregates (e.g., patients likely to present with rest angina or myocardial infarction) might be expected to develop restenosis more frequently than those patients without these features; reducing the "thrombotic load" prior to angioplasty may reduce the restenosis risk. In one recent study (69) patients with refractory angina for 24 hours prior to PTCA were found to be at high risk for restenosis. This may have important implications for the medical management of patients prior to balloon angioplasty, although any delays may be costly. Clearly, the angioplasty procedure itself can result in the formation of thrombus and platelet aggregates, so differences between stable and unstable patients may not be entirely clear. Nonetheless, most observations indicate that patients with acute ischemic coronary syndromes, especially when coupled with angiographic evidence of intracoronary thrombus, are at increased risk for restenosis (35–37).

Table 3.2. Variables That May Be Associated with Restenosis

CHARACTER-ISTICS	ASSOCIATION WITH RESTENOSIS		
	OFTEN	OCASIONALLY	NONE
Patient	Male sex	Unstable angina	Age
	Diabetes	Anginal class	Hypertension
	Variant angina	No previous MI	
	New onset angina	Cholesterol	
Angiographic	Severe stenoses	Eccentric stenoses	Stenosis length
	Prox. LAD stenoses		Dist. anastamosis
	Spasm		Multivessel disease
	Chronic occlusions		LV function
	Branch point stenoses		
	SVG ostial or graft body lesions		
Procedural	High residual stenosis	Low balloon/ artery ratio	Number of balloon inflations
	High initial gradient	Inflation duration	Inflation pressure
	High final gradient		
	Absence of int. tear		
Post-PTCA		Smoking	Calcium antagonists
			Warfarin
			Heparin
			Aspirin

Adapted by permission from Rose and Pepine. Restenosis following coronary artery angioplasty: patterns, recognition, and results of repeat angioplasty. Cardiovasc Clin 1988;19:233–251
Dist. = distal; Int. = intimal; LAD = left anterior descending artery; LV = left ventricle; MI = myocardial infarction; Prox. = proximal; SVG = saphenous vein bypass graft.

Procedural Characteristics

Little can generally be done to meaningfully alter most clinical risk factors when catheter-based intervention is being considered. However, the angioplasty procedure could be modified if certain practices are identified with an increased restenosis risk.

Balloon Catheter Selection and Handling: Catheters with inflated balloon diameters approximately 10% smaller than the reference segment of the treated vessel (i.e., the least diseased arterial segment near the lesion to be dilated) are associated with an increased risk of restenosis (70,71). This is most likely related to inadequate initial dilatation. A large residual stenosis after balloon angioplasty is independently predictive of an increased restenosis risk in some patient groups (36,61,72), and morphologic studies indicate that inadequate dilatation or remodeling contributes to restenosis in lesions with high residual stenoses (73). If a lesion is not sufficiently dilated, elastic recoil (chiefly from medial and adventitial tissues) will tend to restore the lumen size and shape to preangioplasty dimensions. In fibrotic and calcific lesions, elastic recoil may be less of a problem, but the noncompliant characteristics of these lesions (which can extend into the subintimal tissues) may result in poor dilatation results.

Although undersized balloon catheters yield poor initial results and perhaps increased restenosis, the use of oversized balloons does not help. Balloon catheters with diameters exceeding the reference segment diameter by more than 10% are associated with an increased risk of excessive intimal tearing and abrupt closure (70,71) and may also be associated with higher restenosis rates (71). These findings have led to the recommendation that balloon catheters be used to match (or slightly exceed) the target vessel diameter (70). Although this suggests that a more exact method for balloon sizing than simple visual assessment is needed, a convenient and reliable on-line technique for accurately measuring vessel diameter is not available to most operators.

The number of balloon inflations made, the maximum inflation pressure used, and the duration of balloon inflation (maximum single inflation time and total inflation time) may influence restenosis. A larger number of balloon inflations required to achieve a satisfactory result has been associated with increased restenosis in some patient subsets (36,74). However, a gradual increase in balloon inflation pressure up to that required to fully expand the artery is considered proper technique

(75); this may require several balloon inflations, depending on the operator's perception of the adequacy of dilatation at low balloon inflation pressures. Most operators do not perform additional balloon inflations in the vessel once an adequate lumen has been achieved; therefore, the number of balloon inflations may be related both to inherent lesion characteristics and operator preference. High balloon inflation pressures are generally avoided unless necessary to "crack" a resistant plaque. Excessive radial barotrauma may cause excessive medial (and perhaps atherointimal) smooth muscle cell injury and proliferation, as discussed above. It seems likely, then, that high inflation pressures would be correlated with increased restenosis; this has been identified as an independent risk factor (61) but not universally so (36). Prolonged balloon inflations were initially expected to reduce restenosis risk (18,76), but observational evidence indicates that long inflation times may have a deleterious effect on restenosis rates (36); one small randomized trial found no difference in rates of restenosis between patients undergoing 1-minute versus 5-minute balloon inflations (77).

Lesion Characteristics: Recently, lesion morphology has been the principal focus of restenosis studies. The assumption that the local environment could have a substantial impact on subsequent local healing after balloon dilatation seems reasonable and is increasingly supported by clinical, angiographic, biochemical, and animal studies.

Left anterior descending artery lesions are generally thought to be associated with a greater risk of restenosis than right coronary artery lesions or left circumflex artery lesions (53,72,78). However, at least one large retrospective study did not confirm this finding (60) and several multivariate analyses have failed to identify vessel location as a variable independently predictive of restenosis. The location within the coronary artery of a lesion may be important: lesions at the ostium of a coronary artery seem to develop restenosis more frequently than lesions in the body of a coronary artery; this seems to be particularly true for ostial left anterior descending artery lesions (79) and ostial right coronary lesions (80). Lesions located at bend points in an artery ($\geq$ 45° angle between proximal and distal arterial segment) have an increased risk of restenosis (81).

Lesion-specific morphologic features may be critical in estimating the risk of both acute complications and subsequent restenosis events following balloon dilatation. Lesion calcification, particularly dense calcification, is associated with higher restenosis rates (54,82), probably due to suboptimal dilatation results often encountered in rigid vascular segments. Some investigators, however, believe that balloon dilatation is akin to "breaking the bridge" that keeps the vessel narrowed and prevents vasomotion (83). The bulk of pathologic and animal data suggest that successful balloon dilatation involves stretching of compliant intimal and subintimal tissues. Since intimal calcification is associated with thinning and fibrosis or calcification of media, the subintimal tissues immediately beneath calcified atheromas are probably less compliant than normal subintimal tissues. Elastic recoil properties in such lesions are poorly understood.

Stenosis severity, whether measured by preangioplasty stenosis dimension (36,47,72) or by translesion pressure gradient (53), is a predictor of restenosis. Because atheromatous material must be displaced to improve the lumen area, it is clear that to attain a given final lumen area (or diameter), a larger tissue mass must be moved outward given a more severe lesion, resulting in greater stretch injury to the adjacent subintimal tissues. If vascular injury is related to restenosis, then more severe lesions could reasonably be expected to be associated with more restenosis than less severe lesions.

Angiographically evident intraluminal thrombus (84) has been associated with restenosis; the reasons for this have been discussed. Long lesions, particularly those greater than 20 mm in length, have an increased risk of acute complications and high restenosis rates (82,85), and diffuse or complex lesions seem to be at especially high risk of restenosis (79,86). Insufficient dilatation, elastic recoil and poor local hemorrheologic characteristics probably all contribute to restenosis in these lesions.

Lesions at branch vessel bifurcations may have an increased restenosis risk, but at least one study suggests that the restenosis rate of such lesions is the same as for unmatched nonbifurcation lesions (87). High local shear stress at branch points, which tends to increase platelet deposition at a given flow rate compared to a low shear stress environment, and perhaps a greater likelihood of excessive intimal tearing may increase the risk of restenosis in these lesions.

Dilatation of eccentric lesions can be problematic. Because the relatively noncompressible atheroma is organized to one side of the vessel lumen, symmetrically applied radial distending forces will tend to preferentially dilate the less diseased vessel wall opposite to the atheroma (Figure 3.5). This can result in overstretch of the less diseased vessel wall with an increased risk of intimal tearing and excessive injury to

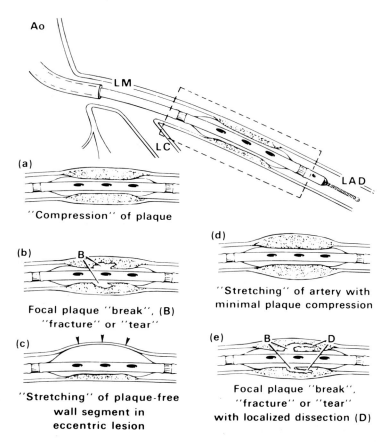

Figure 3.5. Possible mechanisms of balloon dilatation. Mechanisms that appear to be involved in successful balloon angioplasty include compression of atheromatous elements, stretch of underlying vessel wall, and formation of intimal tears (B) with focal dissections (D). Note also that dilatation of eccentric lesions may result in excessive stretch of the less diseased portion of the vessel, with relatively little change in the plaque. (Adapted by permission from Waller BF. Coronary lumen shape and the arc of the disease-free wall: morphologic observations and clinical relevance. J Am Coll Cardiol 1985;6:1100.)

medial smooth muscle cells (88). It is not surprising, then, that eccentric lesions can be associated with increased restenosis (82).

The issue of arterial dissection after balloon dilatation is complex. Certainly, large tears can result in acutely obstructive tissue flaps, which probably account for most unsuccessful balloon angioplasty attempts that result in acute myocardial infarction or urgent coronary bypass surgery. Large tears that do not cause immediate obstruction can still result in subacute ischemic complications or symptoms that may require further intervention. In such patients, the degree of luminal compromise and the presence of persistent intramural staining may identify patients at high risk of abrupt closure with repeated angioplasty attempts (89). These patients ought to be considered as having subacute intimal dissection rather that restenosis, since the biology and morphology of the lesion involved appears distinct from the intimal fibroplasia of typical restenosis. Patients with angiographically evident arterial dissections after balloon angioplasty were initially thought to have an increased risk of restenosis (11,90,91). It is clear, however, that dissections are an essential element in the mechanism of balloon angioplasty and are not associated with increased restenosis if such dissections occur in an otherwise satisfactory angioplasty (92,93). The distinction between a sufficient intimal tear and an excessive but nonobstructive intimal tear is indeed a fine line and currently defies a uniformly accepted definition.

Total occlusion of a coronary artery before angioplasty is a risk factor for restenosis (72,94–96). The impact of total occlusion seems variable (Table 3.3); reported restenosis rates have ranged from 20% to nearly 80% (72,94). Since total occlusions are, by definition, the most severe lesions possible, the increased risk of restenosis may be an extension of the observation that tighter narrowings have more restenosis than less severe narrowings. Although the incidence of restenosis in nontotal occlusions tends to plateau at about 3 to 6 months after dilatation (49), totally occluded coronary arterial lesions may continue to develop restenosis at a significant rate for a longer period of time (72; Figure 3.6).

These lesion characteristics seem to have a common element of increased risk of mechanical injury or biologic reactivity after (and perhaps before) balloon dilatation. If the degree of vascular injury resulting from dilatation is related to subsequent thrombin activation, platelet aggregation, release of growth mediators and vasoconstrictors, and consequently abundant cellular infiltration and replication, then morphologic features such as lesion severity, eccentricity, and angulation are of obvious concern. Similarly, diffuse or complex lesions, and especially those associated with preexisting intraluminal thrombus, will likely have less favorable local blood flow characteristics after balloon angioplasty. Hemorrheologic conditions after balloon dilatation are

Table 3.3. Restenosis After Successful Balloon Angioplasty of Total Coronary Occlusions

INVESTIGATOR	YEAR	PATIENTS (NO.)	ANGIOGRAPHIC FOLLOW-UP (%)	FOLLOW-UP PERIOD (MO.)	RESTENOSIS RATE (%)	RESTENOSIS DEFINITION
Clark (188)	1985	45	36	≥6	56	Unk
Holmes (189)	1985	13	77	7	20	4
Libow (190)	1985	53	79	6	43	3
DiSciascio (95)	1986	29	100	4–12	48	Unk
Melchior (96)	1987	40	71	1–48	55	9
Ellis (72)	1989	484	53	6	41	2
"	"	"	"	12	66	"
"	"	"	"	24	77	"

Adapted by permission from Laarman, Plante and de Feyter: PTCA of chronically occluded coronary arteries. Am Heart J 1990;119:1153–1160.

Restenosis definitions as for Table 3.1, except 9 = ≥ 60% diameter stenosis.

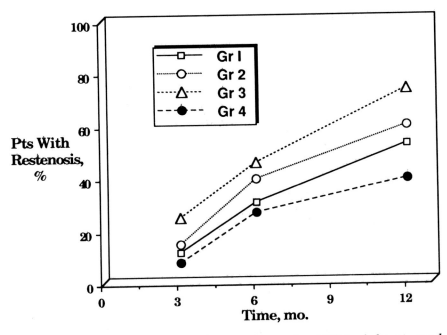

Figure 3.6. Incidence of angiographic restenosis after PTCA of chronic total coronary occlusions. Patients with successful PTCA of chronic total coronary occlusions having post-PTCA residual stenoses of less than 10% (Gr 1), 11% to 20% (Gr 2), or greater than 20% (Gr 3) were compared to patients with subtotal occlusions having final stenoses of 0% to 49% (Gr 4). Restenosis rate was higher for all total occlusion groups (1–3) compared to the subtotal occlusion group (4) at 12 months ($p < 0.01$, log rank analysis). Restenosis rate was also higher for those patients with total occlusions and a greater residual stenosis after PTCA ($p < 0.001$ comparing groups 1–3, life table analysis). (Adapted by permission from Ellis et al. Restenosis after excellent angiographic angioplasty result for chronic total coronary occlusion—implications for newer percutaneous revascularization devices. Am J Cardiol 1989;64:667–668.)

thought to have a profound influence on subsequent vascular healing (3,14). Intimal dissections associated with a low translesional pressure gradient and mildly abnormal filling patterns are probably different in some manner from those with high gradients or angiographic filling defects; the differences in restenosis rates between lesions in these two groups may well be related to differences in the degree of vascular injury occurring at the time of angioplasty.

A final technical component that is independent of the degree of injury done and yet may influence restenosis is coronary collateral circulation. Collateral blood flow may compete with normal anterograde blood flow after angioplasty, resulting in reduced blood flow over the dilated segment. Arteriographically evident collateral blood flow has been associated with a greater restenosis risk (97); reduction in the number of visible collateral vessels after angioplasty is believed to be an indicator of a successful dilatation (98), but the long-term impact of this finding is unknown. The presence and extent of collateral blood flow to the myocardial bed distal to the lesion undergoing dilatation can be measured nonarteriographically by means of the coronary artery wedge pressure, which is the pressure measured distal to the balloon catheter when the angioplasty balloon is inflated (99). Lesions with high coronary wedge pressures ($\geq$ 30 mm Hg) have been observed to have a higher restenosis rate than lesions with low pressures (100); it is unclear how the coronary artery wedge pressure should be integrated with the translesion pressure gradient in predicting likelihood of restenosis. Furthermore, with the current emphasis on low profile catheter systems, gradient measurement is increasingly uncommon.

Although helpful in risk assessment, knowledge of the relative role of lesion morphology in restenosis is actually of limited value currently, because the decision to proceed with balloon intervention is more likely to be based on immediate risk and benefit rather than the more remote risk of potential future events. Furthermore, since many clinical and technical factors seem to be associated with restenosis, the probability that a patient will have at least one risk factor for restenosis is high. Nonetheless, identification of a patient at very high risk for restenosis may influence decisions regarding the appropriateness of coronary bypass surgery or medical therapies instead of catheter-based revascularization. Some characteristics, particularly lesion morphologic features, may in the future dictate which adjunctive medical therapies should be used in conjunction with balloon angioplasty or aid in the choice of interventional device used.

Multivessel Angioplasty: Since both systemic factors and local effects may play a role in the development of fibrointimal hyperplasia, estimating the potential outcome after multivessel balloon dilation is a complex task. Meier has pointed out that, if all lesions in a patient behave similarly after dilatation, then the cumulative risk of restenosis after multivessel angioplasty (assuming an expected restenosis rate of 33%) could be described by a simple mathematical relationship (101):

$$\text{Restenosis rate} = (3 \times 3^{n-1} - 2 \times 2^{n-1})/3^n \times 100\%,$$

where n is the number of lesions dilated. However, as discussed above, restenosis is likely to be greatly influenced by technical and local factors that may have an impact on this equation in significant and unmeasurable ways. In a retrospective analysis of restenosis in 451 patients undergoing multivessel balloon dilatation at Mayo Clinic, the percentage of segments that developed restenosis was similar regardless of the number of vessels dilated (102). The relative risk of restenosis per patient increased modestly as the number of segments dilated increased, with patients undergoing dilatation of multiple segments of at least one coronary artery plus dilatation of at least one segment of another coronary artery at the highest relative risk of restenosis (1.77). This supports the argument that lesion characteristics are more important than patient characteristics in predicting restenosis.

Management of Restenosis Lesions

Animal models have been used chiefly to evaluate the potential for restenosis development and the effect of various therapeutics on restenosis after an initial balloon angioplasty procedure. Little work has been done to elucidate the effect of catheter interventions on restenotic lesions, that is, the effect of second or subsequent angioplasties. Thus, no foundation of animal research exists to direct decisions regarding the feasibility, efficacy, or appropriateness of repeat balloon angioplasty (or any other manner of treatment) in patients who develop restenosis lesions.

Despite this, a large clinical experience has shown that repeat balloon dilatation can be effective in managing patients with restenosis. An early (1984) report on the clinical efficacy of repeat PTCA from Emory University indicated that sustained patency could be obtained in some patients with restenosis if a second or third angioplasty was performed (101,103). Using a strategy of repeated balloon dilatation, continued clinical success was attained in 78% of treated patients without the need for coronary bypass surgery. This study also highlighted the high success rates (> 99%) possible with repeat balloon dilatation procedures. A multicenter experience from the same period confirmed these findings (104). Since then, several centers have reported high success rates and low complication states with PTCA performed for a second and a third time (105–107). Generally, restenosis rates following second or third balloon dilatations have been similar to the rates reported for a first angioplasty (103,104,106), although some have found that the risk of restenosis is higher among patients requiring multiple interventions (108). Most practitioners believe that patients requiring more than three or four catheter interventions are likely to need bypass surgery for successful long-term management.

Several studies have identified clinical and procedural features that may be related to restenosis after multiple balloon angioplasty procedures. A characteristic consistently related to restenosis is a short time interval from original to subsequent dilatation (105–107,109). Pathologic observations in patients dying late after repeat PTCA procedures confirm that a new layer of fibrointimal hyperplasia develops with each procedure (110), similar in morphology to the hyperplastic cell layers found in primary atheromatous tissues. These latter probably develop after spontaneous plaque ruptures (111,112). Robust smooth muscle cell and myofibroblast activation may occur when repeat balloon dilatation is undertaken in a relatively young fibrous restenosis lesion (when the constituent cells are in a synthetic, rather than quiescent, phase). In this setting, further stimulation of the already active cells may result in a greater proliferative response to stretch than would stimulation of quiescent cells. Electron microscopic studies indicate that recruitment of a larger number of fibromuscular cells from the underlying media and from the fibrous portion of the atheromatous intima will occur when PTCA is repeated after a short interval from a first dilatation than when repeated after a long interval (113). Therefore, restenosis after multiple PTCA procedures may be related not only to the extent of vascular injury that occurs, but also to the biologic responsiveness of the cells in the neointima and media of the dilated segment.

No method is currently available to assess the biologic responsiveness of vascular smooth muscle cells. Also lacking are effective therapies to limit the responsiveness of cells stimulated by circumferential barotrauma. Newer interventional devices have focused on the means of reducing obstructive vascular tissue elements without (or with minimal) barotrauma to reduce the stimulus for smooth muscle cell replication.

Table 3.4. Restenosis After Angioplasty of Saphenous Vein Bypass Grafts

INVESTIGATOR	YEAR	PATIENTS (NO.)	ANGIOGRAPHIC FOLLOW-UP (%)	FOLLOW-UP PERIOD (MO.)	RESTENOSIS RATE (%)	RESTENOSIS DEFINITION
Douglas (180)	1983	58	62	6	24	Unk
Block (181)	1984	31	71	8	39	Unk
El Gamal (182)	1984	24	79	26	54	Unk
Corbelli (183)	1985	43	100	8	30	Unk
Dorros (184)	1985	74	Unk	12	20	Unk
Reeder (185)	1986	16	69	20	50	4
Cote (186)	1987	76	57	8	19	3
Ernst (187)	1987	32	49	19	31	3

Adapted by permission from Klein and Rosenblum: Restenosis after successful percutaneous transluminal coronary angioplasty. Prog Cardiovasc Dis 1990; 32:365–382.
Restenosis definitions as for Table 3.1.

Restenosis in Saphenous Vein and Internal Mammary Bypass Grafts

Aortocoronary artery bypass surgery is of proven utility in patients with ischemic syndromes not sufficiently managed with other means. However, an accelerated form of atherosclerosis has been observed in arterialized segments of saphenous vein that can limit the durability of vein bypass grafts. Only 50% to 60% of saphenous vein bypass grafts are patent 10 years after surgery, and of those remaining patent, half will have significant atheromatous disease (114,115) and may require catheter-based treatment or surgical replacement. In addition to the increased risk of acute complications (especially embolization of atheromatous material) during balloon dilatation, vein graft lesions have a high rate of restenosis: the American College of Cardiology/American Heart Association Task Force on the Assessment of Diagnostic and Therapeutic Cardiovascular Procedures (Subcommittee on PTCA) places lesions in old, friable vein grafts in a higher risk category for balloon dilatation (type C) and states that 50% of treated vein graft lesions will restenose (116). Several studies involving relatively small numbers of patients have reported restenosis rates ranging from 19% to 54% (Table 3.4); as has been pointed out, these studies suffer from a broad range of follow-up times (6–26 months) and some have a low follow-up angiographic study rate (75). Lesions at the aortic anastamosis and within the body of vein grafts are expected to have a 50% incidence of restenosis, whereas lesions at the distal anastamoses seem to have an incidence of restenosis of about 37%, which is similar to that of native coronary arteries (117). The reasons for these differences are not clear.

Internal mammary artery grafts survive longer without the development of obstructive atheromatous disease, but many of these grafts may also require attention. Angioplasty of internal mammary artery grafts can now be managed reasonably well, and lesions dilated in these grafts appear to have an incidence of restenosis similar to that reported for native coronary arteries (37%; 117,118).

Impact of Newer Interventional Devices

Balloon angioplasty has been approved for general use for more than a decade, and extensive experience has been gained in its use in a wide variety of clinical settings. Despite this, significant limitations remain for the technique. Restenosis is arguably the most serious remaining limitation to angioplasty because it affects such a large proportion of patients undergoing the procedure. With this in mind, several physician–inventors have devised new tools to open obstructed coronary arteries that might reduce the incidence of restenosis.

Directional Coronary Atherectomy

Simpson coined the term "atherectomy" to describe a procedure in which obstructive atheroma was removed rather than remodeled. He developed a directional coronary atherectomy (DCA) catheter that can be advanced across a coronary lesion and can resect diseased tissues that block the vessel lumen (Figure 3.7). Because a low residual stenosis with a relatively smooth luminal surface is the expected result of the procedure and because barotrauma to the underlying media should be less than with balloon angioplasty, DCA was expected to reduce restenosis rates. Early data from the United States Directional Coronary Atherectomy Investigator Group indicated, however, that restenosis occurs after DCA with a frequency similar to that reported for balloon angioplasty (119). Restenosis after DCA appears to be increased if the treated lesion is in a vessel with a lumen less than 3.0 mm, is at an ostial location, is in a saphenous vein bypass graft, or is initially a postballoon angioplasty restenosis lesion (119–121).

Because resection of media and adventitia is not uncommon with DCA (23,122), it is reasonable to question whether the occurrence of subintimal resection has an impact on restenosis events. Some investi-

Figure 3.7. Directional coronary atherectomy. Rather than remodeling the diseased coronary artery, the AtheroCath[TM] directional atherectomy device (DVI, Redwood City, Calif.) resects tissues obstructing the coronary lumen. A rotating cup-shaped cutter shaves tissues prolapsing into the cutter housing and collects excised tissues into a distal nosecone chamber. Turning the catheter redirects the cutter housing toward other areas needing treatment (reproduced with permission from Mayo Clinic proceedings).

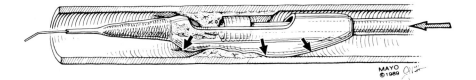

MAYO
©1989

gators have speculated that medial resection might reduce restenosis events because the media is believed to be a primary source of smooth muscle cells that proliferate after coronary intervention (123). However, we have found that restenosis rates increase somewhat with deeper tissue resection (26). Whether this represents a stronger stimulus to cellular proliferation with deeper vascular wall excision or reflects greater barotrauma due to higher balloon inflation pressures or other technical considerations remains unclear. A recent report argues that subintimal tissue resection does not appreciably increase restenosis after DCA (124). Limited autopsy data from the few patients who have died after directional atherectomy (26) suggest that intimal hyperplasia is most abundant in areas with the deepest vessel wall excision (Figure 3.8).

Currently, a randomized clinical trial is underway to compare restenosis rates after balloon angioplasty or directional coronary atherectomy of lesions in native coronary arteries (the Coronary Angioplasty Versus Ex-

Figure 3.8. Intimal hyperplasia following directional coronary atherectomy. Cross section of a saphenous vein graft treated with directional atherectomy 85 days prior to death. Atherectomy treatment sites are evident as focal defects in the atheromatous intima that have filled in with myofibroblasts. The most abundant cellular proliferation has occurred at the sites of deepest (subintimal) tissue excision. Hematoxylin–eosin, 25 × .

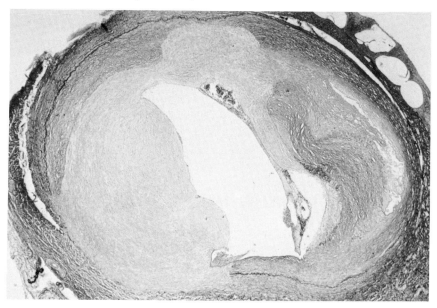

cisional Atherectomy Trial—CAVEAT). This trial will be the first to directly compare outcome in patients treated with a new interventional device to those treated with conventional angioplasty. A limb of this trial (CAVEAT–SVG) will compare PTCA and DCA in saphenous vein graft lesions.

Rotational Atherectomy Devices

Several moderate- or high-speed rotating catheter systems intended to pulverize atheromatous tissue into particles small enough to be removed by aspiration or to pass harmlessly through capillary beds are under development. The transluminal endarterectomy–extraction catheter (TEC) uses a guidewire-directed rotating blade to pulverize tissues into microscopic fragments (125,126). Saline is injected through the catheter to wash over the treatment area and is then aspirated into a vacuum bottle. Particulate material generated by the action of the blades is thereby removed from the artery. Because this device should generate less barotrauma than balloon catheter systems, restenosis may be decreased. This device may find particular application in long, diffusely diseased segments or other "unfavorable" lesions in which conventional angioplasty has a lower probability of success and a higher risk of restenosis (127,128). The TEC device has also been advocated for use in treatment of diffusely diseased saphenous vein grafts, particularly those with evidence of intraluminal thrombus (129).

The Rotablator is another rotational atherectomy catheter that uses a guidewire-directed high-speed rotating burr coated with industrial-grade diamond chips that micropulverize atheroma (130). Most particulate debris generated with this device is less than 10 μ in diameter and is expected to pass through distal capillary beds without causing obstruction (131,132). Treatment of extremely long lesions, however, may generate such a large amount of debris that distall capillary beds are filled, resulting in regional myocardial dysfunction or infarction (132,133). Again, this device results in less barotrauma than PTCA and may overcome elastic recoil problems that could contribute to restenosis (130).

These devices are early in their development, and only preliminary data are available regarding restenosis events. These data involve limited numbers of patients and incomplete angiographic follow-up. According to the most current information, none of the atherectomy devices has yet demonstrated restenosis risk below that expected after balloon angioplasty (134–137).

Laser Systems

Several laser devices are now under study. Infrared lasers are associated with high temperatures and produce significant thermal injury when applied to biologic tissues. Ultraviolet lasers generate much less heat; they appear to cause tissue destruction by exciting the electrons participating in chemical bonds sufficiently to cause the bonds to break, resulting in tissue ablation with minimal thermal injury at the treatment site (138,139). A laser system of particular interest is the excimer ("excited-dimer") laser, which uses a xenon–chloride source to create laser energy in the ultraviolet range. Since this "cold" laser creates injury that is associated with less platelet deposition than "hot" lasers (140), there may be a less potent stimulus for intimal hyperplasia. The excimer laser has been applied successfully to native coronary and saphenous vein graft lesions using flexible fiberoptic delivery systems and is being investigated in several medical centers (141–143). As with rotational atherectomy devices, only early data are available pertaining to restenosis, but preliminary reports indicate that restenosis probably occurs at a rate similar to that reported for balloon angioplasty (141,144). Although investigators initially felt that restenosis may be increased when balloon angioplasty is used in conjunction with excimer laser therapy compared with "stand-alone" excimer laser (145), recent data indicate that restenosis after excimer laser treatment is not increased by use of adjunctive balloon angioplasty (146). Autopsy analysis of one man who died after successful excimer laser suggested that incomplete atheroma ablation may contribute to subsequent restenosis (147). The relationship between postlaser angioplasty restenosis rates and technical aspects of the laser procedure is yet to be established.

Low-range ultraviolet laser energy (266 nm wavelength) appears to be cytotoxic to vascular smooth muscle cells when cells are irradiated during a rapid growth phase (148). This observation suggests that laser irradiation, perhaps a short time after balloon angioplasty, may be beneficial in reducing restenosis.

A true laser–balloon angioplasty (LBA) catheter has been developed that diffuses laser energy through the balloon catheter when the balloon is inflated (149). This results in transient superheating of surrounding tissues and "welding" of the vessel wall in a configuration that conforms to the shape of the inflated balloon (150,151). Thermal ablation of surrounding smooth muscle cells was postulated to reduce the risk of excessive intimal hyperplasia (152). Also, LBA is believed to seal intimal tears and dessicate thrombus, thereby producing a smoother luminal surface. Although initial results are good, a high rate of restenosis has been associated with this device (151). A recent report on a randomized multicenter pilot study to compare LBA with PTCA found no significant difference in 6-month restenosis rates (153). This finding has limited subsequent development of this device.

Stents

Intracoronary stents may reduce restenosis by overcoming elastic recoil and physically supporting the arterial wall, resulting in a predictable and persisting luminal dimension after therapy. Sigwart has reported that the incidence of restenosis after placement of the self-expanding Wallstent in human coronary arteries is significantly less than that associated with balloon angioplasty and has indicated that stents may be a useful treatment modality for restenosis (154,155). In a recent report on the first 56 patients (96% with follow-up angiography) to receive the Wallstent, angiographically documented restenosis (lesion ≥ 50%) was found in only 5 (9%) of patients (156). However, 8 patients (14%) had apparent thrombotic occlusion but were not considered to have restenosis, even though the occlusion may have occurred as late as 8 months after stent implantation. The best results seem to occur when the stent is used in large vessels (vein grafts or coronary arteries ≥ 3.5 mm diameter). Some data suggest that arterial lumen dimensions may be sustained and perhaps even improved over time with use of coronary stents (157,158).

The Palmaz–Schatz stent consists of a rigid slotted metallic tube that is fitted over an angioplasty balloon catheter and delivered by inflation of the balloon (159). A low restenosis rate following coronary implantation of the Palmaz–Schatz stent has been observed (160,161). Overall restenosis rates of about 20% are reported, and restenosis rates as low as 7% may be achieved in some patient subsets. It should be noted, however, that currently this stent is being deployed on an elective basis and has not been used to treat abrupt vascular closure after balloon angioplasty. Also, only relatively large diameter vessels have been treated with this stent. Thrombotic occlusions and technical issues related to placement of a rigid stent are limitations to this device.

The Gianturco–Roubin stent is balloon-expandable and consists of a thin stainless steel filament wrapped in a back-and-forth serpentine fashion around a special angioplasty balloon catheter. This design allows the stent to be extremely flexible, which may facilitate its placement in tortuous vascular segments. Recent multicenter data suggest that this stent may have a restenosis rate ($\geq$ 50% stenosis) of about 35% (162); this figure is likely to be influenced by the indication for stent placement because the Gianturco–Roubin stent has been placed for vascular disruption as well as for postangioplasty restenosis. A similar stent, the Wiktor stent, has a continuous circumferential pattern of wrapping around its deployment balloon and is made of tantalum, which greatly improves visibility under fluoroscopy. At this time, no clinical data exist pertaining to restenosis with use of this stent.

Comparisons between different stent designs are not possible at this time because the patient selection criteria, lesion morphologic features, medical protocols, and follow-up characteristics vary significantly for each stent under study. A broader experience with each of these stents will be required to determine actual restenosis rates and to identify technical variables that have an impact on restenosis after stent placement. Then, randomized trials will be required to determine if one stent design is better than another in the treatment of specified patient subsets.

Although several drugs are known to reduce intimal hyperplasia after balloon angioplasty in animal models, the potential development of toxic side effects from high systemic levels of these drugs remains a limitation to the pharmaceutical treatment of restenosis in patients. Efforts are currently aimed at developing nonmetallic stents that might be capable of delivering drugs locally at the site of stent deployment. In this way, high concentrations of drugs could be achieved at the treatment site while systemic effects of a drug could be avoided or minimized. Also, coating of stents with cultured endothelial cells or modified myofibroblasts before placement of the stent may limit subsequent intimal hyperplasia (163).

Although intracoronary stents have several attractive features that should have an impact on restenosis, the development of intimal hyperplastic tissues through stents sufficient to cause clinical symptoms has been observed; optimal management of this situation is still uncertain, but balloon dilatation of these lesions is possible in some patients (164).

New Imaging Modalities

Coronary arteriography provides a silhouette of the intravascular space of coronary arteries. Unfortunately, many important features of a lesion that could influence restenosis development after intervention may not be identifiable with coronary arteriography alone.

Angioscopy allows an operator to visualize directly the interior of the vessel. Flexible fiberoptic catheters can be passed percutaneously into coronary arteries to illuminate the lumen surface (165). The interior of the vessel can be seen through the fiberoptic eyepiece, or, using electronic chip camera technology, an image of the vascular lumen can be displayed on a color monitor. The ability to see the vessel to be treated allows improved understanding of the pathophysiology of coronary syndromes (166–173) and may identify the presence of morphologic features, such as thrombus or mural hemorrhage, that might aid in predicting the risk of restenosis or help in deciding which interventional tool would be most appropriate (174,175). Angioscopy may reveal important information about the restenosis lesion itself (176). However, angioscopy can delineate only surface characteristics (Figure 3.9).

Intravascular ultrasound can be performed with miniaturized ultrasonic transducers that can be introduced over guidewires. These devices generate a transaxial image of the vessel (Figure 3.10) and can delineate

Figure 3.9. Intraoperative angioscopy of coronary artery after unsuccessful balloon angioplasty. An irregular luminal surface is apparent as a result of atherosclerotic disease. Attempted balloon angioplasty has resulted in disruption of atheroma that protrudes into lumen. Such disruptions may appear angiographically as luminal haziness. Small black dots are artifacts due to optical fiber failure. (Courtesy of Dr. T. Sherman, U.C.L.A. Medical Center, Los Angeles, Calif.)

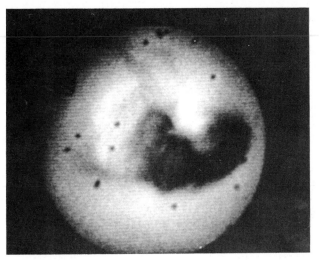

not only surface features but deeper vascular characteristics as well (177). Atheroma can be interrogated thoroughly to reveal the nature of the lesion (e.g., soft with high lipid content or fibrotic and calcified) and results of intervention (178); this information may assist in selecting the treatment modality best able to predict restenosis risk. Currently, these devices are available only to clinical investigators for use in coronary arteries.

Summary and Expectations

The development of balloon angioplasty techniques was a milestone in the continuum of progress in coronary disease treatment. The safety and efficacy of PTCA are excellent, and new devices are likely to have similar, possibly better characteristics as they are developed and refined. Were it not for the problem of restenosis, it is reasonable to claim

Figure 3.10. Intravascular ultrasound image of an atheromatous artery before and after balloon angioplasty. Before dilatation (baseline), atheromatous intima is encroaching upon the vessel lumen, and alterations of the medial area are evident as well. The true lumen is highlighted by white dashes. Following balloon dilatation (8 mm PTA), enlargement of the vascular lumen is evident. Disruption of the intimal plaque that has extended into the underlying media is apparent (white arrows).

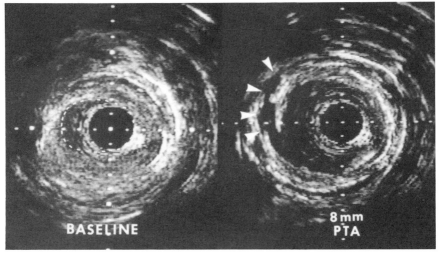

that a majority of patients with coronary disease who have 1) symptoms of myocardial ischemia despite medical therapy, 2) large amounts of myocardium at jeopardy of infarction, 3) critical disease in a vessel following nontransmural myocardial infarction, or 4) unstable ischemic syndromes could be treated promptly with catheter-based techniques. However, the impact of restenosis on the long-term efficacy of catheter-based revascularization, the cumulative risk of multiple catheter procedures, the financial costs, and the psychologic costs (for both patient and practitioner) have been enormous.

From the interventionalist's perspective, restenosis represents the largest hurdle to overcome in effective "less invasive" revascularization of coronary obstructions. Certainly, some patients would be better served with bypass surgery than repeated attempts at balloon angioplasty. However, since it is not possible to prospectively separate those patients who will develop restenosis from those who will not and since the majority of patients are successfully treated with angioplasty, it seems reasonable to offer catheter-based revascularization to most patients who are suitable candidates.

With the huge amounts of time, energy, and money currently being spent on restenosis research, one must be optimistic that some solution, either partial or complete, will soon be found. It does appear that restenosis is a tissue response to vascular injury and is, therefore, unlikely to be overcome by the newer revascularization devices; continued use of new devices should be scrutinized with this in mind. However, inroads are being made in identifying promising medical therapies, and current wisdom has it that the answer to restenosis will be found in the pharmacy rather than in the tool box. Ultimately, the mating of intracoronary delivery devices with medical therapies may be required to attain the best relief from restenosis after intervention.

References

1. Faxon DP. The impact of interventional techniques on the practice of cardiology. Keio J Med 1989;38:60–64.
2. Califf RM, Fortan DF, Frid DJ, et al. Restenosis after coronary angioplasty: an overview. J Am Coll Cardiol 1991;17:2B–13B.
3. Liu MW, Roubin GS, King SB. Restenosis after coronary angioplasty: potential biologic determinants and role of intimal hyperplasia. Circulation 1989;79:1374–1387.

4. Leisch F, Kerschner K, Harringer W, Schutzenberger W. Coronary angioplasty after intravenous streptokinase in acute myocardial infarction: influence of restenosis on clinical outcome and left ventricular function. Clin Cardiol 1990;13:253–259.

5. Reeder G, Krishan T, Nobrega F, et al. Is percutaneous coronary angioplasty less expensive than bypass surgery? N Engl J Med 1984;311: 1157–1162.

6. Ross R. Glomset J. The pathogenesis of atherosclerosis. N Engl J Med 1976;295:420–425.

7. Rose B, Pepine CJ. Restenosis following coronary artery angioplasty: patterns, recognition, and results of repeat angioplasty. Cardiovasc Clin 1988;19:233–251.

8. Faxon D, Sanborn S, Weber V, et al. Restenosis following transluminal angioplasty in experimental atherosclerosis. Arteriosclerosis 1984;4: 189–195.

9. Ip JH, Fuster V, Badimon L, et al. Syndromes of accelerated atherosclerosis: role of vascular injury and smooth muscle cell proliferation. J Am Coll Cardiol 1990;15:1667–1687.

10. Austin G, Ratliff N, Hollman J, et al. Intimal proliferation of smooth muscle cells as an explanation for recurrent coronary artery stenosis after percutaneous transluminal coronary angioplasty. J Am Coll Cardiol 1985;6:369–375.

11. Essed C, Van den Brand M, Becker A. Transluminal coronary angioplasty and early restenosis: Fibrocellular occlusion after wall laceration. Br Heart J 1983;49:393–396.

12. Block PC. Restenosis after percutaneous transluminal coronary angioplasty—anatomic and pathophysiological mechanisms. Strategies for prevention. Circulation 1990;81(suppl IV):2–4.

13. Cequier A, Bonan R, Crepeau J, et al. Restenosis and progression of coronary atherosclerosis after coronary angioplasty. J Am Coll Cardiol 1988;12:49–55.

14. Forrester JS, Fishbein M, Helfant R, Fagin J. A paradigm for restenosis based on cell biology: clues for the development of new preventive therapies. J Am Coll Cardiol 1991;17:758–769.

15. Giraldo A, Esposo O, Meis J. Intimal hyperplasia as a cause of restenosis after percutaneous transluminal coronary angioplasty. Arch Pathol Lab Med 1985;109:173–175.

16. Hwang MH, Sihdu P, Pacold I, et al. Progression of coronary artery disease after percutaneous transluminal coronary angioplasty. Am Heart J 1988;115:297–301.

17. Karsch KR, Haase KK, Wehrmann M, et al. Smooth muscle cell prolif-

eration and restenosis after stand alone coronary excimer laser angioplasty. J Am Coll Cardiol 1991;17:991–994.

18. King JF, Manley JC, Al-Wathiqui MH. Restenosis after angioplasty: mechanisms and clinical experience. Cardiol Clin 1989;7:853–864.

19. Morimoto S, Mizuno Y, Hiramitsu S, et al. Restenosis after percutaneous transluminal coronary angioplasty—a histopathological study using autopsied hearts. Jpn Circ J 1990;54:43–56.

20. Nobuyoshi M, Kimura T, Ohishi H, et al. Restenosis after percutaneous transluminal coronary angioplasty: pathologic observations in 20 patients. J Am Coll Cardiol 1991;17:433–439.

21. Steele P, Chesebro J, Stanson A, et al. Balloon angioplasty: natural history of the pathophysiologic response to injury in a pig model. Circ Res 1985;57:105–112.

22. Ueda M, Becker AE, Tsukada T, et al. Fibrocellular tissue response after percutaneous transluminal coronary angioplasty. An immunocytochemical analysis of the cellular composition. Circulation 1991;83: 1327–1332.

23. Garratt KN, Edwards WD, Kaufmann U, et al. Differential histopathology of primary atherosclerotic and restenotic lesions from coronary arteries and saphenous vein bypass grafts in tissue obtained from 73 patients by percutaneous atherectomy. J Am Coll Cardiol 1991; 17:442–448.

24. Heras M, Chesebro J, Penny W, et al. Importance of adequate heparin dosage in arterial angioplasty in a porcine model. Circulation 1988;78: 654–660.

25. Gal D, Rongione A, Slovenkal G, et al. Atherosclerotic Yucatan microswine: an animal model with high-grade, fibrocalcific, nonfatty lesions suitable for testing catheter-based interventions. Am Heart J 1990;119:291–300.

26. Garratt KN, Edwards WD, Vlietstra RE, et al. Coronary morphology after percutaneous directional coronary atherectomy in humans: autopsy analysis of three patients. J Am Coll Cardiol 1990;16:1432–1436.

27. Nawroth P, Kisiel W, Stern D. The role of endothelium in the homeostatic balance of haemostasis. Clin Haematol 1985;14:531–546.

28. Harker L, Schwartz S. Endothelium and arteriosclerosis. Clin Haematol 1981;10:283–296.

29. Scharf R, Harker L. Thrombosis and atherosclerosis: regulatory role of interactions among blood components and endothelium. Blut 1987;55:131–144.

30. Chesebro J, Lam J, Badimon L, Fuster V. Restenosis after arterial an-

gioplasty: a hemorrheologic response to injury. Am J Cardiol 1987;60 (suppl B):10B–16B.

31. Nieuwenhuis H, Akkerman J, Houdijk W, Sixma J. Human blood platelets showing no response to collagen fail to express glycoprotein Ia. Nature 1985;318:470–472.

32. Wilcox J, Smith K, Williams L, et al. Platelet-derived growth factor mRNA detection in human atherosclerotic plaques by in situ hybridization. J Clin Invest 1988;82:1134–1143.

33. Mann K, Tracy P, Nesheim M. Assembly and function of prothrombinase complex on synthetic and natural membranes. In: Oates J, Hawiger J, Ross R, eds. Interactions of platelets with the vessel wall. Washington, DC: American Physiologic Society, 1985:47–57.

34. Monsen CH, Adams PC, Badimon L, et al. Platelet–vessel wall interactions in the development of restenosis after coronary angioplasty. Z Kardiol 1987;6:23–28.

35. Halon DA, Merdler A, Shefer A, et al. Identifying patients at high risk for restenosis after percutaneous transluminal coronary angioplasty for unstable angina pectoris. Am J Cardiol 1989;64:289–293.

36. Rupprecht HJ, Brennecke R, Bernhard G, et al. Analysis of risk factors for restenosis after PTCA. Cathet Cardiovasc Diagn 1990;19:151–159.

37. Johansson SR, Ekstrom L, Emanuelsson H. Higher recurrence rate after coronary angioplasty in unstable angina pectoris. Angiology 1991;42: 273–280.

38. Guyton J, Rosenberg R, Clowes A, Karnovsky M. Inhibition of rat arterial smooth muscle cell proliferation by heparin. In vivo studies with anticoagulant and non-anticoagulant heparin. Circ Res 1980;46:625–634.

39. Clowes A, Karnovsky M. Suppression by heparin of smooth muscle cell proliferation in injured arteries. Nature 1977;265:625–626.

40. Ellis SG, Roubin GS, Wilentz J, et al. Effect of 18- to 24-hour heparin administration for prevention of restenosis after uncomplicated coronary angioplasty. Am Heart J 1989;117:777–782.

41. Schwartz L, Bourassa MG, Lesperance J, et al. Aspirin and dipyridamole in the prevention of restenosis after percutaneous transluminal coronary angioplasty. N Engl J Med 1988;318:1714–1719.

42. Thornton M, Gruentzig A, Hollman J, et al. Coumadin and aspirin in the prevention of recurrence after transluminal coronary angioplasty. Circulation 1984;69:721–727.

43. Gruentzig A. Results from coronary angioplasty and implications for the future. Am Heart J 1982;103:779–782.

44. Meier B, Gruentzig A, Goebel N, et al. Assessment of stenoses in coro-

nary angioplasty: inter- and intra-observer variability. Int J Cardiol 1983;3:159–169.

45. Blackshear J, O'Callaghan W, Califf R. Medical approaches to prevention of restenosis after coronary angioplasty. J Am Coll Cardiol 1987;9: 834–848.

46. Finci L, Meier B, De Bruyne B, et al. Angiographic follow-up after multivessel percutaneous transluminal coronary angioplasty. Am J Cardiol 1987;60:467–470.

47. Holmes DR Jr, Vlietstra RE, Smith HC, et al. Restenosis after percutaneous transluminal coronary angioplasty (PTCA): a report from the PTCA Registry of the National Heart, Lung and Blood Institute. Am J Cardiol 1984;53:77C–81C.

48. King SI, Weintraub W, Tao X, et al. Bimodal distribution of diameter stenosis 4–12 months after angioplasty: implications for definitions and interpretation of restenosis (abstr). J Am Coll Cardiol 1991;17 (suppl A):345A.

49. Nobuyoshi M, Kimura T, Nosaka H, et al. Restenosis after successful percutaneous transluminal coronary angioplasty: serial angiographic follow-up of 229 patients. J Am Coll Cardiol 1988;12:616–623.

50. Kaltenbach M, Keber G, Scherer D, et al. Recurrence rate after successful coronary angioplasty. Eur Heart J 1985;6:276–281.

51. Meyer J, Schmitz H, Kiesslich T, et al. Percutaneous transluminal coronary angioplasty in patients with stable and unstable angina pectoris: analysis of early and late results. Am Heart J 1983;106:973–980.

52. de Feyter P, Serruys P, van den Brand M, et al. Emergency coronary angioplasty in refractory unstable angina. N Engl J Med 1985;313:342–346.

53. Leimgruber P, Roubin G, Hollman J, et al. Restenosis after successful coronary angioplasty in patients with single vessel disease. Circulation 1986;73:710–717.

54. Ernst S, van der Feltz T, Bal E, et al. Long term angiographic follow up, cardiac events, and survival in patients undergoing percutaneous transluminal coronary angioplasty. Br Heart J 1987;7:220–225.

55. Guiteras VP, Bourassa MG, David PR, et al. Restenosis after successful percutaneous transluminal coronary angioplasty: the Montreal Heart Institute experience. Am J Cardiol 1987;60:50B–55B.

56. Mabin T, Holmes DR Jr, Smith H, et al. Follow-up clinical results in patients undergoing percutaneous transluminal coronary angioplasty. Circulation 1985;71:754–760.

57. Levine S, Ewels C, Rosing D, Kent K. Coronary angioplasty: clinical and angiographic follow-up. Am J Cardiol 1985;55:673–676.

58. Serruys PW, Luijten HE, Beatt KJ, et al. Incidence of restenosis after

successful coronary angioplasty: a time-related phenomenon. A quantitative angiographic study in 342 consecutive patients at 1, 2, 3, and 4 months. Circulation 1988;77:361–371.

59. Cowley M, Mullins S, Kelsey S, et al. Sex differences in early and long term results of coronary angioplasty in the National Heart, Lung and Blood Percutaneous Transluminal Coronary Angioplasty Registry. Circulation 1985;71:90–97.

60. Myler R, Topol E, Shaw R, et al. Multiple vessel coronary angioplasty: classification, results, and patterns of restenosis in 494 consecutive patients. Cathet Cardiovasc Diagn 1987;13:1–15.

61. Rapold HJ, David PR, Guiteras VP, et al. Restenosis and its determinants in first and repeat coronary angioplasty. Eur Heart J 1987;8:575–586.

62. Raizner A, Hust R, Lewis J, et al. Transluminal coronary angioplasty in the elderly. Am J Cardiol 1986;57:29–32.

63. Mock M, Holmes DR Jr, Vlietstra R, et al. Percutaneous transluminal coronary angioplasty in elderly patients: experience in the National Heart, Lung and Blood Institute Percutaneous Transluminal Coronary Angioplasty Registry. Am J Cardiol 1984;53:89C–91C.

64. Hollman J, Gruentzig A, Meier B, et al. Factors affecting recurrence after successful coronary angioplasty (abstr). J Am Coll Cardiol 1983; 1:644.

65. Quigley PJ, Hlatky MA, Hinohara T, et al. Repeat percutaneous transluminal coronary angioplasty and predictors of recurrent restenosis. Am J Cardiol 1989;63:409–413.

66. Margolis J, Krieger R, Glamser E. Coronary angioplasty: increased restenosis risk in insulin dependent diabetics (abstr). Circulation 1984; 70:176.

67. Arora RR, Konrad K, Badhwar K, Hollman J. Restenosis after transluminal coronary angioplasty: a risk factor analysis. Cathet Cardiovasc Diagn 1990;19:17–22.

68. Macdonald RG, Henderson MA, Hirshfeld JW Jr, et al. Patient-related variables and restenosis after percutaneous transluminal coronary angioplasty—a report from the M-HEART Group. Am J Cardiol 1990; 66:926–931.

69. Laskey MA, Deutsch E, Hirshfeld JW Jr, et al. Influence of heparin therapy on percutaneous transluminal coronary angioplasty outcome in patients with coronary arterial thrombus. Am J Cardiol 1990;65:179–182.

70. Nichols AB, Smith R, Berke AD, et al. Importance of balloon size in coronary angioplasty. J Am Coll Cardiol 1989;13:1094–1100.

71. Roubin GS, Douglas JS Jr, King SB III, et al. Influence of balloon size on

initial success, acute complications, and restenosis after percutaneous transluminal coronary angioplasty. A prospective randomized study. Circulation 1988;78:557–565.

72. Ellis SG, Shaw RE, Gershony G, et al. Risk factors, time course and treatment effect for restenosis after successful percutaneous transluminal coronary angioplasty of chronic total occlusion. Am J Cardiol 1989;63:897–901.

73. Klein LW, Noveck H, Kramer B, et al. Comparative analysis of coronary angiographic morphology following restenosis. Am Heart J 1990;119:35–41.

74. Glazier JJ, Varricchione TR, Ryan TJ, et al. Factors predicting recurrent restenosis after percutaneous transluminal coronary balloon angioplasty. Am J Cardiol 1989;63:902–905.

75. Klein LW, Rosenblum J. Restenosis after successful percutaneous transluminal coronary angioplasty. Prog Cardiovasc Dis 1990;32:365–382.

76. Douglas JS Jr, King SB III, Roubin GS. Influence of the methodology of percutaneous transluminal coronary angioplasty on restenosis. Am J Cardiol 1987;60:29B–33B.

77. DiSciascio G, Vetrovec GW, Lewis SA, et al. Clinical and angiographic recurrence following PTCA for nonacute total occlusions: comparison of one- versus five-minute inflations. Am Heart J 1990;120:529–532.

78. Vandormael MG, Deligonul U, Kern MJ, et al. Multilesion coronary angioplasty: clinical and angiographic follow-up. J Am Coll Cardiol 1987;10:246–252.

79. Roubin GS, King SB III, Douglas JS Jr. Restenosis after percutaneous transluminal coronary angioplasty: the Emory University Hospital experience. Am J Cardiol 1987;60:39B–43B.

80. Topol EJ, Ellis SG, Fishman J, et al. Multicenter study of percutaneous transluminal angioplasty for right coronary artery ostial stenosis. J Am Coll Cardiol 1987;9:1214–1218.

81. Ellis SG, Roubin GS, King SB III, et al. Importance of stenosis morphology in the estimation of restenosis risk after elective percutaneous transluminal coronary angioplasty. Am J Cardiol 1989;63:30–34.

82. Mata L, Bosch X, David P, et al. Clinical and angiographic assessment 6 months after double vessel percutaneous coronary angioplasty. J Am Coll Cardiol 1985;6:1239–1244.

83. Consigny P. Prevention of restenosis after transluminal angioplasty. In: Tulenko TN, Cox RH, eds. Recent advances in arterial diseases: atherosclerosis, hypertension, and vasospasm. New York: Alan R. Liss, 1986:59–73.

84. Bourassa M, Alderman E, Bertrand M, et al. Report of the Joint ISFC/WHO task force on coronary angioplasty. Circulation 1988;78:780–789.

85. Kent K, Bentivoglio L, Block P, et al. Percutaneous transluminal coronary angioplasty: report from the Registry of the National Heart, Lung and Blood Institute. Am J Cardiol 1985;49:2011–2020.

86. Ellis SG, Cowley MJ, DiSciascio G, et al. Determinants of 2-year outcome after coronary angioplasty in patients with multivessel disease on the basis of comprehensive preprocedural evaluation. Implications for patient selection. The Multivessel Angioplasty Prognosis Study Group. Circulation 1991;83:1905–1914.

87. Renkin J, Wijns W, Hanet C, et al. Angioplasty of coronary bifurcation stenoses: immediate and long-term results of the protecting branch technique. Cathet Cardiovasc Diagn 1991;22:167–173.

88. Waller BF. The eccentric coronary atherosclerotic plaque: morphologic observations and clinical relevance. Clin Cardiol 1989;12:14–20.

89. Noveck HD, Klein LW, Kramer B, et al. Balloon dilatation of symptomatic subacute intimal dissection presenting as restenosis. Am J Cardiol 1989;64:980–984.

90. Cowley M, Vetrovec G, Wolfgang T. Efficacy of percutaneous transluminal coronary angioplasty: technique, patient selection, salutary results, limitations and complications. Am Heart J 1981;101:272–280.

91. Block P. Mechanism of transluminal angioplasty. Am J Cardiol 1984; 53:69C.

92. Matthews BJ, Ewels CJ, Kent KM. Coronary dissection: a predictor of restenosis? Am Heart J 1988;115:547–554.

93. Leimgruber P, Roubin G, Anderson H, et al. Influence of intimal dissection on restenosis after successful coronary angioplasty. Circulation 1985;72:530–535.

94. Laarman GJ, Plante S, de Feyter PJ. PTCA of chronically occluded coronary arteries. Am Heart J 1990;119:1153–1160.

95. DiSciascio G, Vetrovec G, Cowley M, Wolfgang T. Early and late outcomes of percutaneous transluminal coronary angioplasty for subacute and chronic total coronary occlusion. Am Heart J 1986;111:833–839.

96. Melchior J, Meier B, Urban P, et al. Percutaneous transluminal coronary angioplasty for chronic total occlusion. Am J Cardiol 1987; 59:535–538.

97. Probst P. "Collateral pressure" (occlusion pressure) during coronary angioplasty in coronary artery disease. In: Serruys P, Meester G, eds. Coronary angioplasty: a controlled model for ischemia. Dordrecht: Martinus Nijhoff, 1986:105–114.

98. Rentrop K, Cohen M, Blanke H, Phillips R. Changes in collateral channel filling immediately after controlled coronary artery occlusion by angioplasty in human subjects. J Am Coll Cardiol 1985;5:587–592.

99. Meier B, Luethy P, Finci L, et al. Coronary wedge pressure in relation to spontaneously visible and recruitable collarterals. Circulation 1987;75:906–913.

100. Urban P, Meier B, Finci L, et al. Coronary wedge pressure: a predictor of restenosis after coronary balloon angioplasty. J Am Coll Cardiol 1987;10:504–509.

101. Meier B. Restenosis after coronary angioplasty: review of the literature. Eur Heart J 1988;9:1–6.

102. Holmes DR Jr, Vlietstra RE, Reeder GS, et al. How cumulative is the risk of restenosis with multilesion dilatation? (abstr). J Am Coll Cardiol 1988;11:235A.

103. Meier B, King S III, Gruentzig A, et al. Repeat coronary angioplasty. J Am Coll Cardiol 1984;4:463–466.

104. Williams D, Gruentzig A, Kent K, et al. Efficacy of repeat percutaneous transluminal coronary angioplasty for coronary restenosis. Am J Cardiol 1984;53:32C–35C.

105. Black AJ, Anderson HV, Roubin GS, et al. Repeat coronary angioplasty: correlates of a second restenosis. J Am Coll Cardiol 1988;11:714–718.

106. Joly P, Bonan R, Palisaitis D, et al. Treatment of recurrent restenosis with repeat percutaneous transluminal coronary angioplasty. Am J Cardiol 1988;61:906–908.

107. Deligonul U, Vandormael M, Kern MJ, Galan K. Repeat coronary angioplasty for restenosis: results and predictors of follow-up clinical events. Am Heart J 1989;117:997–1002.

108. Tierstein P, Hoover C, Ligon B, et al. Repeat restenosis: efficacy of the third and fourth coronary angioplasty (abstr). J Am Coll Cardiol 1987;9:63A.

109. Schweiger MJ, Garb JL, Blank F, et al. Long-term follow-up and influence of symptom-free interval on restenosis after repeat percutaneous transluminal coronary angioplasty. Am J Cardiol 1988;62:476–478.

110. Ueda M, Becker AE, Fujimoto T. Pathological changes induced by repeated percutaneous transluminal coronary angioplasty. Br Heart J 1987;58:635–643.

111. Davies M. Thrombosis and coronary atherosclerosis. In: Julian D, Kubler W, Norris R, Swan H, Collen D, Verstraete M, eds. Thrombolysis in cardiovascular disease. New York: Marcel Dekker, 1989:25–44.

112. Stary H. Evolution and progression of atherosclerotic lesions in coro-

nary arteries of children and young adults. Arteriosclerosis 1989;9:I19–132.

113. Ohara T, Nanto S, Asada S, et al. Electron-microscopical evaluation of repeat PTCA for restenosis (abstr). Circulation 1989;80(suppl II):65.

114. FitzGibbon GM, Leach AJ, Kafka HP, Keon WJ. Coronary bypass graft fate: long-term angiographic study. J Am Coll Cardiol 1991;17:1075–1080.

115. Campeau L, Enjalbert M, Lesperance J, et al. Atherosclerosis and late closure of aortocoronary saphenous vein grafts: sequential angiographic studies at 2 weeks, 1 year, 5 to 7 years, and 10 to 12 years after surgery. Circulation 1983;68 (suppl II):1–7.

116. Guidelines for percutaneous transluminal coronary angioplasty. A report of the American College of Cardiology/American Heart Association Task Force on the Assessment of Diagnostic and Therapeutic Cardiovascular Procedures (Subcommittee on PTCA). Circulation 1988;78:486–502.

117. Pinkerton CA, Slack JD, Orr CM, et al. Percutaneous transluminal angioplasty in patients with prior myocardial revascularization surgery. Am J Cardiol 1988;61:15G–22G.

118. Bell MR, Holmes DR Jr, Vlietstra RE, Bresnahan DR. Percutaneous transluminal angioplasty of left internal mammary artery grafts: 2 years' experience with a femoral approach. Br Heart J 1989;61:417–420.

119. US Directional Coronary Atherectomy Investigators Group. Restenosis following directional coronary atherectomy in a multicenter experience (abstr). Circulation 1990;82(suppl III):679.

120. Holmes DR Jr, Garratt KN, Bell MR. Follow-up events after directional coronary atherectomy (abstr). Circulation 1990;82(suppl III):493.

121. Simpson JB, Robertson GC, Selmon MR, et al. Restenosis following successful directional coronary atherectomy (abstr). Circulation 1989;80(suppl II):582.

122. Garratt KN, Kaufmann UP, Edwards WD, et al. Safety of percutaneous coronary atherectomy with deep arterial resection. Am J Cardiol 1989;64:538–540.

123. Karas S, Santoian E, Gravanis M. Restenosis following coronary angioplasty. Clin Cardiol 1991;14:791–801.

124. Kuntz R, Selmon M, Robertson G, et al. Excision of deep wall components by directional coronary atherectomy does not increase restenosis (abstr). Circulation 1991;84 (suppl II):81.

125. Sketch MJ, Stack R. The transluminal extractional-endarterectomy catheter. In: Holmes DR Jr, Garratt KN, eds. Atherectomy. Boston: Blackwell Scientific, 1992, 61–80.

126. Stack R, Califf R, Phillips H, et al. Advances in cardiovascular technol-

ogies: interventional cardiac catheterization at Duke University. Am J Cardiol 1988;62(suppl F):1F–44F.

127. Leon M, Pichard A, Kramer B, et al. Efficacious and safe transluminal extraction atherectomy in patients with unfavorable coronary lesions (abstr). J Am Coll Cardiol 1991;17:219A.

128. Kramer B, Larkin T, Niemyski P, Parker M. Coronary atherectomy in acute ischemic syndromes: implications of thrombus on treatment outcome (abstr). J Am Coll Cardiol 1991;17:385A.

129. O'Neill W, Meany T, Kramer B, et al. The role of atherectomy in the management of saphenous vein grafts disease. J Am Coll Cardiol 1991;17:384A.

130. O'Neill W, Niazi K. Rotational coronary atherectomy using the rotablator atherectomy device. In: Holmes DR Jr, Garratt KN, eds. Atherectomy. Boston: Blackwell Scientific, 1992, 43–60.

131. Friedman H, Elliott M, Gottlieb G, O'Neill W. Mechanical rotary atherectomy: the effects of microparticulate embolization on myocardial blood flow and function. J Intervent Cardiol 1989;2:77–83.

132. Prevosti L, Cook J, Unger F, et al. Particulate debris from rotational atherectomy: size distribution and physiologic effects (abstr). Circulation 1988;78(suppl II):83.

133. Tierstein P, Ginsburg R, Warth D, et al. Complications of human coronary rotablation. J Am Coll Cardiol 1990;15(suppl A):57A.

134. Selmon M, Hinohara T, Vetter J, et al. Experience of directional coronary atherectomy: 848 procedures over 4 years (abstr). Circulation 1991;84 (suppl II):80.

135. Phillips H, Sketch M, Meany T, et al. Coronary transluminal extraction-endarterectomy: a multicenter experience (abstr). Circulation 1991;84(suppl II):82.

136. Warth D, Bertrand M, Buchbinder M, et al. Percutaneous transluminal coronary rotational ablation: six month restenosis rate (abstr). Circulation 1991;84(suppl II):82.

137. Buchbinder M, Warth D, Zacca N, et al. Multicenter registry of percutaneous coronary rotational ablation using the Rotablator (abstr). Circulation 1991;84(suppl II):82.

138. Wollenek G, Laufer G. Thermal effects of far ultraviolet excimer laser radiation on biologic tissue. Asaio Trans 1986;32:327–329.

139. Isner JM, Donaldson RF, Deckelbaum LI, et al. The excimer laser: gross, light microscopic and ultrastructural analysis of potential advantages for use in laser therapy of cardiovascular disease. J Am Coll Cardiol 1985;6:1102–1109.

140. Sanborn TA, Alexopoulos D, Marmur JD, et al. Coronary excimer laser

angioplasty: reduced complications and indium-111 platelet accumulation compared with thermal laser angioplasty. J Am Coll Cardiol 1990;16:502–506.

141. Sanborn TA, Bittl JA, Hershman RA, Siegel RM. Percutaneous coronary excimer laser-assisted angioplasty: initial multicenter experience in 141 patients. J Am Coll Cardiol 1991;17:169B–173B.

142. Litvack F, Eigler NL, Margolis JR, et al. Percutaneous excimer laser coronary angioplasty. Am J Cardiol 1990;66:1027–1032.

143. Margolis JR, Litvack F, Krauthamer D, et al. Excimer laser coronary angioplasty: American multicenter experience. Herz 1990;15:223–232.

144. Karsch KR, Haase KK, Voelker W, et al. Percutaneous coronary excimer laser angioplasty in patients with stable and unstable angina pectoris. Acute results and incidence of restenosis during 6-month follow-up. Circulation 1990;81:1849–1859.

145. Karsch KR, Haase KK, Mauser M, Voelker W. Initial angiographic results in ablation of atherosclerotic plaque by percutaneous coronary excimer laser angioplasty without subsequent balloon dilatation. Am J Cardiol 1989;64:1253–1257.

146. Kent K, Satler L, Kehoe M, Pichard A. Stand alone excimer laser angioplasty (abstr). Circulation 1991;84 (suppl II):363.

147. Karsch KR, Haase KK, Wehrmann M, et al. Smooth muscle cell proliferation and restenosis after stand alone coronary excimer laser angioplasty. J Am Coll Cardiol 1991;17:991–994.

148. Clarke R, Isner J, Van Tassel R. Wavelength-dependent cytotoxicity of laser light on vascular smooth muscle: implications for restenosis (abstr). Circulation 1991;84 (suppl II):360.

149. Spears JR. Percutaneous laser treatment of atherosclerosis: an overview of emerging techniques. Cardiovasc Intervent Radiol 1986;9:303–312.

150. Jenkins RD, Spears JR. Laser balloon angioplasty. A new approach to abrupt coronary occlusion and chronic restenosis. Circulation 1990;81 (suppl IV):101–108.

151. Reis GJ, Pomerantz RM, Jenkins RD, et al. Laser balloon angioplasty: clinical, angiographic and histologic results. J Am Coll Cardiol 1991;18:193–202.

152. Spears JR. Percutaneous transluminal coronary angioplasty restenosis: potential prevention with laser balloon angioplasty. Am J Cardiol 1987;60:61B–64B.

153. Schwartz L, Andrus S, Sinclair I, et al. Restenosis following laser balloon angioplasty: results of a randomized pilot multicenter trial (abstr). Circulation 1991;84 (suppl II):361.

154. Sigwart U, Puel J, Mirkovitch V, et al. Intravascular stents to prevent occlusion and restenosis after transluminal angioplasty. N Engl J Med 1987;316:701–706.

155. Sigwart U, Kaufmann U, Goy JJ, et al. Prevention of coronary restenosis by stenting. Eur Heart J 1988;9:31–37.

156. Goy JJ, Sigwart U, Vogt P, et al. Long-term follow-up of the first 56 patients treated with intracoronary self-expanding stents (the Lausanne experience). Am J Cardiol 1991;67:569–572.

157. Puel J, Juilliere Y, Bertrand ME, et al. Early and late assessment of stenosis geometry after coronary arterial stenting. Am J Cardiol 1988;61:546–553.

158. Serruys PW, Juilliere Y, Bertrand ME, et al. Additional improvement of stenosis geometry in human coronary arteries by stenting after balloon dilatation. Am J Cardiol 1988;61:71G–76G.

159. Schatz RA. Introduction to intravascular stents. Cardiol Clin 1988;6:357–372.

160. Schatz RA, Baim DS, Leon M, et al. Clinical experience with the Palmaz–Schatz coronary stent. Initial results of a multicenter study. Circulation 1991;83:148–161.

161. Schatz RA, Goldberg S, Leon M, et al. Clinical experience with the Palmaz–Schatz coronary stent. J Am Coll Cardiol 1991;17 (suppl B):155B–159B.

162. Raizner A, Minor S, Pinkerton C, et al. Quantitative assessment of the six month restenosis rates of the Gianturco–Roubin stent (abstr). Circulation 1991;84 (suppl II):589.

163. Graham L, Vinter D, Ford J, et al. Endothelial cell seeding of prosthetic vascular grafts. Arch Surg 1980;115:929–933.

164. Macander P, Agrawal S, Cannon A, et al. Is PTCA within the stenotic coronary stent safer than routine angioplasty (abstr)? Circulation 1991;84 (suppl II):198.

165. Sumida S, Masuda M, Furuyama M. Visualization and recording of intravascular details by fiberoptic angioscopy: the Sumida cardioangioscope. J Cardiovasc Surg (Torino) 1988;29:177–180.

166. Uchida Y, Tomaru T, Nakamura F, et al. Percutaneous coronary angioscopy in patients with ischemic heart disease. Am Heart J 1987;114:1216–1222.

167. Ventura HO, White CJ, Ramee SR, et al. Coronary angioscopy in the diagnosis of graft coronary artery disease in heart transplant recipients. J Heart Lung Transplant 1991;10:488.

168. Susawa T, Yui Y, Hattori R, et al. A white flapping structure in the coronary artery lumen observed by angioscopy after coronary throm-

bolysis—is this the "ruptured atheroma" that initiated the acute myocardial infarction? Jpn Circ J 1988;52:580–582.

169. Sherman CT, Litvack F, Grundfest W, et al. Coronary angioscopy in patients with unstable angina pectoris. N Engl J Med 1986;315:913–919.

170. Mizuno K, Miyamoto A, Satomura K, et al. Angioscopic coronary macromorphology in patients with acute coronary disorders. Lancet 1991;337:809–812.

171. Hombach V, Hoher M, Hopp HW, et al. The clinical significance of coronary angioscopy in patients with coronary heart disease. Surg Endosc 1988;2:1–4.

172. Hombach V, Hoher M, Kochs M, et al. Pathophysiology of unstable angina pectoris—correlations with coronary angioscopic imaging. Eur Heart J 1988;9:40–45.

173. Cohen M, Fuster V. Insights into the pathogenetic mechanisms of unstable angina. Haemostasis 1990;1:102–112.

174. Beyer ESA, Zeitler E. Angioplasty and angioscopy. Curr Opin Radiol 1989;1:183–185.

175. Holmes DR Jr, Bresnahan JF. Interventional cardiology. Cardiol Clin 1991;9:115–134.

176. White CJ, Ramee SR, Mesa JE, Collins TJ. Percutaneous coronary angioscopy in patients with restenosis after coronary angioplasty. J Am Coll Cardiol 1991;17:46B–49B.

177. Yock PG, Fitzgerald PJ, Linker DT, Angelsen BA. Intravascular ultrasound guidance for catheter-based coronary interventions. J Am Coll Cardiol 1991;17:39B–45B.

178. Leon M, Keren G. Intracoronary ultrasound assessment of atherectomy procedures. In: Holmes DR Jr, Garratt KN, eds. Atherectomy. Boston: Blackwell Scientific, 1992, 175–196.

179. Levine S, Ewels G, Rosing D, et al. Restenosis following transluminal coronary angioplasty (abstr). Circulation 1983;96 (suppl III):960.

180. Douglas JS Jr, Gruentzig AR, King SB III, et al. Percutaneous transluminal coronary angioplasty in patients with prior coronary bypass surgery. J Am Coll Cardiol 1983;2:745–754.

181. Block P, Cowley M, Kaltenbach M, et al. Percutaneous angioplasty of stenoses of bypass grafts or of bypass graft anastamotic sites. Am J Cardiol 1984;53:666–668.

182. El Gamal M, Connier H, Michels R, et al. Percutaneous transluminal angioplasty of stenosed aortocoronary bypass grafts. Br Heart J 1984;52:617–620.

183. Corbelli J, Franco I, Hollman J, et al. Percutaneous transluminal an-

gioplasty after previous coronary artery bypass surgery. Am J Cardiol 1985;56:398–403.

184. Dorros G, Janke L. Complex coronary angioplasty in patients with prior coronary artery bypass surgery. Cardiol Clin 1985;3:49–71.

185. Reeder GS, Bresnahan JF, Holmes DR Jr, et al. Angioplasty for aortocoronary bypass graft stenosis. Mayo Clin Proc 1986;61:14–19.

186. Cote G, Myler R, Stertzer S, et al. Percutaneous transluminal angioplasty in patients with stenotic coronary artery bypass grafts: 5 years' experience. J Am Coll Cardiol 1987;9:8–17.

187. Ernst S, van der Feltz F, Ascoop C, et al. Percutaneous transluminal coronary angioplasty in patients with prior coronary artery bypass grafting. Long term results. J Thorac Cardiovasc Surg 1987;93:268–275.

188. Clark D, Wexman MP, Murphy M, et al. Factors predicting recurrence in patients who have had angioplasty (PTCA) of total occluded vessels (abstr). J Am Coll Cardiol 1986;7(suppl A):20A.

189. Holmes DR Jr, Vlietstra RE, Reeder GS, et al. Angioplasty in total coronary artery occlusion. J Am Coll Cardiol 1984;3:845–849.

190. Libow M, Leimgruber P, Roubin G, Gruentzig A. Restenosis after angioplasty (PTCA) in chronic total coronary artery occlusion (abstr). J Am Coll Cardiol 1985;5:445.

· ·

CHAPTER 4

Summary of Previous Restenosis Trials

JAMES H. O'KEEFE, JR.
GEOFFREY O. HARTZLER

IF coronary angioplasty and other methods of percutaneous coronary revascularization are to realize their full potential, the incidence of restenosis will have to be reduced. Restenosis compromises the long-term results of the procedure and negatively influences its cost effectiveness. Coronary restenosis is clearly one of the major issues facing cardiology today.

The number of studies addressing restenosis has grown almost exponentially in recent years as the magnitude of this problem has become apparent to clinical cardiologists. This chapter reviews the basic and clinical restenosis trials performed to date and attempts to "cull out" the meaningful lessons learned from this divergent and often confusing area of investigation.

Omega-3 Fatty Acids (Fish Oils)

Omega-3 fatty acids (the active component of fish oil) are one of only a handful of pharmacologic agents that have shown positive results in randomized restenosis trials in patients. Although the results of the various trials are conflicting, there is reason to hypothesize that fish oil may have activity in preventing restenosis after coronary angioplasty. Omega-3 fatty acids exert an antiplatelet effect by inhibiting the production of thromboxane A_2, resulting in platelet inhibition and vasodilatation (1). However, aspirin is more effective than fish oil in inhibiting eicosanoid (thromboxane and prostacyclin) biosynthesis (2), and aspirin has been shown conclusively to be ineffective in preventing restenosis (3). Therefore, it is unlikely that altered eicosanoid biosynthesis alone could explain any activity fish oil may have in reducing the restenosis rate after angioplasty. Fish oil has also been shown to suppress monocyte-related growth factors and chemotactants that modulate the migration and proliferation of fibroblasts and smooth muscle cells (4,5). Fish oil has also been reported to retard the development of atherosclerosis in experimental animal models (6) and appears to lower mortality related to ischemic heart disease in patients on the basis of epidemiologic (7,8) and prospective randomized trials (9).

The first published study using fish oil after coronary angioplasty in patients suggested that it was effective in reducing restenosis and generated both enthusiasm and skepticism (10). This study by Dehmer and colleagues included 82 patients in a randomized, unblinded study using fish oil commencing 1 week before angioplasty and continuing for 6 months postangioplasty. The per patient restenosis rates in this study were 36% in the control group and 16% in the fish oil group ($p = 0.026$). Subsequently, six studies have been published on the use of fish oil for restenosis. Five of these six studies used angiographic end points for restenosis. The single study (by Slack and colleagues [11]) that utilized clinical criteria alone had a restenosis rate of 35% in treated patients versus 39% in control patients ($p = $ NS). Including the study by Dehmer and colleagues, the six trials with an angiographic end point for restenosis have been combined in a meta-analysis for the purposes of this discussion (10,12–16; Table 4.1) This meta-analysis revealed a restenosis rate of 26% in the 396 patients treated with fish oil compared with 32% in the 374 control patients ($p = 0.095$).

To lower the restenosis rate, it may be necessary to pretreat patients with high-dose omega-3 fatty acids for a prolonged period before angioplasty. Many of the effects of omega-3 fatty acids depend on their incorporation into the cell membrane phospholipid pool. Membrane levels of omega-3 fatty acids adequate to alter platelet and monocyte function and affect eicosanoid metabolism are achieved only after several days to several weeks of fish oil therapy (17,18). The two studies

Table 4.1. Meta-analysis of the Six Fish Oil Restenosis Trials with Angiographic End Points

	PRETREAT-MENT (DAYS)	OMEGA-3* DOSE (G)	RESTENOSIS (TREATED PATIENTS)	RESTENOSIS (CONTROL PATIENTS)
Reis (12)	5	6	42/124 (34%)	14/62 (23%)
Grigg (13)	1	3.0	17/50 (34%)	18/51 (35%)
Dehmer (10)	7	5.4	7/43 (16%)	14/39 (36%)
Milner (14)	0	4.5	15/84 (18%)	22/99 (26%)
Nye (16)	0	N/A	4/35 (11%)	15/64 (23%)
Meyer (15)	21	6.8	18/60 (31%)	28/59 (48%)
Total[†]			104/396 (26%)	119/374 (32%)

*Eicosopentaenoic acid or docosahexaenoic acid
[†]p = 0.095

using the longest pretreatment schedule (Dehmer, 1 week; Meyer, 3 weeks) both showed positive results (10,15). The combined data from these two trials revealed a restenosis rate of 24% in the 103 patients treated with fish oil versus 43% in the 98 control patients ($p = 0.005$). In the remaining four trials utilizing pretreatment of less than 1 week, the restenosis rate in the fish oil treated patients was 27% compared with 28% in the control patients (Table 4.2).

Thus, after seven independent studies assessing the effectiveness of fish oil in the prevention of restenosis after coronary angioplasty, the issue remains largely unsettled. It is likely that if fish oil is effective in preventing restenosis, high-dose therapy with pretreatment for at least 1 to 3 weeks before angioplasty may be necessary. A large National Institutes of Health–supported trial currently underway using fish oil ini-

Table 4.2. Meta-analysis of Fish Oil Trials with Angiographic End Points: Effect of Pretreatment

	FISH OIL RESTENOSIS	CONTROL RESTENOSIS	p VALUE
Trials with pretreatment ≥7 days (Dehmer [10] and Meyer [15])	25/103 (24%)	42/98 (43%)	0.005
No or <7 days pretreatment (12–14,16)	79/293 (27%)	77/276 (28%)	NS

tiated 2 weeks before angioplasty may help clarify this controversy. Unfortunately, the logistics of pretreating patients undergoing elective angioplasty with fish oil for 1 to 3 weeks are difficult and may preclude the widespread use of this therapy, even if it should ultimately prove efficacious.

Calcium Antagonists and β-Adrenergic Blockers

Calcium antagonists are theoretically attractive for use after angioplasty. By reducing smooth muscle contraction at the angioplasty site, calcium antagonists may be useful in minimizing ongoing endothelial trauma and platelet deposition in the early hours after the procedure. Chronic restenosis may be mediated by elastic recoil or vasospasm at the angioplasty site during follow-up (19–21). Evolving evidence also suggests that calcium antagonists may retard the development of atherosclerosis in animal models (22–25). Preliminary evidence suggests that this class of drugs may inhibit the development of new atherosclerotic lesions in patients as well (26,27). Diltiazem and verapamil both have mild antiplatelet activity (28,29) and, as a class, calcium antagonists have been shown to provide cardioprotection during myocardial ischemia (30,31). Although these perceived advantages of calcium antagonists after angioplasty have led to widespread acceptance in this role, clinical data on actual benefits are lacking.

A randomized, placebo-controlled, double-blinded trial evaluating the usefulness of diltiazem in patients after coronary angioplasty was recently reported (32). In this study, 201 patients were randomized to placebo or diltiazem and were pretreated for 24 hours before angioplasty and for 1 year following angioplasty. The angiographic restenosis rate (per patient) in the diltiazem group was 36% versus 32% in the placebo group (p = NS). Additionally, the incidence of late cardiac events (death, Q wave myocardial infarction, recurrent angina, or coronary artery bypass graft surgery) was similar in the treated and untreated patients. Thus, diltiazem appeared to be ineffective for the prevention of restenosis and recurrent events following coronary angioplasty (Figure 4.1).

All but one of the previously reported studies using calcium antagonists for the prevention of restenosis have also been negative. Corcos and colleagues used diltiazem in an earlier study that also showed no reduction in the restenosis rate (33). Whitworth and colleagues used nifedipine after angioplasty with no benefit against restenosis (34). The

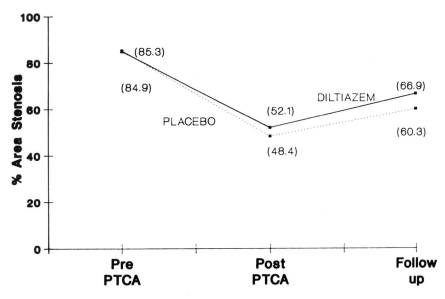

Figure 4.1. Changes in the mean area percent stenosis in the diltiazem (solid line) and placebo (dotted line) groups were similar during the study (*p* = NS).

single study that showed positive results with a calcium antagonist after angioplasty used 480 mg verapamil daily or placebo in 196 patients. The authors reported that no treatment effect was apparent in the 88 patients with unstable angina (restenosis rates: placebo, 62%; verapamil, 56%). An effect was found in the 84 patients with stable angina pectoris (placebo, 63%; verapamil, 38%; *p* = 0.04; 35). Although the authors concluded that verapamil reduced restenosis in patients with stable angina pectoris undergoing angioplasty, the use of subgroup analysis to show positive results raises questions about this interpretation.

Coronary vasospasm in the dilated segment in the early hours after angioplasty is a common problem and may be underappreciated by many clinicians. In a study using quantitative angiography at frequent intervals during the first 12 hours after angioplasty, predictable progressive coronary vasoconstriction was noted in the dilated segments (36). This vasospasm occurred even in patients pretreated with calcium antagonists, suggesting that it is a result of a direct receptor-mediated or myogenic response to arterial injury. This reflex vasoconstriction can be reversed or prevented by nitroglycerin (36).

Abnormal vasomotion in the dilated coronary segments has been frequently observed for up to 6 months after angioplasty. One study documented an abnormal response to ergonovine provocation in 28% of patients, 4 to 6 months postangioplasty (37). Although the restenosis rate was 50% in patients with provocable coronary spasm, pretreatment with high-dose nifedipine did not prevent the abnormal vasomotor response.

Thus, although calcium antagonists have been used empirically after coronary angioplasty since Gruentzig first introduced the procedure 14 years ago, convincing clinical evidence to support this practice still does not exist. These agents probably do not need to be routinely used postangioplasty unless a distinct indication (angina, hypertension, incomplete revascularization, supraventricular dysrhythmias, etc.) is present. On the other hand, nitrates are probably critically important in preventing acute reocclusion in the acute (72 hours) postangioplasty phase. In patients intolerant to nitroglycerin or in those who develop symptoms despite adequate nitrate therapy, calcium antagonists may be useful. No evidence suggests that calcium antagonists or nitrates modify the chronic restenosis rate.

Most invasive cardiologists consider β-adrenergic blockers (β blockers) to be contraindicated in patients undergoing coronary angioplasty. This belief grew out of theoretical concerns about coronary spasm resulting from unopposed α-adrenergic tone (38). A retrospective analysis of 455 patients who underwent coronary angioplasty while receiving β blockers showed the early complication and success rates in these patients were as good or slightly better than those not receiving β-blocker therapy (39). Indeed, the success rates, 75% versus 69% and the in-hospital mortality rates, 0.7% versus 2.3%, tended to favor the patients treated with β blockers.

β Blockers may inhibit the development of intimal hyperplasia (39) and might be hypothesized to reduce the restenosis rate after angioplasty. The only study to date addressing this question showed restenosis rates of 36% and 38% in patients being treated with and without β blockers, respectively (p = NS; 39).

Corticosteroids

Percutaneous methods of coronary revascularization involve controlled traumatic injury to the vessel wall. The immediate effects of this injury include platelet aggregation at the site of injury and subsequent infiltration by inflammatory cells. It is thought that the inflammatory response mediates the proliferation of smooth muscle that is commonly recognized as the "final common pathway" of restenosis in most cases (40). Corticosteroids possess profound anti-inflammatory and immunosuppressive effects and have been shown to blunt inflammatory cell migration and stabilize lysosomal cell membranes (41). Glucocorticoids also reduce smooth muscle cell growth in culture (42) and possess an antiplatelet effect by inhibiting the formation of platelet-activating factor (43). Additionally, glucocorticoids also interfere with collagen synthesis by fibroblasts in response to injury (44). Thus, it is logical that steroids might possibly be effective agents for reducing restenosis after coronary angioplasty (45).

To date, three studies using steroids following coronary angioplasty have been reported. The first published study enrolled 102 patients in a randomized trial (46). The 52 treated patients received 125 mg methylprednisolone intramuscularly the evening before and the morning of angioplasty. Oral prednisone was continued at a dose of 60 mg/day for the first 7 days postangioplasty. Angiographic follow-up was available in only 54 patients at a mean interval of 6 months. The restenosis rates were 59% in the treated patients and 57% in the control group ($p =$ NS). The largest study to assess the role of steroids after angioplasty was the Multi-Hospital Eastern Atlantic Restenosis Trial (M-HEART) (47). This multicenter study enrolled 915 patients randomly assigned to placebo or 1 g methylprednisolone infused intravenously 2 to 24 hours before angioplasty. Steroids were not continued postangioplasty. The angiographic restenosis rates were 39% in the placebo group and 40% in the steroid group ($p =$ NS). Of interest, retrospective subgroup analysis showed a trend toward a reduced restenosis rate in steroid-treated patients with lesions characterized as low risk for restenosis. The final steroid restenosis study used a 5-day high-dose corticosteroid regimen beginning at the time of angioplasty. This study, involving only 66 patients, had a restenosis rate of 32% in both steroid- and placebo-treated patients (48).

It is possible that a higher dose of corticosteroids given for a more prolonged period of time before and after angioplasty might significantly reduce the restenosis rate. However, the myriads of inevitable adverse side effects of such a regimen makes this a somewhat undesirable option. Perhaps more practical and effective would be local application of potent steroids at the angioplasty site. This may be possible either through the use of a perforated balloon that allows local introduction of drugs into the coronary segment being dilated (49) or through the use of an impregnated biodegradable stent (50).

Antimitotic and Antineoplastic Agents

The essence of restenosis can be summarized as an exuberant vascular reparative response, characterized by overgrowth of smooth muscle cells. All methods of percutaneous coronary revascularization, including balloon dilatation, atherectomy devices, laser photo-ablation, and intraluminal stenting, result in significant endovascular trauma. The stimuli for smooth muscle cell proliferation after such endovascular trauma involve heterogeneous growth factors emanating from inflammatory cells, elements of the coagulation system, and mechanical and rheologic factors (51). The majority of restenosis trials to date have attempted to modify a single component of this complex, redundant system. The failure of any single pharmacologic agent to consistently reduce the restenosis rate is not surprising in this context.

Some investigators have likened the smooth muscle cell proliferation responsible for restenosis to a neoplastic process (52). An analogy to restenosis might be found in the formation of keloid scars from dermal trauma in susceptible individuals (53). In interventional cardiology rapid refractory recurrences after repeated attempts at percutaneous coronary revascularization is referred to as "malignant restenosis" (54). When viewed from this perspective, the use of antimitogenic and antineoplastic agents is perhaps one of the most promising avenues of exploration in the search for a solution to the vexing problem of restenosis.

Colchicine

Colchicine is a plant alkaloid used since the first century A.D. in medicinal applications. Colchicine is an antimitogenic agent that binds to tubulin, disrupting spindle formation and resulting in metaphase arrest of cell division. The principal indication for colchicine in modern medicine is in acute gouty arthritis where it promptly reduces inflammation and pain. In addition to its antimitogenic effects, colchicine inhibits polymorphonuclear leukocytes and chemotaxis (55,56). Colchicine also interferes with collagen formation in response to injury or inflammation (57). In the setting of incipient hepatic cirrhosis, chronic oral colchicine (0.6 mg b.i.d.) improved survival and reduced fibrosis in one clinical study (58).

In experimental animal models, colchicine prevented or reduced the formation of atherosclerotic plaques (59,60). A single study used colchicine for the prevention of intimal thickening after balloon arterial injury in an experimental animal model (61). Currier and colleagues documented a dose-dependent reduction in intimal thickening in atherosclerotic rabbits 4 weeks after iliac balloon dilatation in those rabbits treated with colchicine. However, in this study, the effect was apparent only in animals treated with high-dose (0.2 mg/kg per day), but not low-dose (0.02 mg/kg per day) colchicine (Figure 4.2) In the standard 70-kg man, this dose would translate to 14 mg colchicine daily. Problems with patient tolerance and safety would preclude the use of colchicine at this dosage in a clinical trial.

The first study using colchicine to prevent restenosis in human beings was recently reported (62). This was a placebo-controlled trial that randomized patients in a 2:1 fashion to colchicine 0.6 mg p.o. b.i.d. or placebo. Treatment began within 12 hours of angioplasty and continued

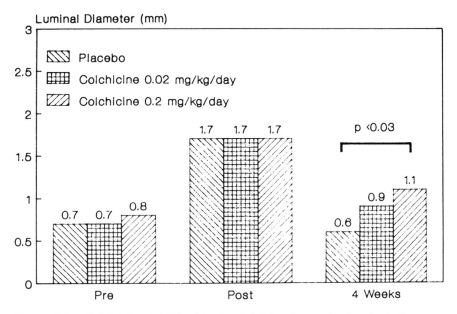

Figure 4.2. Colchicine inhibited intimal thickening and a luminal diameter stenosis in postangioplasty iliac arteries in atherosclerotic rabbits. Significant reduction was apparent only with the higher dose of colchicine.

for 6 months. A total of 197 patients were enrolled in the trial; 130 were randomized to colchicine. This dose (0.6 mg p.o. b.i.d.) was the same as that used in the clinical trial demonstrating the effect of colchicine in preventing progression of cirrhosis of the liver (58). Although this was considered a relatively low dose, side effects (usually diarrhea) resulted in a 7% drop-out rate in the colchicine-treated angioplasty patients. Quantitative angiographic follow-up was available in 145 patients (74%). The restenosis rates were 41% in colchicine-treated patients and 45% in the placebo group (p = NS). When the data were analyzed as a continuous variable, the changes in luminal diameter stenosis postangioplasty were nearly identical in colchicine and placebo-treated patients (Figure 4.3).

Antineoplastic Agents

Application of antineoplastic agents in the treatment of restenosis has been limited to experimental animal models. Restenosis in human beings can be a frustrating and expensive clinical problem, but it is gener-

Figure 4.3. The mean luminal diameter stenoses were essentially identical in colchicine and placebo-treated lesions before, immediately after, and at 6 months following coronary angioplasty.

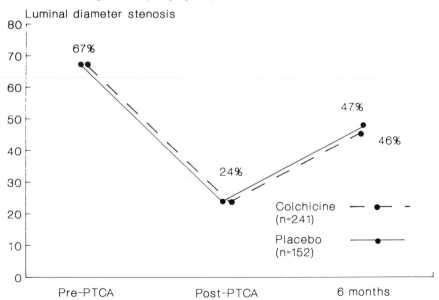

ally benign in its presentation and easily treated with repeat dilatation. Conversely, potent antineoplastic agents have numerous adverse effects, ranging from cosmetic (alopecia) to life-threatening (severe leukopenia), that mitigate against indiscriminate use in this setting. The hyperplastic smooth muscle cells responsible for the restenotic process are of mesenchymal cell origin (63). The agents generally used for tumors arising from mesenchymal cells include methotrexate, vincristine, cyclophosphamide, and anthracycline antibiotics. Accordingly, the antineoplastic agents investigated thus far in animals have been from this group of drugs.

The systemic use of combination therapy with vincristine and actinomycin D has been evaluated in a rabbit aortic model. Short-term therapy (3 days after endothelial denudation) resulted in less smooth muscle cell hyperplasia in the treated animals (64). The intermediate and long-term effects of this therapy were not observed in this study and, thus, the clinical relevance of these findings is entirely circumspect.

Investigators from the University of Michigan evaluated the effectiveness of local methotrexate therapy on intimal proliferation after balloon arterial injury, which was induced in the porcine carotid artery model (65). The antimetabolite methotrexate was administered locally through a Wolinsky coronary infusion balloon catheter (49). This local methotrexate infusion did not abolish or even attenuate intimal proliferation in this model. The question of antineoplastic agents for restenosis was also addressed by Murphy and colleagues from the Mayo Clinic (66). Their restenosis model was created by oversized coils (stents) placed in the porcine coronary artery. In this study, the use of oral or intramuscular methotrexate or azathioprine did not inhibit porcine intimal proliferation and restenosis.

To summarize, the use of antineoplastic and antimitogenic agents in the prevention of restenosis after coronary angioplasty has thus far been disappointing. Although this approach does merit further consideration on theoretical grounds, the use of high-dose, potent agents will be limited by the inevitable myriads of troublesome and even life-threatening side effects inherent in such regimens. As is the case with potent corticosteroids, a more acceptable approach might involve the sustained local administration of cytotoxic or antineoplastic agents at the site of balloon injury. This may be feasible through the use of impregnated, biodegradable stents or perfusion balloon catheters. These technologies are currently being evaluated in their early stages and certainly warrant further investigation.

Lipid-Lowering Therapy

The role of elevated lipid levels in the progression of atherosclerotic coronary artery disease is now firmly established. Several studies have also shown it is possible to halt the progression of coronary artery disease or even reverse established lesions by aggressive lipid-lowering therapy (67–69). The importance of hypercholesterolemia in restenosis after coronary angioplasty is controversial, although some studies have shown a relationship between lipid levels and restenosis (70,71).

In long-term follow-up after angioplasty, recurrent coronary events or death are commonly due to progression of coronary atherosclerosis in nondilated segments rather than restenosis after angioplasty (72,73). The only pharmacologic intervention to date documented to halt progression of coronary disease is aggressive low-density lipoprotein (LDL) cholesterol lowering. Thus, even if lipid-lowering agents do not diminish or abolish the restenosis rate after coronary angioplasty, they may significantly improve the long-term follow-up in these patients. A recent study has shown that the cholesterol levels in patients with preexisting cardiovascular disease are much more powerful predictors of future cardiac events than in those without coronary disease as baseline (74). Additionally, evidence suggests that some of the available lipid-lowering agents may have an impact on the restenosis rates by methods independent of their lipid-lowering activity.

Lovastatin is an HMG-CoA reductase inhibitor that is potent in the reduction of LDL cholesterol levels (67). Typical LDL cholesterol reductions range from 24% to 40% with lovastatin alone (75). Previous reports have suggested that lovastatin may be useful to prevent restenosis after coronary angioplasty. Gellman and colleagues found that lovastatin reduced intimal hyperplasia following balloon injury of the femoral artery in the atherosclerotic rabbit (76). Positive results also were reported using lovastatin after coronary angioplasty in human beings as well (77). In this trial, 157 patients, who underwent successful coronary angioplasty, were randomized to lovastatin 20 to 40 mg daily or conventional therapy (control group). Unfortunately, this study was flawed by inconsistent angiographic follow-up. Follow-up quantitative coronary angiography was performed in 50 of the 79 patients (63%) in the lovastatin group versus only 29 of the 78 patients (37%) in the control group. The reasons for this inequity were not clarified. In the lovastatin group, only 6 of the 50 patients (12%) had restenosis compared with 13 of the 29 patients (45%) in the control group ($p < 0.001$). The authors concluded that lovastatin following angioplasty reduced the incidence of restenosis.

Fascinating data from investigators at the University of Washington have recently shown it is possible to regress established restenotic lesions with HMG–CoA reductase inhibitors or niacin (78). In this trial, 16 patients with 18 restenotic lesions underwent coronary angiography at 7 months and 2.5 years postangioplasty. These patients were among those enrolled in the FATS trial (67) who were randomly assigned to lovastatin plus colestipol, niacin plus colestipol, or placebo therapy. A mean regression of 14% was noted in the restenotic lesions in patients treated with lovastatin or niacin compared with a mean lesion progression of 1% in the placebo-treated patients. The frequency of definite regression in the restenotic lesions over the 2-year interval between angiograms was 0% in the placebo-treated patients compared with 69% in the lovastatin- or niacin-treated patients. This was compared to only 11% of the nonangioplasty lesions that regressed in these same aggressively treated patients.

These authors concluded that intensive lipid-lowering therapy with lovastatin or niacin in combination with bile acid sequestrants can effectively diminish established restenotic lesions dramatically (78). In patients who received this aggressive lipid-lowering therapy, the restenotic lesions were, in fact, much more likely to regress than the nondilated lesions. The mechanisms of action of aggressive lipid-lowering therapy in decreasing restenotic lesions are somewhat speculative. The restenotic lesions are generally newer and perhaps more susceptible to dramatic changes in the biochemical milieu than are older, more established lesions.

Probucol is another lipid-lowering agent with unique properties that may render it useful in preventing restenosis. This moderately active lipid-lowering agent typically reduces total cholesterol by 15% to 20%. The reduction in total cholesterol is achieved by modest reductions of LDL with striking reductions of high-density lipoprotein (HDL) cholesterol levels (20% to 25%). The clinical use of probucol has waned in recent years due to this apparent counterproductive HDL cholesterol-lowering effect. Paradoxically, probucol appears to markedly enhance the reverse cholesterol transport system, thereby facilitating mobilization of cholesterol from vascular plaques and transport back to the liver (79, 80) Probucol is a powerful antioxidant and was originally developed by Marion Merrell Dow (Kansas City, Missouri) approximately 30 years ago in an attempt to formulate a compound to maximize airplane tire rubber longevity. Before LDL cholesterol becomes atherogenic, it must undergo oxidative modification. Oxidized LDL then facilitates the production of interleukin-1 by foam cells and becomes a strong chemotactic agent for the recruitment of monocytes and macrophages. These activities may account for the striking ability to halt progression and often induce regression of atherosclerosis in probucol-treated animals (81,82).

A recent retrospective study evaluated the effects of probucol or pravastatin (an HMG-CoA reductase inhibitor) on restenosis after angioplasty (83). This trial included 111 patients pretreated for 3 to 30 days with probucol or pravastatin. Probucol lowered LDL levels to a lesser extent and HDL levels to a greater extent than pravastatin in this trial. However, the only subset showing a significant reduction in restenosis was the probucol group pretreated for 30 days preangioplasty. In this group, a restenosis rate of 8.3% was noted (Figure 4.4). Although these results are intriguing, this was a small retrospective study that will require confirmation and clarification with randomized controlled trials.

Emory University is currently conducting a multicenter, randomized

Figure 4.4. The restenosis rate following coronary angioplasty was significantly reduced only in patients pretreated with probucol for 30 days preangioplasty. This trial involved very small sample sizes.

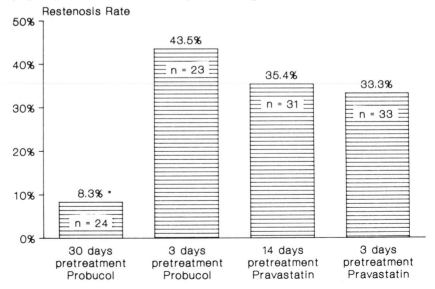

*p <0.05

trial using lovastatin for the prevention of restenosis. Additionally, the Mid America Heart Institute is initiating a multicenter, randomized trial assessing the effectiveness of high-dose lovastatin in combination with probucol in the prevention of restenosis and long-term recurrent coronary events after angioplasty.

Angiotensin-Converting Enzyme Inhibitors and Angiopeptin

The use of angiotensin-converting enzyme (ACE) inhibitors in clinical cardiovascular medicine has grown rapidly since these agents were introduced over 10 years ago. ACE inhibitors are effective and well tolerated in treating hypertension and congestive heart failure. This class of drugs has several important mechanisms of action, including inhibiting the conversion of angiotensin-I to angiotensin-II. Angiotensin-II is a potent vasoconstrictor peptide that may have growth-promoting activity as well (84,85). ACE inhibitors also block the degradation of bradykinin and appear to down-regulate the sympathetic nervous system (86).

ACE inhibitors markedly suppress the proliferative response to balloon angioplasty-induced vascular trauma in the rat carotid artery (87). These investigators pretreated the animals with cilazapril or captopril with supraphysiologic doses for 6 days before balloon angioplasty and for 2 weeks following the procedure, at which time the animals were euthanized and examined. A dose-dependent inhibition of neointimal thickening was seen in treated animals. The cross-sectional area of neointimal thickening was reduced by approximately 70% to 80% in treated animals compared with the placebo group. Although pretreatment with ACE inhibitors for 6 days was most effective in inhibiting the neointimal proliferation, animals started on cilazapril at the time of angioplasty and treated for 2 weeks also showed a significant (60%) reduction in the intimal thickening.

In a more recent publication, the same investigators (Powell and colleagues) tested the combination of cilazapril and heparin in the same rat carotid model (88). When used alone, heparin suppressed neointimal proliferation about as effectively as cilazapril alone. An additive effect was noted when cilazapril and heparin were used in combination, resulting in a 90% reduction in neointimal thickening. Bilizarian and colleagues also reported a modest antiproliferative effect with high-dose cilazapril in a rabbit iliac artery angioplasty model (89).

Little information exists regarding the utility of ACE inhibitors in patients after coronary angioplasty. A retrospective study assessing the role of ACE inhibitors in preventing restenosis after coronary angioplasty was recently reported. This trial evaluated 322 patients who underwent elective coronary angioplasty; 36 of these patients were being treated coincidently with an ACE inhibitor (generally for congestive heart failure or hypertension) at the time of the procedure (90). Restenosis was defined as the appearance of angina within 6 months after angioplasty. Angiographic end points were not used. The restenosis rate in patients on ACE inhibitors was 3%, compared with 30% in the 286 patients not receiving ACE inhibitors ($p < 0.05$). The obvious limitations of this trial include the small sample size, the retrospective nature of the data, and the lack of angiographic end points for restenosis. Additionally, the patients on ACE inhibitors were those with congestive heart failure and hypertension and on this basis alone they were probably more likely to be inactive or experience silent ischemia. The definition of restenosis as simply the appearance of angina during the first 6 months postangioplasty in this study renders the data essentially meaningless.

Several trials using ACE inhibitors in the prevention of restenosis in patients are also underway. Early results from these trials indicate little effect. It seems likely that the modest antiproliferative effect of ACE inhibitors when used alone will prove ineffective in reducing the restenosis rate in patients. Nonetheless, it ultimately may be found to have an adjunctive role in this scenario.

Angiopeptin is an analogue of somatostatin. Smooth muscle cell proliferation in vivo appears to be stimulated in part by platelet-derived growth factor and insulin-like growth factor-1 (also known as somatomedin C) (91). Native somatostatin inhibits release of insulin-like growth factor-1 (by reducing growth hormone release). By inhibiting insulin-like growth factor-1, somatostatin appears to possess potent antiproliferative activity (92).

Exogenously administered angiopeptin, like somatostatin, will inhibit growth hormone release and insulin-like growth factor-1 production. In a rat model of endothelial injury, subcutaneous angiopeptin inhibited subsequent neointimal proliferation in animals treated from 2 days or 30 minutes before injury (93). Angiopeptin has also been investigated in a rabbit model. Rabbit aorta and iliac arteries were deendothelialized with a balloon catheter (94). Angiopeptin significantly inhibited neointimal proliferation in response to the balloon trauma in this model.

Clinical studies using angiopeptin in patients undergoing angioplasty have not been performed. Although the animal studies using angiopeptin have been promising, they may have little or no relevance to the pathophysiologic processes responsible for restenosis after percutaneous revascularization in human beings. A multicenter, double-blind controlled clinical trial evaluating the effectiveness of angiopeptin on restenosis in patients is currently underway (93).

Anticoagulants

Heparin, like aspirin, is accepted as essential during and in the early hours after angioplasty to prevent acute reocclusion. Heparin has also been hypothesized to be a possible agent in the prevention of late restenosis after coronary angioplasty. Endogenous heparin-like molecules are produced by endothelial and smooth muscle cells and appear to be growth inhibitory (95,96). The mechanism of action of heparin in preventing smooth muscle cell proliferation is uncertain. Heparin modifies smooth muscle cells, making them unresponsive to growth factor stimuli in the milieu of an injured vessel (97). Heparin also causes a dose-dependent inhibition of smooth muscle cell proliferation in cultured cells from human, bovine, rat, and rabbit tissues (97).

Heparin and heparinoids (heparin fragments without anticoagulant activity) have been investigated for potential activity in the inhibition of smooth muscle cells in animal angioplasty models. Heparin inhibits myointimal proliferation in a rabbit iliac balloon injury model (98) and a rat carotid balloon injury model (99). This ability to blunt neointimal hyperplasia following balloon injury has been noted with both anticoagulant and nonanticoagulant heparins (100).

The clinical studies using heparin after angioplasty for the prevention of restenosis are less encouraging. One retrospective study, however, did find a restenosis rate of 44% in 36 patients, who were treated with heparin for only a mean of 2.5 hours postangioplasty compared with a restenosis rate of 26% in 138 patients treated for a mean of 21 hours postangioplasty (101).

One large clinical trial using heparin to prevent restenosis after coronary angioplasty has been reported. This trial included 416 patients, who were randomized to receive heparin or dextrose intravenously for 18 to 24 hours postangioplasty (102). All patients received 10,000 to 15,000 U heparin during the procedure. The angiographic restenosis rates at 6 months were 41% in the heparin-treated group and 37% in the placebo-treated group (p = NS). A small randomized trial using heparin chronically after coronary angioplasty reported a paradoxic increase in the restenosis rate in treated patients (103). This study, however, included only 23 patients and was terminated early due to the apparent adverse effect of chronic heparin postangioplasty.

A prospective, multicenter trial is currently ongoing, using a low molecular weight heparin (enoxaparin) administered subcutaneously for 1 month postangioplasty. Results from this trial are not yet available.

Warfarin has also been investigated for its potential activity in preventing restenosis after angioplasty. The first trial assessing this question involved 248 patients randomized to either aspirin or warfarin chronically after successful elective coronary angioplasty (104). The restenosis rates in the aspirin- and warfarin-treated patients were 27% and 36%, respectively (p = NS). A more recent study of warfarin and verapamil versus verapamil alone in a randomized trial involved 110 patients (105). The per patient restenosis rates in the warfarin and verapamil group versus the verapamil alone group were 29% and 37%, respectively (p = NS).

To summarize, the use of warfarin postangioplasty for the prevention of restenosis is unlikely to be effective. Although some theoretical and animal evidence suggests that heparin may be effective in this application, human studies to date do not support this. Still, the definitive studies using heparin and heparin fragments for the prevention of restenosis after angioplasty in patients have not been reported. These results are awaited with interest.

Antiplatelet Agents

Platelet interaction with the vascular wall appears to play a significant role in the development of atherosclerosis (106). Platelet activation at the site of angioplasty-induced endothelial injury is also a major factor in the occurrence of acute vessel closure and subsequent angioplasty complications. Several studies have documented a role for antiplatelet agents, specifically aspirin, in reducing the incidence of acute vessel closure in the early postangioplasty hours (107,108). On the other hand, aspirin with or without dipyridamole does not reduce the restenosis rate after angioplasty in patients (3,109–111). Schwartz and colleagues conducted a randomized, blinded, placebo-controlled trial of chronic oral aspirin (330 mg t.i.d.) and dipyridamole (75 mg t.i.d.) in postangioplasty patients (3). Follow-up angiography at approximately 6 months revealed a restenosis rate of 38% in treated patients and 39% in the placebo group.

Aspirin and dipyridamole do not completely inhibit platelet aggregation at the site of angioplasty (112). Newer agents, like ticlopidine, capable of more complete platelet inhibition have been found to be equally ineffective at preventing restenosis (109). The use of monoclonal antibodies directed at the glycoprotein receptor IIb/IIIa has also been endorsed as a possible solution to the restenosis problem (113). Platelet aggregation occurs as a result of the linking of two platelets by fibrinogen bound to the platelet glycoprotein IIb/IIIa receptors. This glycoprotein complex is the most abundant platelet cell surface protein. Monoclonal antibodies to the glycoprotein IIb/IIIa receptor have been found to markedly reduce platelet aggregation (beyond that seen with aspirin alone) in experimental coronary angioplasty animal models (114).

The early clinical experience with monoclonal platelet antibodies has shown a marked dose-dependent inhibition of platelet function that dissipates within 24 hours. Concerns have been raised about potential bleeding complications associated with monoclonal platelet antibodies. The first reported clinical experience did not substantiate these worries (115). This study, involving 27 patients who received the 7E3 plaetelet antibody, reported no major bleeding episodes (although patients were screened and excluded from the study if they were at increased risk for hemorrhage).

It is conceivable that the use of monoclonal platelet antibodies will reduce the incidence of acute thrombotic reocclusion after coronary angioplasty. The likelihood that these agents will have an impact on the restenosis rate is much lower, owing to the complex, redundant pathophysiologic processes that are responsible for renarrowing of the vessel after percutaneous revascularization. Trials assessing the utility of monoclonal platelet antibodies in these settings are currently underway.

Prostacyclin analogues have also been evaluated for their activity in preventing restenosis after angioplasty. Preliminary results with ciprostene (a prostacyclin analogue) showed a trend toward less restenosis in a study involving 311 patients (116). More recently, Knudtson and colleagues reported that the restenosis rates in patients treated with prostacyclin (27%) and placebo (32%) were similar ($p = $ NS; 117).

A final agent in this drug class that has shown promise in preventing thrombus formation and subsequent smooth muscle cell proliferation after angioplasty is hirudin. Hirudin decreases platelet and fibrinogen deposition and abolishes mural thrombus formation in the pig carotid angioplasty model (118,119). Minimization of platelet and thrombus deposition at the angioplasty site should reduce chemotaxis, inflammation, growth factor release, and the like (120). This agent has also yet to be tested in human clinical trials.

Devices and Restenosis

Analysis of the restenosis data on the newer devices for percutaneous revascularization is somewhat difficult. The major impetus for the development of these new devices has been the problem of chronic restenosis after balloon coronary angioplasty. However, most of the early reports on the use of these technologies have, for logistic considerations, focused mainly on feasibility and acute results. Data on the restenosis rates with these newer devices is now beginning to emerge and with one notable exception have looked disappointingly familiar.

Laser-Assisted Angioplasty

Several forms of laser-assisted percutaneous coronary revascularization have been studied over the past several years. The two modalities that have been shown to be safe and practical enough to warrant clinical application are the excimer laser (121) and the Spears laser balloon (122).

The largest series to date assessing the question of restenosis after excimer laser coronary angioplasty was recently reported (123). This study included the first 958 patients (1151 lesions) to undergo excimer laser angioplasty. In this series, 446 patients had completed the first 6 months of follow-up. Repeat percutaneous revascularization or coronary artery bypass graft surgery was required in 129 patients (29%). Additionally, seven myocardial infarctions and six late deaths were noted. Of those without cardiac events during the first 6 months of follow-up, 189 underwent elective follow-up coronary arteriography at 6 months. The restenosis rate in this group was 32%. Thus, restenosis or recurrent cardiac events occurred in approximately 45% of the first 446 patients to complete 6 months of follow-up after excimer laser coronary angioplasty (123).

These data were corroborated by restenosis results with excimer laser coronary angioplasty from a single center (124). In this series reported by Rothbaum and colleagues, the angiographic restenosis rate at 6 months was 47% in 57 patients. Restenosis rates were similar in patients treated with excimer laser angioplasty alone (52%) and those who underwent laser therapy with adjunctive balloon coronary angioplasty (43%). Finally, Sanborn and colleagues reported an angiographic restenosis rate of 40% in 74 patients who underwent excimer laser angioplasty (125).

The follow-up results after laser balloon angioplasty (with the Spears balloon) have been equally disappointing. Mast and colleagues reported angiographic restenosis rates between 38% and 100% at 6 months in 34 patients with follow-up angiography (126). The restenosis rates in this study seemed to increase in direct proportion to the amount of laser energy used. A second small study documented angiographic restenosis at 6 months in 8 of the 15 patients to undergo laser balloon angioplasty (53%; 127).

Atherectomy Devices

Various atherectomy devices are currently under investigation for potential use in percutaneous coronary revascularization. The device with the largest clinical experience and the only one approved by the Food and Drug Administration for use in human beings is the Simpson Atherocath (directional atherectomy). Although this device is useful for debulking large plaques in the native coronaries as well as in vein bypass grafts, it too appears to be plagued by relatively high restenosis rates. Garratt and colleagues from the Mayo Clinic reported an overall restenosis rate of 50% (37 of 74 lesions) at the time of follow-up angiography at 6 months after directional atherectomy (128). Subsequent studies have confirmed these results, showing restenosis rates of 36% (129) to 58% with the Simpson Atherocath (130). These studies generally documented a higher restenosis rate in restenotic versus previously undilated (de novo) lesions.

The Rotablator is a mechanical rotational atherectomy device that is also currently under clinical investigation. Restenosis rates in 60 lesions treated with the rotablator were recently reported to range between 29% and 69%, depending on the lesion characteristics (saphenous vein bypass grafts, de novo lesions, left anterior descending location, etc.) (131).

The transluminal extraction catheter is another atherectomy device being used for percutaneous coronary revascularization. The angiographic restenosis rate following the use of the transluminal extraction atherectomy catheter in a series of 281 patients was approximately 43% and was similar to the restenosis rate seen with balloon angioplasty in these patients (132).

Stents

Coronary stenting involves the placement of any one of a growing number of endoluminal vascular prostheses. The first report on the deployment of stents in human coronary arteries was published in 1987 by Sigwart and colleagues (133). In this initial report, coronary stenting was touted as a potential solution to the problem of restenosis. Now, almost 5 years later, coronary stenting has clearly emerged as the only device that has shown potential in the prevention of restenosis, although its exact role in this application has yet to be defined.

Several mechanisms may be responsible for potential effectiveness of stenting in reducing the incidence of late restenosis after coronary angioplasty. The tendency for the dilated segment of the vessel wall to return to its predilated state immediately after angioplasty is referred to as elastic recoil. Elastic recoil predictably narrows the cross-sectional area of the dilated segment by almost 50% in the first few hours after angioplasty (134). Coronary stenting has been demonstrated to mitigate the effects of elastic recoil postangioplasty. The radial forces exerted by the coronary stent overcome the effects of elastic recoil and, thereby, optimize vessel caliber in the early postangioplasty state (135). The placement of a coronary stent probably has little to no effect on the subsequent smooth muscle proliferation that is generally responsible for restenosis after angioplasty (135). Indeed, the animal model that most closely simulates human coronary restenosis is produced by deploying metal coils or stents with grossly oversized angioplasty balloons deep into the media of porcine coronary arteries, resulting in exuberant smooth muscle proliferation (136). Thus, the key to any potential activity coronary stents have in preventing restenosis lies not in the ability to blunt the subsequent myointimal proliferation, but rather by diminishing the functional significance of the hyperplasia. A suboptimal immediate postangioplasty result with a residual luminal diameter stenosis of greater than 35% to 40% has been frequently identified as a major risk factor for the subsequent development of restenosis (137,138). Following stent deployment, the same degree of neointimal proliferation that might have resulted in a hemodynamically significant lesion in a patient treated with conventional balloon angioplasty might not sufficiently encroach on the lumen in the stented segment to impair blood flow.

Several varieties of coronary stents are currently being investigated in clinical trials. The largest reported clinical experience thus far has been with the Palmaz–Schatz coronary stent, developed by Johnson and Johnson Interventional Systems (139). The angiographic restenosis rate in a series of 247 patients who underwent elective stenting of native coronary arteries with a single Palmaz–Schatz stent was 20% (103 of 247 patients) (139). In this series, the restenosis rate of a single stent in the 45 patients without previous angioplasty was only 7% compared with 27% in the 91 patients with prior angioplasty. The use of multiple stents markedly increases the risk of restenosis following deployment. In a series of 37 patients reported by Levine and colleagues, the restenosis rate was 17% in patients with a single stent and 57% in patients with multiple stents (140).

The French experience with the Palmaz–Schatz stent has been similar to that described above. Fajadet and colleagues reported an angiographic restenosis rate of 23% in 122 patients who underwent successful Palmaz–Schatz stent implantation (141). These investigators found a restenosis rate of 19% in patients with a single stent versus 58% in those with multiple stents. The restenosis rates following stent deployment in the specific coronary arteries were as follows: left anterior descending, 24%; left circumflex, 20%; right coronary, 8%. These investigators found no difference in the incidence of restenosis following stent placement in patients with previous angioplasty (18%) and those with de novo lesions (19%).

Much of the published European stent experience has been with the use of the Wallstent, manufactured by Medinvent. This is a self-expanding, stainless-steel, woven-mesh prosthesis that is positioned in the coronary artery using a guiding catheter. A report of angiographic follow-up at 6 months on 117 patients to receive the Wallstent was published recently (142). Angiographic restenosis (defined as a return to a luminal diameter stenosis of $\geq 50\%$ at follow-up) occurred in 14% of patent stents. Complete occlusion at 6 months was noted in an additional 24% of stents.

Thus, the early experience with coronary stenting suggests that this modality may reduce the restenosis rate to 20% to 25%. Definitive answers on this question will require randomized, controlled trials. With the current state of the art, it appears that a toll is exacted for this potential reduction in the restenosis rate. Acute coronary occlusion in the stented segment occurs despite aggressive antiplatelet and anticoagulant therapy in approximately 24% of the Wallstents and approximately 4% to 7% of Palmaz–Schatz stents (143–145). Another stent in early stages of clinical evaluation, the Cook stent, has been reported to have an 8% incidence of acute thrombosis of the stented segment (146).

An exciting potential solution to the restenosis problem involves the use of the most promising mechanical and pharmacologic approaches in a synergistic fashion. A biodegradable stent with minimal thrombogenecity could allow for optimization of the early postangioplasty luminal result. Impregnation of these stents with potent steroids, antimitogenic, or growth factor inhibitory agents could allow for local suppression of the proliferative response. Stents with some of these characteristics are in the early stages of development (50).

Conclusion

Although the search for the "magic bullet" for restenosis continues, the likelihood that we will find a simple solution that completely abolishes the process seems unlikely. The studies to date, though largely negative, do provide important insight into the pathophysiology of restenosis. Additionally, several approaches have demonstrated potential activity against restenosis. If these modest successes can be substantiated and their mechanisms of action elucidated, they may provide a foundation on which more substantial inroads into the process of restenosis can be built. The ultimate solution may entail a multipronged approach to counter the multifactorial nature of the restenotic process. Even a partial solution to the problem of restenosis will have major ramifications on the long-term results and cost effectiveness of coronary angioplasty.

References

1. Knapp HR, Reilly IAG, Alessandrini P, et al. In vivo indexes of platelet and vascular function during fish-oil administration in patients with atherosclerosis. N Engl J Med 1986;314:937–942.

2. Braden GA, Knapp HR, Fitzgerald GA. Suppression of eicosanoid biosynthesis during coronary angioplasty by fish oil and aspirin (abstr). J Am Coll Cardiol 1991;17:180A.

3. Schwartz L, Bourassa MG, Lesperance J, et al. Aspirin and dipyridamole in the prevention of restenosis after percutaneous transluminal coronary angioplasty. N Engl J Med 1988;318:1714–1719.

4. Lee TH, Hoover RL, Williams JD. Effect of dietary enrichment with fish oils on monocyte and neutrophil function. N Engl J Med 1985;312:1217.

5. Endres S, Ghorbani R, Kelley VE, et al. The effect of dietary supplementation with n-3 polyunsaturated fatty acids on the synthesis of interleukin-1 and tumor necrosis factor by mononuclear cells. N Engl J Med 1989;320:265–271.

6. Davis HR, Bridentstine RT, Vesselinovitch D, et al. Fish oil inhibits development of atherosclerosis in rhesus monkeys. Arteriosclerosis 1987;7:441–449.

7. Kromhout D, Bosschieter EB, Coulander C. The inverse relation between fish consumption and 20-year mortality from coronary heart disease. N Engl J Med 1985;312:1205–1209.

8. Shekelle RB, Missell L, Paul O, et al. Fish consumption and mortality from coronary heart disease. N Engl J Med 1985;313:820.

9. Burr ML, Gilbert JF, Holliday RM, et al. Effects of changes in fat, fish, and fibre intakes on death and myocardial reinfarction: diet and reinfarction trial (DART). Lancet 1989;September 30:757–761.

10. Dehmer GJ, Popma JJ, Van den Berg EK, et al. Reduction in the rate of early restenosis after coronary angioplasty by a diet supplemented with n-3 fatty acids. N Engl J Med 1988;319:733–740.

11. Slack JD, Pinkerton CA, Van Tassel J, et al. Can oral fish oil supplement minimize restenosis after percutaneous transluminal coronary angioplasty (abstr)? J Am Coll Cardiol 1987;9:64A.

12. Reis GJ, Sipperly ME, Boucher TM, et al. Randomised trial of fish oil for prevention of restenosis after coronary angioplasty. Lancet 1989; 2:177–181.

13. Grigg LE, Kay TWH, Valentine PA, et al. Determinants of restenosis and lack of effect of dietary supplementation with eicosapentaneoic acid on incidence of coronary artery restenosis after angioplasty. J Am Coll Cardiol 1988;12:1073–1078.

14. Milner MR, Gallino RA, Leffingwell A, et al. Usefulness of fish oil supplements in preventing clinical evidence of restenosis after percutaneous transluminal angioplasty. Am J Cardiol 1989;64:294–299.

15. Meyer F, Bairati I, Roy L. Effects of fish oil supplements and fish con-

sumption in the prevention of restenosis after coronary angioplasty (abstr). Am Soc Clin Nutrition 1991;May Annual Meeting;24.

16. Nye ER, Ilsley CDJ, Ablett MB, et al. Effect of eicosapentaneoic acid on restenosis rate, clinical course and blood lipids in patients after percutaneous transluminal coronary angioplasty. Aust NZ J Med 1990; 20:549–552.

17. Von Schacky C, Fisher S, Weber PC. Long-term effects of dietary omega-3 fatty acids upon plasma and cellular lipids, platelet function, and eicosanoid formation in man. J Clin Invest 1985;76:1626–1631.

18. Von Schacky C, Weber PC. Metabolism and effects on platelet function of the purified eicosapentaneoic and docasohexaneoic acids in humans. J Clin Invest 1985;76:2446–2450.

19. Hollman J, Austin GE, Gruentzig AR, et al. Coronary artery spasm at the site of angioplasty in the first 2 months after successful PTCA. J Am Coll Cardiol 1983;2:1039–1045.

20. Waller BF, Pinkerton CA. Cutters, scoopers, shavers and scrapers: the importance of atherectomy devices and clinical relevance of tissue removed. J Am Coll Cardiol 1990;15:426–428.

21. Waller BF, Pinkerton CA. Coronary balloon angioplasty restenosis: pathogenesis and treatment strategies from a morphological perspective. J Invasive Cardiol 1989;2:167–178.

22. Henry PD, Bentley KI. Suppression of atherogenesis in cholesterol-fed rabbits treated with nifedipine. J Clin Invest 1981;68:1366–1369.

23. Rouleau JL, Parmley WW, Stevens J, et al. Verapamil suppressed atherosclerosis in cholesterol-fed rabbits. J Am Coll Cardiol 1983;1:1453–1460.

24. Stein O, Halperin G, Stein Y. Long-term effects of verapamil on aortic smooth muscle cells cultured in the presence of hypercholesterolemic serum. Arteriosclerosis 1987;7:585–592.

25. Sugano M, Nakashima Y, Matsushima T, et al. Suppression of atherosclerosis in cholesterol-fed rabbits by diltiazem injection. Arteriosclerosis 1986;6:237–241.

26. Lichtlen PR, Hugenholtz PG, Rafflenbeul W, et al. Retardation of angiographic progression of coronary artery disease by nifedipine. Lancet 1990;335:1109–1113.

27. Waters D, Lesperance J, Theroux P, et al. Prevention of progression of minimal coronary lesions with a calcium channel blocker (abstr). J Am Coll Cardiol 1990;15:116A.

28. Ikeda Y, Kikuchi M, Toyama K, et al. Inhibition of human platelet functions by verapamil. Thromb Haemost 1981;45:158–161.

29. Kiyomoto A, Sasaki Y, Odawara A, et al. Inhibition of platelet aggrega-

tion by diltiazem. Comparison with verapamil and nifedipine and inhibitory potencies of diltiazem metabolites. Circ Res 1983;52(suppl I): 115–119.

30. Mehta P, Mehta J, Ostrowski N, et al. Inhibitory effects of diltiazem on platelet activation caused by ionosphore A23187 plus ADP or epinephrine in subthreshold concentrations. J Lab Clin Med 1983;102:332–339.

31. Garcia-Dorado D, Theroux P, Fernandez-Aviles F, et al. Diltiazem and progression of myocardial ischemic damage during coronary artery occlusion and reperfusion in porcine hearts. J Am Coll Cardiol 1987;10:906–911.

32. O'Keefe JH Jr, Giorgi LV, Hartzler GO, et al. Effects of diltiazem on complications and restenosis after coronary angioplasty. Am J Cardiol 1991;67:373–376.

33. Corcos T, David PR, Val PG, et al. Failure of diltiazem to prevent restenosis after percutaneous transluminal coronary angioplasty. Am Heart J 1985;109:926–931.

34. Whitworth HB, Roubin GS, Hollman J, et al. Effect of nifedipine on recurrent restenosis after percutaneous transluminal coronary angioplasty. J Am Coll Cardiol 1986;8:1271–1276.

35. Hoberg E, Schwarz F, Schomig A, et al. Prevention of restenosis by verapamil: the verapamil angioplasty study (VAS) (abstr). Circulation 1990;82(suppl III):428.

36. Fischell TA, Derby G, Tse TM, et al. Coronary artery vasoconstriction routinely occurs after percutaneous transluminal coronary angioplasty: a quantitative arteriographic analysis. Circulation 1988;78:1323–1334.

37. Bertrand ME, Lablanche JM, Fourrier JL, et al. Relation to restenosis after percutaneous transluminal coronary angioplasty to vasomotion of the dilated coronary arterial segment. Am J Cardiol 1989;63:277–281.

38. Kern MJ, Ganz P, Horowitz JD, et al. Potentiation of coronary vasoconstriction by beta-adrenergic blockade in patients with coronary artery disease. Circulation 1983;67:1178–1185.

39. Johansson SR, Lamm C, Bondjers G, et al. Role of beta-adrenergic blockers after percutaneous transluminal coronary angioplasty. Am J Cardiol 1990;66:915–920.

40. Nobuyoshi M, Kimura T, Ohishi H, et al. Restenosis after percutaneous transluminal coronary angioplasty: pathologic observations in 20 patients. J Am Coll Cardiol 1991;17:433–439.

41. Parrillo JE, Fauci AS. Mechanism of glucocorticoid action on immune response. Annu Rev Pharmacol Toxicol 1979;19:179–201.

42. Longenecker JP, Kilty LA, Johnson LK. Glucocorticoid influence on growth of vascular wall cells in culture. J Cell Physiol 1982;113:197–202.

43. Parente L, Fitzgerald MF, Flower RJ, et al. The effect of glucocorticoids on lyso-PAF formation in vitro and in vivo. Agents Actions 1985;17:312–313.

44. Krane SM, Amento EP. Glucocorticoids and collagen disease. Adv Exp Med Biol 1984;171:61–71.

45. MacDonald RG, Panush RS, Pepine CJ. Rationale for use of glucocorticoids in modification of restenosis after percutaneous transluminal coronary angioplasty. Am J Cardiol 1987;60:56B–60B.

46. Stone GW, Rutherford BD, McConahay DR, et al. A randomized trial of corticosteroids for the prevention of restenosis in 102 patients undergoing repeat coronary angioplasty. Cathet Cardiovasc Diagn 1989;18:227–231.

47. Pepine CJ, Hirshfeld JW, MacDonald RG, et al. A controlled trial of corticosteroids to prevent restenosis after coronary angioplasty. Circulation 1990;81:1753–1761.

48. Rose TE, Beauchamp BG. Short term high dose steroid treatment to prevent restenosis in PTCA. Circulation 1987;76(suppl IV):371.

49. Wolinsky H, Lin CS. Use of the perforated balloon catheter to infuse marker substances into diseased coronary artery walls after experimental postmortem angioplasty. J Am Coll Cardiol 1991;17:174B–178B.

50. Gammon RS, Chapman GD, Agrawal GM, et al. Mechanical features of the Duke biodegradable intravascular stent (abstr). J Am Coll Cardiol 1991;17:235A.

51. Muller DWM, Ellis SG, Topol EJ. Colchicine and antineoplastic therapy for the prevention of restenosis after percutaneous coronary interventions. J Am Coll Cardiol 1991;17:126B–131B.

52. Waterfield MD, Scrace GT, Whittle N, et al. Platelet-derived growth factor is structurally related to the putative transforming protein p28[sis] of simian sarcoma virus. Nature 1982;304:35–39.

53. Russell SB, Trupin KM, Rodriguez-Eaton S, et al. Reduced growth-factor requirement of keloid-derived fibroblasts may account for tumor growth. Proc Natl Acad Sci USA 1988;85:587–591.

54. Buchwald A, Werner G, Unterberg C, et al. Malignant restenosis after primary successful excimer laser coronary angioplasty. Clin Cardiol 1990;13:397–400.

55. Ehrenfeld M, Levy M, Bar Eli M. Effect of colchicine on PMN's in human volunteers. Br J Clin Pharm 1980;10:297–300.

56. Caner JE. Colchicine inhibition of chemotaxis. Arthritis Rheum 1965;8:757–764.

57. Ehelich HP. Microtubules in transcellular movement of procollagen. Nature 1972;238:257–260.

58. Kershenobich D, Vargas F, Tsao GG, et al. Colchicine in the treatment of cirrhosis of the liver. N Engl J Med 1988;318:1709–1713.

59. Godeau G, Lagrue G, Wegrowski J, et al. Effect of colchicine on atherosclerosis. Clin Physiol Biochem 1985;3:221–239.

60. Hollander W, Paddock J, Nagrat S, et al. Effects of anticalcifying and antifibrotic drugs on pre-established atherosclerosis in the rabbit. Atherosclerosis 1979;33:111–123.

61. Currier JW, Pow TK, Minihan AC, et al. Colchicine inhibits restenosis after iliac angioplasty in the atherosclerotic rabbit (abstr). Circulation 1989;80(suppl II):66.

62. O'Keefe JH, McCallister BD, Bateman TM, et al. Colchicine for the prevention of restenosis after coronary angioplasty (abstr). J Am Coll Cardiol 1991;17:181A.

63. Beranek J. Possible and up-to-now not-exploited treatment of restenosis (letter). Circulation 1989;80:1924.

64. Barath P, Arakawa K, Cao J, et al. Low dose of antitumor agents prevents smooth muscle cell proliferation after endothelial injury (abstr). J Am Coll Cardiol 1989;13:252A.

65. Muller DWM, Topol EJ, Abrams G, et al. Intramural methotrexate therapy for the prevention of intimal proliferation following porcine carotid balloon angioplasty (abstr). Circulation 1990;82(suppl III):429.

66. Murphy JG, Schwartz RS, Edwards WD, et al. Methotrexate and azathioprine fail to inhibit porcine coronary restenosis (abstr). Circulation 1990;82(suppl III):429.

67. Brown G, Albers JJ, Fisher LD, et al. Regression of coronary artery disease as a result of intensive lipid-lowering therapy in men with high levels of apolipoprotein B. N Engl J Med 1990;323:1289–1298.

68. Blankenhorn DH, Nessin SA, Johnson RL, et al. Beneficial effects of combined colestipol-niacin on coronary atherosclerosis and coronary venous bypass grafts. J Am Med Assoc 1987;275:3233–3240.

69. Hahmann HW, Bunte T, Hellwig N, et al. Progression and regression of minor coronary arterial narrowings by quantitative angiography after fenofibrate therapy. Am J Cardiol 1991;67:957–961.

70. Hamm C, Kupper W, Thief W, et al. Factors predicting recurrent stenosis in patients with successful angioplasty. J Am Coll Cardiol 1985;5:518–523.

71. Reis GJ, Silverman DI, Boucher TM, et al. Do serum lipid levels predict restenosis after coronary angioplasty (PTCA) (abstr)? Circulation 1990; 82(suppl III):427.

72. O'Keefe JH Jr, Rutherford BD, McConahay DR, et al. Multivessel coronary angioplasty from 1980 to 1989: procedural results and long-term outcome. J Am Coll Cardiol 1990;16:1097–1102.

73. Benchimol D, Benchimol H, Bonnet J, et al. Risk factors for progression of atherosclerosis six months after balloon angioplasty of coronary stenosis. Am J Cardiol 1990;65:980–985.

74. Pekkanen J, Linn S, Heiss G, et al. Ten-year mortality from cardiovascular disease in relation to cholesterol level among men with and without preexisting cardiovascular disease. N Engl J Med 1990;322:1700–1707.

75. Bradford RG, Shear CL, Chremos AN, et al. Expanded clinical evaluation of lovastatin (EXCEL) study results. Arch Intern Med 1991;151:43–49.

76. Gellman J, Ezekowitz MD, Sarembock IJ, et al. Effect of lovastatin on intimal hyperplasia after balloon angioplasty: a study in an atherosclerotic hypercholesterolemic rabbit. J Am Coll Cardiol 1991;17:251–259.

77. Sahni R, Maniet AR, Voci G, et al. Prevention of restenosis by lovastatin after successful coronary angioplasty. Am Heart J 1991;121:1600–1608.

78. Zhao XQ, Flygenring BP, Stewart DK, et al. Increased potential for regression of post-PTCA restenosis using intensive lipid-altering therapy: comparison with matched non-PTCA lesions (abstr). J Am Coll Cardiol 1991;17:230A.

79. Jamanoto A, Hara H, Takaichi S, et al. Effect of probucol on macrophages, leading to regression of xanthomas and atheromatous vascular lesions. Am J Cardiol 1988;62:31B–35B.

80. Sirtori CR, Sirtori M, Calabresi L, et al. Changes in high-density lipoprotein subfraction distribution and increased cholesteryl ester transfer after probucol. Am J Cardiol 1988;62:73B–75B.

81. Ku G, Doherty NS, Wolos JA, et al. Inhibition by probucol of interleukin 1 secretion and its implication in atherosclerosis. Am J Cardiol 1988;62:77B–81B.

82. Kita T, Nagano Y, Yokode M, et al. Probucol prevents the progression of atherosclerosis in Watanabe heritable hyperlipidemic rabbit, an animal model for familial hypercholesterolemia. Proc Natl Acad Sci USA 1987;84:5928–5931.

83. Young JL, Hiroyuki D, Yokoi H, et al. Does lipid lowering therapy prevent early restenosis after coronary angioplasty (abstr)? Presented at

the 9th International Symposium on Atherosclerosis, October 6–11, 1991, Chicago, Illinois.

84. Walker LN, Bowen-Pope DF, Ross R, et al. Production of platelet-derived growth factor-like molecules by cultured arterial smooth muscle cells accompanies proliferation after arterial injury. Proc Natl Acad Sci USA 1983;83:7311–7315.

85. Ehlers MRW, Riordan JF. Angiotensin-converting enzyme: new concepts concerning its biological role. Biochemistry 1989;28:5311–5318.

86. Kohlmann O, Bresnahan M, Gavras H. Central and peripheral indices of sympathetic activity after blood pressure lowering with enalapril and hydralazine in normotensive rats. Hypertension 1984;6:I-1–6.

87. Powell JS, Clozel JP, Muller RKS, et al. Inhibitors of angiotensin-converting enzyme prevent myointimal proliferation after vascular injury. Science 1989;245:186–188.

88. Powell JS, Muller RKM, Baumgartner HR. Suppression of the vascular response to injury: the role of angiotensin-converting enzyme inhibitors. J Am Coll Cardiol 1991;17:137B–142B.

89. Bilazarian SD, Currier JW, Haudenschild CC, et al. Angiotensin converting enzyme inhibition reduces restenosis in experimental angioplasty (abstr). J Am Coll Cardiol 1991;17(2):268A.

90. Brozovich FV, Morganroth J, Gottlieb NB, et al. Effect of angiotensin converting enzyme inhibition on the incidence of restenosis after percutaneous transluminal coronary angioplasty. Cathet Cardiovasc Diagn 1991;23:263–267.

91. Clemmon DR, VanWyk JJ. Evidence for a functional role of endogenously produced somatomedin-like peptides in the regulation of DNA synthesis in cultured human fibroblasts and porcine smooth muscle cells. J Clin Invest 1985;75:1914–1918.

92. Moreau JP, DeFeudis FU. Pharmacologic studies of somatostatin and somatostatin-analogues: therapeutic advances and perspectives. Life Sci 1987;40:419–437.

93. Lundergan CF, Foegh ML, Ramwell PW. Peptide inhibition of myointimal proliferation by angiopeptin, a somatostatin analogue. J Am Coll Cardiol 1991;17:132B–136B.

94. Conte JV, Foegh ML, Calcagno RB, et al. Peptide inhibition of myointimal proliferation following angioplasty in rabbits. Transplant Proc 1989;21:3686–3688.

95. Castellot JJ Jr, Addonizio M, Rosenberg R, et al. Cultured endothelial cells produce a heparin-like inhibitor of smooth muscle cell growth. J Cell Biol 1981;90:372–379.

96. Fritze LMS, Reilly CF, Rosenberg R. An antiproliferative heparin sul-

fate species produced by postconfluent smooth muscle cells. J Cell Biol 1985;100:1041–1049.

97. Berk BC, Gordon JB, Alexander RW. Pharmacologic roles of heparin and glucocorticoids to prevent restenosis after coronary angioplasty. J Am Coll Cardiol 1991;17:111B–117B.

98. Pow TK, Currier JW, Minihan AC, et al. Low molecular weight heparin reduces restenosis after experimental angioplasty (abstr). Circulation 1989;80(suppl II):65.

99. Okada T, Bark DH, Mayberg MR. Localized release of perivascular heparin inhibits intimal proliferation after endothelial injury without systemic anticoagulation. Neuroscience 1989;26:892–897.

100. Guyton J, Rosenberg R, Clowes AW, et al. Inhibition of rat arterial smooth muscle cell proliferation by heparin. I. In vivo studies with anticoagulant and non-anticoagulant heparin. Circ Res 1980;46:625–634.

101. Meier B. Prevention of restenosis after coronary angioplasty: a pharmacological approach. Eur Heart J 1989;10(suppl G):64–68.

102. Ellis SG, Roubin GS, Wilentz J, et al. Effect of 18 to 24-hour heparin administration for prevention of restenosis after uncomplicated coronary angioplasty. Am Heart J 1989;117:777–782.

103. Lehmann KG, Doria RJ, Feuer JM, et al. Paradoxical increase in restenosis rate with chronic heparin use: final results of a randomized trial (abstr). J Am Coll Cardiol 1991;17:181A.

104. Thornton MA, Gruentzig AR, Hollman J, et al. Coumadin and aspirin in the prevention of recurrence after transluminal coronary angioplasty: a randomized study. Circulation 1984;69:721–727.

105. Urban P, Bulen N, Fox K, et al. Lack of effect of warfarin on the restenosis rate or on clinical outcome after balloon angioplasty. Br Heart J 1988;6:485–488.

106. Wilentz JR, Sanborn TA, Hauderschild CC, et al. Platelet accumulation in experimental angioplasty. Circulation 1987;75:636–642.

107. Barnathan ES, Schwartz JS, Taylor L, et al. Aspirin and dipyridamole in the prevention of acute coronary thrombosis complicating coronary angioplasty. Circulation 1987;76:125–134.

108. White CW, Chaitman B, Lasser TA, et al. Antiplatelet agents are effective in reducing the immediate complications of PTCA: results from the ticlopidine multicenter trial (abstr). Circulation 1987;76(suppl IV):400.

109. White CW, Knudson M, Schmidt D, et al. Neither ticlopidine nor aspirin-dipyridamole prevents restenosis post PTCA: results from a randomized placebo-controlled multicenter trial (abstr). Circulation 1987;76(suppl IV):213.

110. Mufson L, Black A, Roubin G, et al. A randomized trial of aspirin in PTCA: effect of high vs low dose aspirin on major complications and restenosis (abstr). J Am Coll Cardiol 1988;11(suppl A):236A.

111. Schanzenbacher P, Grimmer M, Maisch B, et al. Effect of high dose and low dose aspirin on restenosis after primary successful angioplasty (abstr). Circulation 1988;78(suppl II):99.

112. Steele PM, Chesebro JH, Stanson AW, et al. Balloon angioplasty: effect of platelet-inhibitor drugs on platelet-thrombus deposition in a pig model (abstr). J A Coll Cardiol 1984;3:506.

113. Ellis SG, Bates ER, Schaible T, et al. Prospects for the use of antagonists to the platelet glycoprotein IIb/IIIa receptor to prevent postangioplasty restenosis and thrombosis. J Am Coll Cardiol 1991;17:89B–95B.

114. Bates ER, McGillem MJ, Mickelson JK, et al. A monoclonal antibody to the platelet receptor GP IIb/IIIa (7E3) prevents acute thrombosis in a canine model of coronary angioplasty (abstr). Circulation 1988;78 (suppl II):289.

115. Ellis SG, Navetta FI, Tcheng JT, et al. Antiplatelet GP IIb/IIIa (7E3) antibody in elective PTCA; safety and inhibition of platelet function (abstr). Circulation 1990;82(suppl III):191.

116. Raizner A, Hollman J, Demke D, et al. Beneficial effects of ciprostene in PTCA: a multicenter, randomized controlled trial (abstr). Circulation 1988;78(suppl II):276.

117. Knudtson ML, Flintoft VF, Roth DL, et al. Effect of short-term prostacyclin administration on restenosis after percutaneous transluminal coronary angioplasty. J Am Coll Cardiol 1991;15:691–697.

118. Heras M, Chesebro JH, Penny WJ, et al. Effects of thrombin inhibition on the development of acute platelet thrombus deposition during angioplasty in pigs: heparin versus recombinant hirudin, a specific thrombin inhibitor. Circulation 1989;79:657–665.

119. Heras M, Chesebro JH, Webster MWI, et al. Hirudin, heparin, and placebo during deep arterial injury in the pig: the in vivo role of thrombin in platelet-mediated thrombosis. Circulation 1990;82:1476–1484.

120. Ip JH, Fuster V, Israel D, et al. The role of platelets, thrombin and hyperplasia in restenosis after coronary angioplasty. J Am Coll Cardiol 1991;17:77B–88B.

121. Sanborn TA, Bittl JA, Hershman RA, et al. Percutaneous coronary excimer laser-assisted angioplasty: initial multicenter experience in 141 patients. J Am Coll Cardiol 1991;17:169B–173B.

122. Spears JR, Kundu SK, McMath LP. Laser balloon angioplasty: potential for reduction of the thrombogenicity of the injured arterial wall and for

local application of bioprotective materials. J Am Coll Cardiol 1991;17:179B–188B.

123. Margolis JR, Krauthamer D, Litvack F, et al. Six month follow-up of excimer laser coronary angioplasty registry patients (abstr). J Am Coll Cardiol 1991;17:218A.

124. Rothbaum D, Linnemeier T, Landin R, et al. Excimer laser coronary angioplasty: angiographic restenosis rate at six month follow-up (abstr). J Am Coll Cardiol 1991;17:205A.

125. Sanborn TA, Bittl JA, Torre SR. Procedural success, in-hospital events, and follow-up clinical and angiographic results of percutaneous coronary excimer laser-assisted angioplasty (abstr). J Am Coll Cardiol 1991;17:206A.

126. Mast G, Plokker T, Bal E, et al. Laser balloon angioplasty does not reduce restenosis rate in type A and B coronary lesions (abstr). Circulation 1990;82(suppl III):313.

127. Reis GJ, Pomerantz RM, Jenkins RD, et al. Laser balloon angioplasty: clinical, angiographic, and histologic results (abstr). Circulation 1990;82(suppl III):672.

128. Garratt KN, Holmes DR Jr, Bell MR, et al. Restenosis after directional coronary atherectomy: differences between primary atheromatous and restenosis lesions and influence of subintimal tissue resection. J Am Coll Cardiol 1990;16(7):1665–1671.

129. Hinohara T, Selmon MR, Robertson GC, et al. Angiographic predictors of restenosis following directional coronary atherectomy (abstr). J Am Coll Cardiol 1991;17:385A.

130. Ghazzal ZMB, Douglas JS, Holmes DR Jr, et al. Directional coronary atherectomy of saphenous vein grafts: recent multicenter experience (abstr). J Am Coll Cardiol 1991;17:219A.

131. Niazi K, Cragg DR, Strzelecki M, et al. Angiographic risk factors for coronary restenosis following mechanical rotational atherectomy (abstr). J Am Coll Cardiol 1991;17:218A.

132. Leon MB, Pichard AD, Kramer BL, et al. Efficacious and safe transluminal extraction atherectomy in patients with unfavorable coronary lesions (abstr). J Am Coll Cardiol 1991;17:218A.

133. Sigwart U, Puel J, Mirkovitch, et al. Intravascular stents to prevent occlusion and restenosis after transluminal angioplasty. N Engl J Med 1987;316:701–706.

134. Rensing BJ, Hermans WRM, Beatt KJ, et al. Quantitative angiographic assessment of elastic recoil after percutaneous transluminal coronary angioplasty. Am J Cardiol 1990;66:1039–1044.

135. Serruys PW, Strauss BH, Van Beusekon HM, et al. Stenting of coronary

arteries: has a modern pandora's box been opened? J Am Coll Cardiol 1991;17:143B–154B.

136. Schwartz RS, Murphy JG, Edwards WD, et al. Restenosis after balloon angioplasty: a practical proliferative model in porcine coronary arteries. Circulation 1990;82:2190–2200.

137. Leimgruber PP, Roubin GS, Hollman J, et al. Restenosis after successful coronary angioplasty in patients with single-vessel disease. Circulation 1986;73:710–717.

138. Lambert M, Bonan R, Cote G, et al. Multiple coronary angioplasty: a model to discriminate systemic and procedural factors related to restenosis. J Am Coll Cardiol 1988;12:310–314.

139. Schatz RA, Goldberg S, Leon M, et al. Clinical experience with the Palmaz–Schatz coronary stent. J Am Coll Cardiol 1991;17:155B–159B.

140. Levine MJ, Leonard BM, Burke JA, et al. Clinical and angiographic results of balloon-expandable intracoronary stents in right coronary artery stenoses. J Am Coll Cardiol 1990;16:332–339.

141. Fajadet JC, Marco J, Cassagneau BG, et al. Restenosis following successful Palmaz–Schatz intracoronary stent implantation (abstr). J Am Coll Cardiol 1991;17:346A.

142. Serruys PW, Strauss BH, Beatt KJ, et al. Angiographic follow-up after placement of a self-expanding coronary artery stent. N Engl J Med 1991;324:13–17.

143. Ver Lee PN, Muller DWM, Popma JJ, et al. Coronary stenting for abrupt closure vs elective stenting for refractory restenosis: clinical and quantitative angiographic outcomes (abstr). J Am Coll Cardiol 1991;17:280A.

144. Teirstein PS, Schatz RA, Leon MB, et al. Should patients with discrete, de novo coronary stenoses undergo stenting as a primary procedure? Risk vs. benefit (abstr). J Am Coll Cardiol 1991;17:280A.

145. Cleman MW, Cabin HS, Leon M, et al. Major complications associated with intracoronary delivery with the Palmaz–Schatz stent (abstr). J Am Coll Cardiol 1991;17:280A.

146. Roubin GS, Agrawal S, Dean LS, et al. What are the predictors of acute complications following coronary artery stenting? Single institutional experience (abstr). J Am Coll Cardiol 1991;17:281A.

. . . .

CHAPTER 5

Trial Design in Restenosis: Problems and Solutions

DAVID W. M. MULLER
ERIC J. TOPOL

RECURRENT stenosis following mechanical interventions for obstructive coronary arterial stenoses remains one of the foremost challenges for investigative and clinical cardiologists. The failure of new percutaneous devices, such as atherectomy catheters, intravascular stents, and laser ablation devices, to eliminate or to even significantly reduce the 30% to 40% incidence of restenosis that follows percutaneous transluminal coronary angioplasty (PTCA) has again focused attention on the need for well-controlled, adequately powered clinical trials. Several large, multicenter, randomized trials, examining the impact of pharmacologic and mechanical therapies on the incidence of restenosis, are currently in progress. The scale of these trials, in terms of financial resources and personnel, is considerably greater than has been previously committed to clinical restenosis trials. This commitment is clearly warranted because, in addition to its associated morbidity and potential mortality, restenosis represents a substantial drain on limited national fiscal resources. Even a modest reduction in the incidence of restenosis could, therefore, have a major impact on the costs of providing health care (1). Clearly, the question of optimal trial design is timely and relevant to the interpretation of the findings of these ongoing trials.

Although many smaller, randomized clinical studies have been performed over the past decade, no pharmacologic therapy has yet consistently reduced the incidence of recurrent stenosis. In contrast, multiple therapies have been reported to inhibit the development of neointimal thickening in experimental models of coronary restenosis (2). The explanation for this discrepancy is unclear. Although it may indicate that the animal models poorly reflect the pathogenesis of restenosis in man, an alternative, and perhaps equally likely, explanation is that the design of the clinical trials has been suboptimal, with a majority having inadequate statistical power to detect a potentially valuable, if modest, therapeutic influence of individual drug therapies. With this discrepancy in mind, this chapter reviews the important considerations in the design of clinical and experimental trials for the study of restenosis, with particular attention to the use of animal models for initial drug screening, the selection of end points for clinical trials, sample size and statistical considerations, the interpretation of published pharmacologic studies, and the prospects for identification of effective therapies in ongoing randomized trials.

Experimental Models of Coronary Restenosis

Over the past 40 to 50 years, several animal species have been used to investigate the events that characterize the development of atherosclerosis (3–6), and more recently, to identify pharmacologic inhibitors of intimal proliferation (2). Based on the "response to injury" hypothesis of spontaneous atherosclerosis (7,8), these models have used one of a variety of arterial injuries (including balloon dilatation, air drying, and the use of in-dwelling arterial catheters) often in combination with dietary manipulation to achieve concomitant hypercholesterolemia. The sequence of events that follows balloon injury in these models has been well characterized and is similar for all species examined (9–12). Balloon dilatation is associated with extensive endothelial denudation and necrosis of a variable thickness of the underlying medial smooth muscle cell layer. The injury is followed by rapid deposition of circulating platelets, thrombin formation, release of chemotactic and mitogenic growth factors, and migration and proliferation of smooth muscle cells from the remaining viable media. Neointimal thickening then develops as a result of increasing cell number in association with new connective tissue matrix production. Depending on the model, incorporation of thrombus and the deposition of intramural lipid have variable roles in the formation of the neointima.

The animal models have been used for studying the biology of the arterial response to injury and for identifying pharmacologic therapies that inhibit this response. In contrast to clinical restenosis trials, the use of animal models is relatively inexpensive. Moreover, the use of an animal model allows determination of angiographic minimal luminal diameter (MLD) and direct measurement of absolute neointimal thickness and lumen–intimal area ratio in the entire study population. These measurements can be performed as continuous variables, thereby minimizing the sample size required to demonstrate a therapeutic effect. There are, however, several important limitations to the use and interpretation of data from animal models (2). First, the histopathology of neointimal thickening varies significantly among respective models. In the balloon-injured rat carotid artery, for example, the neointima consists predominantly of smooth muscle cells and a loose connective tissue matrix. There is little evidence of an inflammatory cell infiltrate, incorporation of mural thrombus, or lipid deposition (9,10). In the atherosclerotic rabbit iliac artery, on the other hand, lipid plays an important role in the genesis of both the primary lesion and the neointimal thickening that follows balloon dilatation; lipid-laden macrophages or "foam" cells constitute a large proportion of the cells in both lesions (11). In the pig, the histopathologic appearances are more consistent with those seen in human restenosis with a predominance of smooth muscle cells in the neointima but with evidence of an important role for platelet aggregates and thrombus and with occasional inflammatory cell infiltrates (12). A second limitation is that, apart from the atherosclerotic rabbit model, the arteries of the commonly used models are nondiseased. In these arteries, balloon dilation is associated with complete endothelial denudation followed by rapid endothelial regeneration within 5 to 7 days. The inhibitory effects of the regenerated endothelium on smooth muscle cell proliferation have been well studied in the rat carotid model (9). Few data are available, however, on the rate of endothelial regeneration following balloon injury of diseased arteries in man, but the metallic struts of resected intracoronary stents have been observed to remain without regeneration as long as 5 weeks after stent implantation (13). Third, in some models, the injury may cause an inconsistent degree of vascular mural damage, and, therefore, a variable degree of stimulation of medial smooth muscle cell proliferation. This variability can result in the need for large sample sizes to show a significant therapeutic effect. To some extent, this limitation has been overcome in the porcine model by using oversized stent implantation to create a controlled injury. In this model, the depth of mural penetration of the metal struts correlates with the subsequent thickness of the neointima (14). The intimal thickness can be corrected for the degree of arterial injury, thereby eliminating much of the variability in response. Finally, and perhaps most importantly, undoubtedly significant differences among animal species in drug metabolism and distribution do not allow direct correlation of drug dosages on a weighted basis. Thus, drugs effective in the rat or rabbit, for example, cannot be assumed to be effective in man at the same dose per kilogram body weight. Ideally, therefore, some index of the therapeutic effect of the drug should be measured in the animal model and, if possible, the drug dose should be titrated to achieve a comparable effect in man.

Despite these limitations, drug screening in animal models remains a valuable means of studying the biology of the vascular response to injury and of identifying potentially valuable strategies for preventing restenosis following balloon angioplasty. The optimal model remains debatable because no single model has been predictive of the effects of a therapeutic intervention in man. Regardless of the model chosen, it is important that an attempt be made to achieve a consistent, and preferably quantifiable, degree of arterial injury; that the sample size be adequate to avoid a type II statistical error (i.e., a false negative study); that the extent of intimal proliferation be carefully measured over the full length of the injured arterial segment; and if possible, that some index of the therapeutic effect of the chosen drug be quantified to permit evaluation of the agent in other animal species using a comparable drug dose. Ideally, in addition to histopathologic assessment, contrast angiography should also be performed to allow differentiation between the effects on arterial luminal caliber of neointimal thickening and changes in vasomotor tone.

Clinical Trials

The most notable feature of the published clinical restenosis trials is the striking lack of uniformity among study protocols. Not only has there been little consensus in recent years on questions as fundamental as the definition of restenosis, but study protocols have differed in the timing of initiation of study drug administration, the time at which randomization is performed, patient inclusion and exclusion criteria, the duration of treatment, the duration of follow-up, the methods of angiographic assessment, and the use of intention-to-treat versus treatment-received analysis. For example, to date, the results of six randomized studies examining the effects of oral fish oil supplementation on the incidence of restenosis have been published in peer reviewed journals (15–19) or as a preliminary communication (20). Four studies (16,18–20) showed a significant reduction in the incidence of restenosis and two (15,17) showed no benefit (Figure 5.1; Table 5.1). Comparison of the six study protocols shows such a considerable difference in design that no meaningful conclusions about the efficacy of fish oil supplementation can yet be reached (see Table 5.1). The patient sample size, for example, ranged from 82 to 194 randomized patients. Assuming a restenosis rate of 33% in the control population, three of the studies had a power of less than 60% to detect a 50% reduction in the incidence of restenosis (see Figure 5.1). Randomization was performed prior to PTCA in only three studies (15–17), and in these, treatment was initi-

Figure 5.1. The effects of oral fish oil supplementation on the incidence of restenosis after PTCA. Results are shown as the odds ratio with 95% confidence limits. An effective therapy has an odds ratio less than 1; this effect is statistically significant at the $p < 0.05$ level if the confidence interval (horizontal line) does not cross the vertical line (odds ratio = 1).

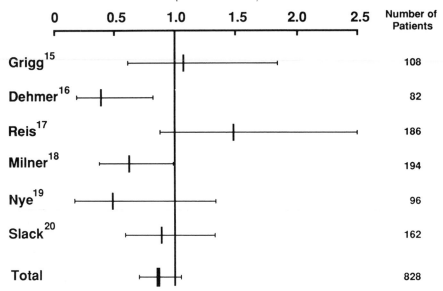

Table 5.1. Comparison of the Study Protocols for the Six Reported Fish Oil Restenosis Studies

PARAMETER	GRIGG (15)	DEHMER (16)	REIS (17)	MILNER (18)	NYE (19)	SLACK (20)
Sample size	108	82	186	194	108	162
Randomization pre-PTCA	Yes	Yes	Yes	No	NR	NR
Treatment ≥24 h pre-PTCA	Yes	Yes	Yes		No	NR
Placebo controlled	Yes	No	Yes	No	Yes	No
N3FA dose (g/day)	3.0	5.4	6.0	4.5	2.2	2.7
Angiographic end point (>80% pts)	Yes	Yes	No	No	Yes	No
Quantitative angiography	Yes	Yes	No	NA	NR	NA
Restenosis definition*	4,5	5	2	5	4	NR
Compliance check/lipid testing	Yes	Yes	Yes	No	Yes	Yes
Interim analysis/early cessation	No	Yes	Yes	No	No	NR
Intention-to-treat analysis	Yes	NR	Yes	Yes	NR	NR

*Definitions of restenosis:
1. An increase in diameter stenosis of ≥ 30% from immediately post-PTCA to the time of follow-up (NHLBI 1).
2. An immediate post-PTCA diameter stenosis of <50% increasing to ≥ 70% at follow-up (NHLBI 2).
3. An increase in stenosis severity to within 10% of the diameter stenosis before PTCA at the time of follow-up (NHLBI 3).
4. A loss of ≥ 50% of the gain in luminal diameter achieved immediately post-PTCA (NHLBI 4).
5. An increase in diameter stenosis from < 50% immediately after PTCA to > 50% at follow-up.
NA = not applicable; NHLBI = National Heart, Lung, and Blood Institute; NR = not recorded.

ated between 1 and 7 days prior to the interventional procedure. Only three of the studies were placebo-controlled (15,17,19). Angiographic analysis was performed routinely at the time of follow-up in only three studies (15,16,19). The severity of the recurrent stenosis was measured by calipers in two of these angiographic studies (in the single tightest view in one and averaged in two orthogonal views in the other), and was measured visually in the third; angiographic restenosis was defined using three different definitions (see Table 5.1). Two of the trials were discontinued early following interim analysis of the data (16,17), and only three stated that data analysis was performed on both an intention-to-treat and a treatment-received basis. This comparison highlights the need for a more rational and consistent approach to the clinical evaluation of interventions to reduce the incidence of restenosis. The following section examines the study protocol design issues that should be considered in planning or critically evaluating clinical restenosis trials.

Patient Inclusion Criteria

Patients undergoing percutaneous coronary interventions are not a homogeneous group. Rather, they consist of a diverse population of patients whose risk of restenosis may range from as low as 20% to as high as 60%. These patients can, however, be loosely grouped into those at relatively low risk and those at relatively high risk of recurrent stenosis (1). The low-risk group consists of patients undergoing elective PTCA of primary stenoses in the right coronary artery, the circumflex coronary, or the mid or distal segments of the left anterior descending artery for chronic stable anginal symptoms. Patients in the high-risk group include those undergoing PTCA of recurrent coronary stenoses, ostial or proximal left anterior descending artery stenoses, lesions in saphenous vein grafts, and chronic total occlusions, and those with unstable or early postinfarction angina. Conventionally, patients in the relatively high-risk category have been excluded from most restenosis trials to minimize disparities in baseline characteristics between the control and treated groups. A more rational approach may be to include all patients undergoing a given interventional procedure but to stratify randomized patients into low-risk and high-risk subgroups. The principal advantage of this approach is that the overall restenosis rate is increased for the entire population, thereby reducing the sample size of the study population necessary to demonstrate a therapeutic drug effect. In addition, therapies shown to be effective in these studies could legitimately then be applied to all patients undergoing the procedure rather than to selected subgroups of patients in whom one mechanism of restenosis may predominate.

A second consideration in the selection of patients relates to the timing of randomization. Most studies performed to date have randomized patients after successful completion of the dilatation procedure. Although this approach does minimize the number of patients who are randomized but are then ineligible for follow-up because of an unsuccessful coronary angioplasty, it does introduce the potential for bias in patient selection. By excluding patients with suboptimal angiographic results after PTCA, post-PTCA randomization may select a group of patients with a relatively low risk of restenosis that is not truly representative of the total population. Clearly, when drug therapy must be initiated before PTCA, randomization must also be performed before PTCA. A case can also be made, however, for randomization of all patients prior to the interventional procedure and the inclusion of all patients in whom the procedure is considered successful by prospectively defined criteria.

Timing and Administration of Drug Therapy

Several of the studies performed in recent years have been criticized because the study drug was not initiated early enough to have achieved the required therapeutic effect or because the duration of administration was insufficient to have covered the period during which the arterial healing response is most active. In experimental models of arterial injury, balloon dilatation is followed within minutes by platelet adherence and activation at the site of injury (12). Maximal thrombus formation occurs during the first 24 to 48 hours and is thereafter followed by the stimulation of smooth muscle cell mitogenesis and migration from the media to the intima. In the rat, smooth muscle cell activation and proliferation begins between 24 and 36 hours after injury and reaches a peak at 5 to 7 days (9). A similar time course is apparent in other animal models. Collagen synthesis and deposition accounts for the majority of the increase in neointimal thickness that occurs after the first 14 days. If a similar time course occurs in man, it follows that pharmacologic interventions that interfere with platelet activation or thrombus formation, including fish oil supplements, thromboxane and serotonin antagonists, and thrombin inhibitors, must be maximally active at the time of the injury and should probably be continued after the procedure in high doses for a period of at least 5 to 7 days. Agents that interfere primarily with the smooth muscle cell proliferative phase or with connective tissue matrix production need not be administered before the procedure but should be continued for several weeks to months. Data from experimental studies suggest, for example, that cessation of inhibitors of proliferation within 2 weeks of balloon arterial injury may postpone rather than prevent neointimal thickening (J. Powell, personal communication).

A second consideration is the adequacy of drug dosing. One possible explanation for the discrepancy between the experimental and clinical studies is that equivalent drug doses were not used in the clinical trials. Unfortunately, there is no simple way to directly extrapolate a drug dose shown to be effective in a rat carotid model, for example, to the clinical situation because drug absorption, distribution, and metabolism are likely to be different. Ideally, a measure of drug effect (such as platelet aggregation studies, serum lipid levels, or angiotensin levels) should be performed to confirm the adequacy of the selected drug dose. Clearly, this is more readily achieved for drugs with systemic effects than for those with local inhibitory activity such as the inhibitors of individual growth factors or of their cell receptors. When no end point of drug effect is available, dose-ranging studies should be considered as a means of ensuring that an adequate but tolerable drug dose is achieved. This situation will become more complex once studies are initiated with patients randomized to more than one drug therapy, given the potential for additive, synergistic, or adverse drug interactions. It is possible that a significant reduction in the incidence of restenosis will be achieved only with a combination of potent antithrombotic and antiproliferative therapies. Such a study would require a factorial design, careful attention to the dosing adequacy of each drug, and a very large patient sample size.

Although generally considered mandatory for scientific validity, the use of placebo therapy in the control group has not been consistent in recent clinical trials (see Table 5.1). In part, this has arisen because of difficulties encountered in adequately disguising the taste or odor of active drug therapies (such as fish oil supplements) or because of concerns that the placebo therapies (such as corn oil or olive oil) may actually exert some therapeutic effect on platelet function or atherogenesis. Although these are valid concerns, trials without a placebo arm will be criticized. A final consideration in drug dosing and administration is the adequacy of patient compliance with the study protocol. Every effort should be made to ensure that the study medications are taken as prescribed throughout the study period. This is best achieved by regular outpatient visits and the use of labelled packs for study medications with tablet count monitoring at each outpatient visit. When possible, serum drug levels should also be measured at the time of these visits.

Selection of Trial End Points

Coronary Angiography

One of the greatest inconsistencies among the published clinical restenosis trials has been the choice of trial end points. Although most used angiographic assessment of stenosis severity immediately post-PTCA and at 6 months, many relied on clinical end points such as recurrence of anginal symptoms, exercise-induced myocardial ischemia, and the need for repeat revascularization procedures. In recent years, greater attention has been paid to the optimal use of coronary angiography as a means of providing an objective, reproducible, and clinically relevant end point. Stenosis severity can be assessed visually, by hand-held calipers, or by computerized, digitized, quantitative analysis systems. Although used in some clinical restenosis studies, visual evaluation of stenosis severity has been associated with a high degree of interobserver and intraobserver variability, particularly for stenoses of intermediate severity [21–23]. The variability associated with the detection of small changes in lesion severity appears to be particularly high [24]. Moreover, a major limitation of this approach is its ability to express lesion severity only in terms of the percentage diameter stenosis, a parameter whose clinical relevance has been questioned recently [25–27]. The simplest and least expensive method of quantitatively measuring stenosis severity is by hand-held caliper measurement [28–30]. Digital electronic calipers provide precise measurements, but the accuracy of the technique still depends on the visual interpretation of the angiogram. Validation studies have suggested that when used for the measurement of coronary stenoses that have not been dilated, the standard deviation for multiple measurements of percent diameter stenosis is approximately ± 6% and for measurements of MLD it is ± 0.18 mm [28]. Although some studies have shown a good overall correlation between caliper measurements and computerized quantitative analysis systems [28,

29), others have questioned the superiority of caliper measurements over visual assessment (30). In contrast to visual estimates, caliper measurements appear to underestimate stenosis severity for lesions of 75% or more and to overestimate the severity of less significant stenoses (29).

The new "gold" standard for coronary restenosis studies and for atherosclerosis progression or regression trials is computer-assisted quantitative analysis of stenosis severity. Several approaches, including computerized analysis of hand-drawn arterial borders (31), computerized edge-detection and analysis (32–34), and videodensitometric analysis (35–37), have been evaluated. The accuracy and precision of automated edge-detection systems have been well validated in experimental models and in vivo. In one study, the variability in measurement of absolute MLD was 0.36 mm for analyses of coronary angiograms performed 90 days apart (34). The variabilities in reference diameter and percentage diameter stenosis were 0.66 mm and 6.5% respectively. Importantly, these measurements were made on nondilated stenoses with no attempt to reduce potential sources of variability such as the volume, rate, or choice of contrast agent, the technical characteristics of the x-ray system, or changes in vasomotor tone. Thus, although not validated for dilated stenoses, these values have been taken to represent the largest standard deviation for repeated measures of coronary stenoses performed under controlled conditions in the setting of a clinical restenosis trial.

Although automated edge-detection represents a significant improvement in the accuracy and precision of measurement of stenosis severity, it has several important limitations. Because many arterial stenoses are eccentric, complete analysis requires the determination of MLD in orthogonal projections and the calculation of minimal luminal area. However, orthogonal projections that adequately show the stenosis at end diastole without foreshortening or side-branch overlap are not always possible. Second, although automated, a significant degree of operator-induced variability is possible. Variations may occur in the choice of angiographic projection and of end-diastolic cine frame, the selection of reference arterial segments and of center positions, and the manual correction of detected contours, particularly for the complex coronary morphology that may follow balloon arterial dilatation. Videodensitometry has been proposed as a means of overcoming some of these limitations. In particular, densitometric analysis, which assumes that the intraluminal content of contrast medium is directly proportional to the lumen cross-sectional area, may obviate the need for orthogonal projections by effectively providing a three-dimensional analysis from a two-dimensional image. In practice, however, videodensitometry has not yet proved to be practical for large volume studies, and it appears to be limited by many of the same variables as edge-detection techniques. Whether it will ultimately prove to be more reliable than edge-detection methods in the assessment of the physiologic significance of residual stenoses after PTCA remains to be determined (36,37).

Angiographic Definitions of Restenosis

After a method for angiographic analysis is selected, it is necessary to decide what to measure and how to define restenosis. Conventionally, restenosis has been defined on the basis of arbitrarily selected changes in the percentage luminal diameter stenosis; at least five different definitions have been used in clinical restenosis trials (see Table 5.1). As noted previously (38), the apparent restenosis rate may vary considerably depending on the definition chosen. Serruys and colleagues, for example, restudied four groups of patients at 30 days, 60 days, 90 days, or 120 days after balloon dilatation (38). The discrepancy between the definitions increased progressively such that, in the 120-day follow-up group, the incidence of restenosis ranged from 2.8% (NHLBI 2) to 30.2% (NHLBI 4; Figures 5.2 and 5.3).

In addition to the arbitrary values used for these definitions, other concerns have been raised about the utility of angiographic diameter stenosis. First, the percentage diameter stenosis may be a poor index of the physiologic significance of a luminal narrowing. Histopathologic studies (both experimental and clinical) have shown, for example, that coronary angiography greatly underestimates the severity of diffuse atherosclerotic disease (39,40). Thus, a lesion measured angiographically to be 50% in diameter stenosis (which, in experimental studies represents the point at which coronary flow reserve begins to decline; 41,42) may actually be narrowed by more than 75% when examined histologically (39). More importantly, measurements of changes in percent diameter stenosis assumes no change has occurred in caliber of the reference arterial segment. Careful angiographic studies have shown, however, that this is not a valid assumption. In a study by Beatt and colleagues, for example, the mean diameter of the reference arterial segment decreased by 0.17 mm at 90 days and by 0.26 mm at 120 days (43). Thus, calculation of the percent diameter stenosis may underestimate

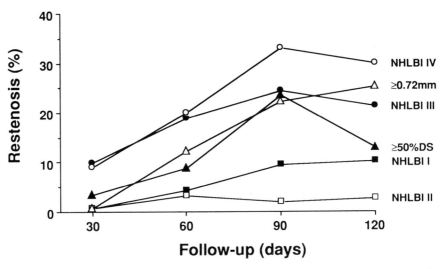

Figure 5.2. Incidence of restenosis in four groups of patients in one study according to six different angiographic definitions. (Reproduced with permission of the American Heart Association from ref. 38.)

changes in luminal caliber at the site of balloon dilatation if significant changes in the caliber of the reference segment have also occurred. Finally, selection of a single arbitrary cutoff, such as a 50% or greater diameter stenosis, does not consider the adequacy of the initial dilatation procedure. Rather, patients with a considerable degree of neointimal thickening following an optimal PTCA result may be excluded, whereas those with only a mild degree of thickening following a suboptimal result may be included.

These concerns have led to the proposal of absolute MLD as an alternative index of restenosis (38, 43–45). This has the considerable advantage of including all patients with a significant change in luminal caliber at the site of dilatation and is independent of changes in caliber of the proximal reference segment. To ensure reliable measurements, angiography should be performed in the same projection, with the same contrast medium, after intravenous nitroglycerin to eliminate changes in vasomotor tone. The selected image diameter can be converted to an absolute diameter by using a calibration factor, in millimeters per pixel, derived from measurement of the image of the angiographic catheter before contrast injection. To minimize errors associated with variation in the caliber of the catheters, many investigators now require that the

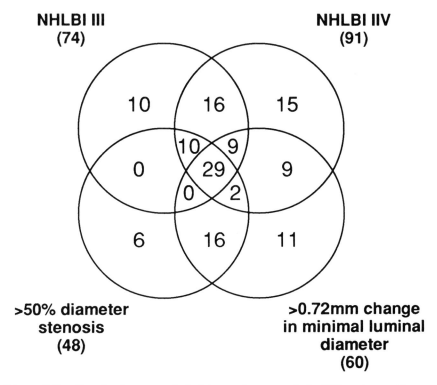

NHLBI III
(74)

NHLBI IIV
(91)

10   16   15

10   9

0   29   9

0   2

6   16   11

>50% diameter
stenosis
(48)

>0.72mm change
in minimal luminal
diameter
(60)

Figure 5.3.   Overlap between definitions of restenosis in 273 patients. (Reproduced with permission of the American Heart Association from ref. 38.)

segment of catheter used for calibration be forwarded to the core angiographic laboratory for ex vivo measurement. Using this parameter, angiographic studies have shown that, as in animal models (2), restenosis is not a dichotomous event. Rather, most angioplasty sites develop some degree of recurrent narrowing and the degree of change is normally distributed about a mean value which, in one study, was 0.42 mm at 120 days (43). Using this approach, the incidence of restenosis, if defined as a categorical variable, again depends on the selected cutoff for the degree of change in MLD. Rather than selecting an arbitrary value, however, investigators have used a value that is twice the standard deviation for repeated measures of luminal caliber for the quantitative angiographic system, thereby ensuring a false positive rate of only 2.5% (38,44). Thus, Serruys and colleagues (38) have used a change in MLD of more than 0.72 mm as the cutoff, and Nobuyoshi and colleagues (44) have used 0.50 mm. A further potential advantage of this approach is that the end point is expressed as a continuous variable rather than a binary outcome, thereby offering the possibility of considerably reduced sample sizes.

Measurement of MLD on its own is not, however, entirely free of limitations. First, the variabilities reported for repeated measures of coronary stenosis severity were determined for nondilated stenoses (34,44). This value has not been validated for lesions with complex geometry because of intimal dissection after balloon dilatation. Second, without comparison with the caliber of the reference segment, the absolute change in MLD has no physiologic meaning. Clearly, a change of 0.72 mm in a 1.5-mm vessel is of considerably greater significance than the same absolute change in a 4.0-mm vessel. Similarly, like percentage diameter stenosis measurements and all single dimensional measurements, the MLD does not allow for other changes in lesion morphology, such as the length of the lesion, its geometric regularity, and its entrance and exit angles, that may have a considerable impact on its hemodynamic significance.

A recent detailed analysis of the procedural factors associated with an increased likelihood of restenosis, as defined first by a change in MLD of 0.72 mm or greater and second by the presence of a lesion with 50% or more luminal diameter stenosis has shed some light on the importance of distinguishing between these two definitions (45). In this study of 500 patients, the major procedural risk factor for restenosis, as defined by the former definition, was the degree of improvement in MLD at the time of balloon dilatation. Thus, the greater the improvement and the better the final angiographic result, the greater the magnitude of the subsequent deterioration in luminal caliber. On the other hand, using the second definition, a different population of patients was identified as having "restenosed." In these patients, the predominant procedural risk factor for restenosis was a suboptimal angiographic result ($\geq 35\%$ residual diameter stenosis). The authors concluded that it is important to distinguish between the incidence of clinically relevant restenosis and the "restenosis process." Thus, it is likely that a combination of absolute change in MLD, final percentage diameter (or area) stenosis, and lesion morphology will be necessary to fully describe the changes in angiographic appearance and functional significance of the stenosis from immediately post-PTCA to the time of follow-up.

Clinical End Points

Although the above angiographic comparisons are undoubtedly the simplest and most logistically feasible end points for restenosis studies, it is the clinical outcome that matters most to the clinician performing the procedure and to the patient on whom it is performed. The angiographic and clinical restenosis rates are likely to be somewhat discordant. It is possible, for example, that a given pharmacologic intervention might not prevent "restenosis" as judged angiographically by changes in MLD or percent diameter stenosis, but might change the natural history of the recurrent lesion (for example by reducing its propensity to progress to complete occlusion) so that its clinical relevance is reduced. Similarly, it has been suggested that some mechanical interventions, such as intracoronary stenting, might improve clinical outcome not by altering the biologic process of restenosis, but by limiting its physiologic significance by providing a greater immediate postinterventional luminal caliber (46). Finally, patients with clinical restenosis will include a proportion with progression of disease in nondilated arteries rather than recurrent stenosis of previously dilated lesions.

In previous studies, the major difficulties in comparing clinical outcomes has been the low incidence in study populations of objective end points, such as death or myocardial infarction. Most studies have relied, therefore, on the evaluation of recurrent anginal symptoms and noninvasive testing as indices of coronary restenosis. However, recurrent chest pain has been shown in many studies to be poorly discriminatory for the presence of recurrent stenosis. In the NHLBI Registry (47), for example, the incidence of angiographic restenosis at 6 months was only 56% in patients with typical angina compared with 14% in asymptomatic patients. Conversely, 24% of patients with angiographically documented restenosis were free of recurrent chest pain. Similarly, the reliability of exercise treadmill testing (48–51), radionuclide angiography (49–50,52), and thallium scintigraphy (48–50) has been suboptimal. The positive predictive value for treadmill exercise-induced ischemia 6 months after PTCA has ranged from 39% to 64%, and the negative predictive value has ranged from 50% to 95% (48–51). For exercise radionuclide ventriculography, the positive predictive value has ranged from 15% to 54%, and the negative predictive value has ranged from 50% to 100% (49,50,52); the values for exercise thallium studies performed 6 months after PTCA have ranged from 37% to 100% and from 75% to

100%, respectively (48–50). Noninvasive studies performed in the first few days after PTCA have yielded conflicting results. Although several studies have suggested that recurrent stenosis may be predicted within the first few days after PTCA by exercise treadmill testing (53) or exercise thallium scintigraphy (54,55), others have suggested that thallium perfusion defects noted in the first few days after PTCA may resolve completely within the first 3 months (56). The findings of the latter study are consistent with the observations that recovery in coronary flow reserve following balloon dilatation of coronary stenoses may also be delayed (57–59). These findings have been attributed to changes in vasomotor tone of the distal vascular bed and to delayed recovery of myocardial function following a period of chronic myocardial ischemia (56,57).

The low frequency of objective clinical end points and poor predictive values of both recurrent symptoms and exercise stress testing after PTCA have led some investigators (60) to recommend that clinical outcome be expressed as a composite end point with weighted adjustment for clinical events. Table 5.2 describes the frequency of clinical events 6 months after PTCA from the least desirable to least significant adverse outcomes, based on data from the Duke University and University of Michigan Medical Centers, and outlines a proposed ordinal event ranking scheme based on the clinical significance of each event. Although

Table 5.2. Composite Ordinal Ranking of Adverse Clinical Events After PTCA in Descending Order of Clinical Significance

EVENT	EVENT FREQUENCY*	CUMULATIVE EVENT FREQUENCY	COMPOSITE RANKING
Death	2.7	2.7	1
Myocardial infarction	3.5	6.2	2
Emergency CABG	0.9	7.1	3
Elective CABG	1.3	8.4	4
Emergency PTCA	1.4	9.8	5
Elective PTCA	9.6	19.4	6
Recurrent chest pain	15.5	34.9	7
Positive ETT	12.6	47.5	8
Angiographic restenosis only	10.9	58.4	9

*Events are listed in hierarchical order with each patient counted only once.
CABG = coronary artery bypass graft surgery; ETT = exercise tolerance test; PTCA = percutaneous transluminal coronary angioplasty.
Reproduced with permission of the American Heart Association from reference 60.

this approach has not yet been prospectively validated, it does promise to be a useful means of combining clinical outcome data with angiographic data to provide a meaningful composite outcome index for comparison in clinical trials using manageable patient population sizes.

Statistical Issues

Sample Size Estimates

As noted previously, the vast majority of clinical studies performed to date have enrolled too few patients to reliably detect a meaningful therapeutic effect of a given pharmacologic intervention on the incidence of restenosis when measured as a binary outcome. Several factors must be considered in determining the optimal sample size for a clinical restenosis trial. First, it is necessary to have a reliable estimate of the incidence of restenosis in the control population. Most previous and several ongoing studies have assumed a control incidence of between 20% and 30%. The control incidence will depend, however, on the patient inclusion criteria and the method of angiographic assessment. The incidence of restenosis will be higher, for example, if patients with prior restenosis, total occlusions, or saphenous vein graft stenoses are included. The restenosis rate in the larger published trials has ranged from 13% to 43% at 3 months and from 16% to 43% at 6 months (Table 5.3;38,44, 45,47,61–68). Although much of this variability may be due to differences in angiographic definitions of restenosis, it is also likely to be associated with differences in patient selection criteria.

The second question in determining sample size is: what degree of reduction in the incidence of restenosis is clinically meaningful? For example, is it necessary to show a 50% reduction in the restenosis rate, or would a therapy be widely accepted if it could be shown to reduce the rate by 25%? To some extent, this will depend on the side effect profile of the therapeutic agent because approximately 60% to 70% of patients do not develop clinically significant recurrent stenoses. Thus, an agent with few side effects could be given to all patients in the hope of achieving a relatively small reduction in the incidence of restenosis (but nonetheless, a potentially large savings in health care costs). On the other hand, therapies with the potential for severe side effects should be expected to show a substantial decrease in the restenosis rate before being

Table 5.3. Reported Restenosis Rates in Control Populations of Studies with More Than 200 Patients and More Than 75% Angiographic Follow-up

STUDY	PATIENTS	ANGIOGRAPHY (%FU)	TIME TO FU (MO)	DEFINITION	RESTENOSIS (%)
Serruys (38)	400	85	4	≥0.72 mm increase	26
Beatt (45)	500	85	3	≥50% diam stenosis	13
Serruys (61)	649	80	6	≥0.72 mm increase	17
Nobuyoshi (44)	219	96	3	≥0.72 mm increase	19
				loss ≥50% initial gain	43
Holmes (47)	665	84	6.2	loss ≥50% initial gain	34
Kaltenbach (62)	356	94	5.6	loss ≥50% initial gain	16
Whitworth (63)	241	82	6.5	loss ≥50% initial gain	30
Rapold (64)	247	94	4.9	≥70% diam stenosis visually	29
Bertrand (65)	266	92	6	loss ≥50% initial gain	41
Frid (66)	396	86	6	≥50% diam stenosis	36
Taylor (67)	216	98	7.4	loss ≥50% gain + ≥50% DS	43
Nelson (68)	2191	84	6	≥50% diam stenosis	37

diam = diameter; DS = diameter stenosis; FU = follow-up; mo = months.

recommended as routine prophylactic therapy. The degree of reduction in restenosis must also be clinically relevant. It might be possible, for example, to show, with a relatively small sample size using a continuous measure of MLD, that a small reduction in the severity of neointimal thickening by a given therapy is statistically significant, but this difference may be of minimal physiologic and clinical significance.

A third important consideration is the adequacy of clinical and angiographic follow-up. Recent analyses of the impact of incomplete angiographic follow-up on estimates of the restenosis rate suggest that the assumption that asymptomatic patients have no restenosis will considerably underestimate the true restenosis rate (69). Similarly, the assumption that symptomatic patients and those with positive functional studies have recurrent stenoses, without angiographic confirmation, will significantly overestimate the true restenosis rate. For this reason, study population sizes should be calculated to include a surplus of approximately 15% to 20% more patients than the estimated sample size to account for patients lost to follow-up. Every effort should be made to ensure as complete an angiographic follow-up rate as possible, and the clinical status of patients who do not have repeat angiography should be reported in detail. The baseline characteristics of patients with and those without follow-up should be compared to ensure that no selection bias is likely by exclusion of the group without angiographic follow-up. Use of a composite clinical end point with weighted adverse clinical outcomes also allows patients dying during the follow-up period to be accounted for without the need to impute the angiographic stenosis severity.

A further consideration is the number of lesions, rather than patients, treated at the time of the interventional procedure. If the probability of restenosis were lesion dependent, as opposed to patient dependent, the sample number could be considerably increased if the population included a large proportion of patients with multilesion or multivessel disease. If the probability of restenosis were the same (for example, 0.4) for each of two dilated stenoses, the overall probability of at least one recurrent stenosis would be 0.64; similarly, for three dilated lesions, the probability of one or more recurrence, assuming independent probabilities, is 0.78. Using an assumed risk of restenosis of 0.35 per lesions, the probabilities of at least one recurrence would be 0.58 and 0.73, respectively. Large data base studies have suggested, however, that although the overall probability of restenosis per patient rises with multilesion angioplasty, restenosis occurs less frequently than might be expected from these calculations (69). This suggests that the phenomenon of restenosis is determined by both patient-related and lesion-dependent factors; it cannot be assumed that the risk of restenosis for each lesion is independent. Sample size estimates for clinical restenosis studies should therefore be based on the number of patients treated, but ideally, restenosis rates should be reported both on a per patient and per lesion basis.

Table 5.4 lists the estimated sample size, assuming 100% follow-up and a categorical definition of restenosis, according to the assumed event rate, the expected impact of the therapeutic agent, and the required statistical power (1-β) (70). It can be seen from the table that the number of patients required to show a 50% reduction in the incidence of restenosis ranges from 182 to 572, depending on the control event rate. To show a 25% reduction in restenosis would require a minimum of 752 patients assuming a control rate of 40%. To date, only two published studies have randomized more than 500 patients (61,71). In the study by Pepine and colleagues (71), 915 patients received intravenous methylprednisolone or placebo within 24 hours of PTCA. Of these, PTCA was successfully performed in 722 patients, and follow-up angiography was performed in 510 (i.e., 73.5% of those eligible for follow-

Table 5.4. Sample Size Calculations by Frequency of End Point and Desired Statistical Power*

α	β	ASSUMED EVENT RATE CONTROL (%)	ASSUMED EVENT RATE TREATMENT (%)	EVENT RATE REDUCTION (%)	SAMPLE SIZE (TOTAL PTS)
0.05	0.10	20	10	50	572
0.05	0.20	20	10	50	438
0.05	0.10	30	20	33	824
0.05	0.20	30	20	33	626
0.05	0.10	30	15	50	348
0.05	0.20	30	15	50	268
0.05	0.10	35	25	29	918
0.05	0.20	35	25	29	696
0.05	0.10	40	30	25	992
0.05	0.20	40	30	25	752
0.05	0.10	40	20	50	236
0.05	0.20	40	20	50	182

*Assuming 100% follow-up, a binary definition of restenosis, and two-tailed probability testing (Adapted from reference 70).

up and 56% of the original study population). In this study, the sample size was estimated assuming a control restenosis rate of 20%, a 50% reduction by methylprednisolone, an α (probability of type 1, false positive study) of 0.05, and a β (probability of type 2, false negative study) of 0.10. It was estimated that 1000 patients would need to be randomized to provide 800 patients with successful PTCA and 600 patients with adequate angiographic follow-up at 6 months. In fact, the incidence of restenosis was 39% in the control group and 40% in the treated group.

A different trial design was used in the Coronary Artery Restenosis Prevention on Repeated Thromboxane-Antagonism (CARPORT) Study (61). In this study, 697 patients were randomly assigned prior to attempted PTCA to either GR32191B, a thromboxane A_2-receptor blocker, or to placebo. Of 649 patients with a successful procedure, 522 (80%) had repeat coronary angiography performed at 6 months. The primary end point for the trial was absolute change in MLD at the site of balloon dilatation for immediately post-PTCA to the time of follow-up angiography as determined by quantitative coronary angiography. Clinical outcome was also reported for each group of patients using an assigned ranking of clinical events. The change in MLD was measured as a continuous rather than a categorical variable. Sample size estimates were based on the assumption of a 30% reduction in the change in diameter from -0.40 ± 0.50 mm in the control group to -0.25 ± 0.50 mm in the treated group. Using these estimates and an α of 0.05 and β of 0.10, the sample size calculated for the study was 466 patients. This is approximately one third of the 1240 patients who would have been required to show a 30% reduction in the incidence of recurrent stenosis if restenosis was defined categorically as a change in MLD of 0.72 mm or greater. The angiographic findings of the study were similar in the two groups. The absolute change in MLD was -0.31 ± 0.54 mm in the control group compared with -0.31 ± 0.55 mm in the treated group (Figures 5.4 and 5.5). When restenosis was defined as a reduction in MLD of 0.72 mm or greater, the incidence of restenosis was 19% in the control group compared with 21% in the treated group (relative risk 1.15; 95% confidence intervals, 0.82 to 1.60; see Figure 5.5). This form of data analysis represents a novel and potentially valuable approach to the description of the angiographic outcome in restenosis trials and, when combined with careful analysis of the frequencies of adverse clinical events and quantitation of the extent of functional myocardial ischemia, should permit a more thorough and reproducible evaluation of pharmacologic and mechanical interventions for the prevention of restenosis.

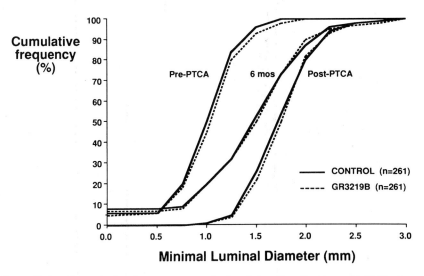

Figure 5.4. Cumulative frequency analysis of the distribution of MLDs determined by quantitative coronary angiography before PTCA, immediately following PTCA, and at 6-month (6 mos) follow-up in 522 patients randomly assigned to thromboxane A$_2$-receptor blocker therapy (GR32191B: Glaxo Group Research Ltd.) or to placebo. (Reproduced with permission of the American Heart Association from ref. 61.)

Figure 5.5. Cumulative frequency analysis of the change in MLD from post-PTCA to 6-month follow-up. The incidence of restenosis, defined as a decrease in MLD of more than 0.72 mm, was 19% in the control group and 21% in the treatment group. (Reproduced with permission of the American Heart Association from ref. 61.)

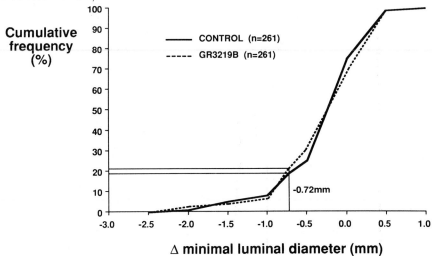

Prospects for Effective Restenosis Therapy from Ongoing Clinical Trials

As noted previously, a large number of clinical pharmacologic restenosis trials are currently in progress; these have been well summarized by Popma and colleagues (60). Of the nine trials listed in Table 5.5, eight will enroll more than 400 patients and each has sufficient statistical power, assuming adequate follow-up, to detect a 33% to 50% reduction in the angiographic incidence of restenosis. However, only the cilazapril study is likely to have sufficient power to detect a 25% reduction using a binary outcome variable, and then only if the control rate is actually 35% to 40%. Approximately half the studies plan to use percent diameter stenosis at follow-up as the primary end point; several will report both percent diameter stenosis and the change in absolute MLD.

One of these large trials might identify a single pharmacologic agent that reduces the incidence of restenosis to a moderately large degree. This assumes, however, that restenosis is due to one predominant mechanism that will be affected by single agent therapy. This in itself could prove a naive assumption. It is more likely that single agent therapy will reduce one component of the restenosis process, such as platelet activation, thrombus formation, or even smooth muscle cell proliferation, without interfering with other components such as interstitial matrix formation or elastic recoil. Other approaches, such as debulking atheromatous lesions or stenting coronary arteries, in combination with single or multidrug therapy warrant careful evaluation. Multicenter trials have been initiated for the randomized comparison of mechanical revascularization strategies (e.g., the 1000 patient Coronary Angioplasty Versus Excisional Atherectomy Trial [CAVEAT]), and for the evaluation of coronary atherectomy with pharmacologic therapies, such as angiopeptin (Henri Beaufort Institute). Other studies using intracoronary stent implantation in combination with a variety of pharmacologic therapies will soon follow.

Over the next few years, therefore, the study of restenosis and the evaluation of mechanical and pharmacologic therapies to combat this problem should reach a new level of complexity and scientific validity. With greater attention to the details of trial design and data analysis, many of the limitations of previous studies will be avoided. Only then will it be possible to legitimately conclude that individual therapies or mechanical devices are truly effective or ineffective for the prevention of restenosis following percutaneous coronary revascularization.

Table 5.5. Sample Size Estimates for Ongoing Multicenter Clinical Restenosis Trials

Agent	α	β	ASSUMED EVENT RATE CONTROL (%)	ASSUMED EVENT RATE TREATMENT (%)	EVENT REDUCTION (%)	ENROLLMENT SIZE	SAMPLE SIZE	RESTENOSIS DEFINITION*
PLATELET INHIBITORS								
Sulotroban	0.05	0.20	30	15	50	800	800	2
Ketanserin	0.05	0.10	NR	NR	NR	600	460	2
Fish oil	0.05	0.20	30	20	33	510	460	1
SMOOTH MUSCLE CELL PROLIFERATION INHIBITORS								
EMPAR trial	0.05	0.10	20	10	50	800	800	3
Lovastatin	0.05	0.10	30	15	50	400	360	1,2
Enoxaparin	0.05	0.20	30	20	33	400	400	2,3
Cilazapril	0.05	0.20	30	20	33	1,400	1,200	2
Fosinopril	0.05	0.20	30	20	33	820	626	4
GROWTH FACTOR INHIBITOR								
Angiopeptin	0.05	0.10	30	15	50	900	900	1 or 3

Enoxaparin/Max-EPA for Prevention of Angioplasty Restenosis trial; NR = not reported.
* 1 = ≥ 50% diameter stenosis at follow up; 2 = change in minimal luminal diameter; 3 = loss of ≥50% of the initial gain in diameter stenosis; 4 = composite clinical outcome.
Adapted with permission of the American Heart Association from ref. 60.

References

1. Califf RM, Ohman EM, Frid DJ, et al. Restenosis: the clinical issues. In: Topol EJ, ed. Textbook of interventional cardiology. Philadelphia: WB Saunders, 1990:363–394.

2. Muller DWM, Ellis SG, Topol EJ. Experimental models of coronary artery restenosis. J Am Coll Cardiol 1992;19:418–432.

3. Faggiotto A, Ross R, Harker L. Studies of hypercholesterolemia in the non-human primate: I. Changes that lead to fatty streak formation. Arteriosclerosis 1984;4:323–340.

4. Faggiotto A, Ross R. Studies of hypercholesterolemia in the non-human primate: II. Fatty streak conversion to fibrous plaque. Arteriosclerosis 1984;4:341–356.

5. Gerrity RG, Naito HK, Richardson M, Schwartz CJ. Dietary induced atherogenesis in swine: morphology of the intima in prelesion stages. Am J Pathol 1979;95:775–792.

6. Rosenfeld ME, Faggiotto A, Ross R. The role of the mononuclear phagocyte in primate and rabbit models of atherosclerosis. In: Van Furth R, ed. Mononuclear phagocytes: characteristics, physiology and function. Martinus Nijhoff, The Hague, Netherlands, 1985:795–801.

7. Virchow R. Der atheromatous Prozess der Arteries. Wien Med Wochenschr 1856;6:825–829.

8. Ross R. The pathogenesis of atherosclerosis—an update. N Engl J Med 1986;314:488–500.

9. Clowes AW, Reidy MA, Clowes MM. Kinetics of cellular proliferation after arterial injury. I. Smooth muscle cell growth in the absence of endothelium. Lab Invest 1983;49:327–333.

10. Clowes AW, Schwartz SM. Significance of quiescent smooth muscle migration in the injured rat carotid artery. Circ Res 1985;56:139–145.

11. Block PC, Baughman KL, Pasternak RC, Fallon JT. Transluminal angioplasty: correlation of morphologic and angiographic findings in an experimental model. Circulation 1980;61:778–785.

12. Steele PM, Chesebro JH, Stanson AW, Holmes Dr, Dewanjee MK, Badimon L, Fuster V. Balloon angioplasty: natural history of the pathophysiological response to injury in a pig model. Circ Res 1985;57:105–112.

13. Buchwald A, Unterberg C, Werner G, Voth E, Kreuzer H, Wiegand V. Initial clinical results with the Wiktor stent: a new balloon-expandable coronary stent. Clin Cardiol 1991;14:374–379.

14. Schwartz RS, Huber KC, Murphy JG, et al. Restenosis and the proportional response to coronary artery injury: results in a porcine model. J Am Coll Cardiol 1992;19:267–274.

15. Grigg LE, Kay TWH, Valentine PA, et al. Determinants of restenosis and lack of effect of dietary supplementation with eicosapentaneoic acid on the incidence of coronary restenosis after angioplasty. J Am Coll Cardiol 1989;13:665–672.

16. Dehmer GJ, Popma JJ, van den Berg EK, et al. Reduction in the rate of early restenosis after coronary angioplasty by a diet supplemented with n-3 fatty acids. N Engl J Med 1988;319:733–740.

17. Reis GJ, Boucher TM, Sipperly ME, et al. Randomised trial of fish oil for prevention of restenosis after coronary angioplasty. Lancet 1989;ii:177–181.

18. Milner MR, Gallino RA, Leffingwell A, et al. Usefulness of fish oil supplements in preventing clinical evidence of restenosis after percutaneous transluminal coronary angioplasty. Am J Cardiol 1989;64:294–299.

19. Nye ER, Ablett MB, Robertson MC, Ilsley CDJ, Sutherland WHF. Effect of eicosapentaneoic acid on restenosis rate, clinical course and blood lipids in patients after percutaneous transluminal coronary angioplasty. Aust NZ J Med 1990;20:549–552.

20. Slack JD, Pinkerton CA, Van Tassel J, et al. Can oral fish oil supplement minimize restenosis after percutaneous transluminal coronary angioplasty? (abstr). J Am Coll Cardiol 1987;9:64A.

21. Detre KM, Wright E, Murphy ML, Takaro T. Observer agreement in evaluating coronary angiograms. Circulation 1977;55:979–983.

22. Zir LM, Miller SW, Dinsmore RE, Gilbert JP, Hawthorne JW. Interobserver variability in coronary angiography. Circulation 1976;53:627–632.

23. DeRouen TA, Murray JA, Owen W. Variability in the analysis of coronary arteriograms. Circulation 1977;55:324–328.

24. Azen SP, Cashin-Hemphill L, Pogoda J, et al Evaluation of human panelists in assessing coronary atherosclerosis. Arteriosclerosis Thromb 1991;11:385–394.

25. White CW, Wright CB, Doty DB, et al. Does the visual interpretation of the coronary arteriogram predict the physiological significance of a coronary stenosis? N Engl J Med 1984;310:819–824.

26. Marcus ML, Skorton DJ, Johnson MR, Collins SM, Harrison DG, Kerber RE. Visual estimates of percent diameter stenosis: a battered gold standard. J Am Coll Cardiol 1988;11:882–885.

27. Gould KL. Percent coronary stenosis: battered gold standard, pernicious relic or clinical practicality? J Am Coll Cardiol 1988;11:886–888.

28. Scoblionko DP, Brown G, Mitten S, et al. A new digital electronic caliper for measurement of coronary artery stenosis: comparison with visual estimates and computer-assisted measurements. Am J Cardiol 1984;53:689–693.

29. Kalbfleisch SJ, McGillem MJ, Pinto IMF, Kavanaugh KM, DeBoe SF, Mancini J. Comparison of automated quantitative coronary angiography with caliper measurements of percent diameter stenosis. Am J Cardiol 1990;65:1181–1184.

30. Holder DA, Johnson AL, Stolberg HO, et al. Inability of caliper measurement to enhance observer agreement in the interpretation of coronary cineangiograms. Can J Cardiol 1985;1:24–29.

31. Brown BG, Bolson E, Frimer M, Dodge HT. Quantitative arteriography: estimation of dimensions, hemodynamic resistance, and atheroma mass of coronary artery lesions using the arteriogram and digital computation. Circulation 1977;55:329–337.

32. Mancini GBJ, Simon SB, McGillem MJ, LeFree MT, Friedman HZ, Vogel RA. Automated quantitative coronary arteriography: morphologic and physiologic validation in vivo of a rapid digital angiographic method. Circulation 1987;75:452–460.

33. Sanz ML, Mancini GBJ, LeFree MT, et al. Variability of quantitative digital subtraction coronary angiography before and after percutaneous transluminal coronary angioplasty. Am J Cardiol 1987;60:55–60.

34. Reiber JHC, Serruys PW, Kooijman CJ, et al. Assessment of short-, medium-, and long-term variations in arterial dimensions from computer-assisted quantification of coronary cineangiograms. Circulation 1985;71:280–288.

35. Johnson MR, McPherson DD, Fleagle SR, et al. Videodensitometric analysis of human coronary stenoses: validation in vivo by intraoperative high-frquency epicardial echocardiography. Circulation 1988;77:328–336.

36. Serruys PW, Reiber JHC, Wijns W, et al. Assessment of percutaneous transluminal coronary angioplasty by quantitative coronary angiography: diameter versus densitometric area measurements. Am J Cardiol 1984;54:482–488.

37. Tobis J, Henry WL. Videodensitometric determination of minimum coronary luminal diameter before and after angioplasty. Am J Cardiol 1987;59:38–44.

38. Serruys PW, Luijten HE, Beatt KJ, et al. Incidence of restenosis after successful coronary angioplasty: a time-related phenomenon. A quantitative angiographic study in 342 consecutive patients at 1, 2, 3, and 4 months. Circulation 1988;77:361–371.

39. Arnett EN, Isner JM, Redwood DR, et al. Coronary artery narrowing in coronary heart disease: comparison of cineangiographic and necropsy findings. Ann Intern Med 1979;91:350–356.

40. Weiner BH, Ockene IS, Jarmolych J, Fritz KE, Daoud AS. Comparison of

pathologic and angiographic findings in a porcine preparation of coronary atherosclerosis. Circulation 1985; 72:1081–1086.

41. Folts JD, Gallagher K, Rowe GG. Hemodynamic effects of controlled degrees of coronary artery stenosis in short-term and long-term studies in dogs. J Thorac Cardiovasc Surg 1977;73:722–727.

42. Gould KL, Kelley KO. Physiological significance of coronary flow velocity and changing stenosis geometry during coronary vasodilation in awake dogs. Circ Res 1982;50:695–704.

43. Beatt KJ, Luyten HE, de Feyter PJ, van den Brand M, Reiber JHC, Serruys PW. Change in diameter of coronary artery segments adjacent to stenosis after PTCA: failure of percent diameter stenosis measurements to reflect morphometric changes induced by balloon dilation. J Am Coll Cardiol 1988;12:315–323.

44. Nobuyoshi M, Kimura T, Nosaka H, et al. Restenosis after successful percutaneous transluminal coronary angioplasty: serial angiographic follow-up of 299 patients. J Am Coll Cardiol 1988;12:616–623.

45. Beatt KJ, Serruys PW, Luijten HE, et al. Restenosis following coronary angioplasty: the paradox of improvement in lumen diameter and restenosis. J Am Coll Cardiol 1991;19:258–266.

46. Ellis SG, Savage M, Baim D, et al. Intracoronary stenting to prevent restenosis: preliminary results of a multicenter study using the Palmaz–Schatz stent suggest benefit in selected high risk patients (abstr). J Am Coll Cardiol 1990;15:118A.

47. Holmes DR Jr, Vlietstra RE, Smith HC, et al. Restenosis after percutaneous transluminal coronary angioplasty: a report from the PTCA Registry of the National Heart, Lung, and Blood Institute. Am J Cardiol 1984;53:77C–81C.

48. Scholl JM, Chaitman BR, David PR, et al. Exercise electrocardiography and myocardial scintigraphy in the serial evaluation of the results of percutaneous transluminal coronary angioplasty. Circulation 1982;66:380–390.

49. Rosing DR, van Raden MJ, Mincemoyer RM, et al. Exercise, electrocardiographic and functional responses after percutaneous transluminal coronary angioplasty. Am J Cardiol 1984;53:36C–41C.

50. Ernst SM, Hillebrand FA, Klein B, Ascoop CA, van Tellingen C, Plokker HW. The value of exercise tests in the follow-up of patients who underwent transluminal coronary angioplasty. Int J Cardiol 1985;7:267–279.

51. Bengston JR, Mark DB, Honan MB, et al. Detection of restenosis after elective coronary angioplasty using the exercise treadmill test. Am J Cardiol 1990;65:28–34.

52. DePuey EG, Leatherman LL, Leachman RD, et al. Restenosis after trans-

luminal coronary angioplasty detected with exercise-gated radionuclide ventriculography. J Am Coll Cardiol 1984;4:1103–1113.

53. El-Tamimi H, Davies GJ, Hackett D, Fragasso G, Crea F, Maseri A. Very early prediction of restenosis after successful coronary angioplasty: anatomic and functional assessment. J Am Coll Cardiol 1990;15:259–264.

54. Wijns W, Serruys PW, Reiber JHC, et al. Early detection of restenosis after successful percutaneous transluminal coronary angioplasty by exercise-redistribution thallium scintigraphy. Am J Cardiol 1985; 55:357–361.

55. Hardoff R, Shefer A, Gips S, et al. Predicting late restenosis after coronary angioplasty by very early (12 to 24 H) thallium-201 scintigraphy: implications with regard to mechanisms of late coronary restenosis. J Am Coll Cardiol 1990;15:1486–1492.

56. Manyari DE, Knudtson M, Kolber R, Roth D. Sequential thallium-201 myocardial perfusion studies after successful percutaneous transluminal coronary angioplasty: delayed resolution of exercise-induced scintigraphic abnormalities. Circulation 1988;77:86–95.

57. Popma JJ, Dehmer GJ, Eichhorn EJ. Variability of coronary flow reserve obtained immediately after coronary angioplasty. Int J Card Imaging 1991;6:31–38.

58. Zijlstra F, Reiber JC, Juilliere Y, Serruys PW. Normalization of coronary flow reserve by percutaneous transluminal coronary angioplasty. Am J Cardiol 1988;61:55–60.

59. Wilson RF, Johnson MR, Marcus ML, et al. The effect of coronary angioplasty on coronary flow reserve. Circulation 1988;77:873–885.

60. Popma JJ, Califf RM, Topol EJ. Clinical trials of restenosis after coronary angioplasty. Circulation 1991;84:1426–1436.

61. Serruys PW, Rutsch W, Heyndrickx GR, et al., for the Coronary Artery Restenosis Prevention on Repeated Thromboxane-Antagonism Study Group (CARPORT). Prevention of restenosis after percutaneous transluminal coronary angioplasty with thromboxane A_2-receptor blockade: a randomized, double-blind, placebo-controlled trial. Circulation 1991; 84:1568–1580.

62. Kaltenbach M, Kober G, Scherer D, Vallbracht C. Recurrence rate after successful coronary angioplasty. Eur Heart J 1985;6:276–281.

63. Whitworth HB, Roubin GS, Hollman J, et al. Effect of nifedipine on recurrent stenosis after percutaneous transluminal coronary angioplasty. J Am Coll Cardiol 1986;8:1271–1276.

64. Rapold HJ, David PR, Val PG, Mata AL, Crean PA, Bourassa MG. Restenosis and its determinants in first and repeat coronary angioplasty. Eur Heart J 1987;8:575–586.

65. Bertrand ME, Allain H, LaBlanche JM. Results of a randomized trial of ticlopidine versus placebo for prevention of acute closure and restenosis after coronary angioplasty (PTCA). The TACT Study (abstr). Circulation 1990;82(suppl III):190.

66. Frid DJ, Fortin DF, Lam LC, et al. Effects of unstable symptoms on restenosis (abstr). Circulation 1990;82(suppl III):427.

67. Taylor RR, Gibbons FA, Cope GD, Cumpston GN, Mews GC, Luke P. Effects of low-dose aspirin on restenosis after coronary angioplasty. Am J Cardiol 1991;68:874–878.

68. Nelson CL, Tcheng JE, Frid DJ, et al. Incomplete angiographic followup results in significant underestimation of true restenosis rates after PTCA (abstr). Circulation 1990;82(suppl III):312.

69. Tcheng JE, Fortin DF, Frid DJ, et al. Conditional probabilities of restenosis following coronary angioplasty (abstr). Circulation 1990;82(suppl III):1.

70. Fleiss JL. Statistical methods for rates and proportions. New York: John Wiley and Sons. 1981:261–267.

71. Pepine CJ, Hirshfeld LW, Macdonald RG, et al., for the M-HEART Group. A controlled trial of corticosteroids to prevent restenosis after coronary angioplasty. Circulation 1990;81:1753–1761.

· ·

CHAPTER 6

Clinical and Angiographic Definitions of Restenosis: Recommendations for Clinical Trials

WILLEM J. VAN DER GIESSEN
WALTER R. M. HERMANS
BENNO J. RENSING
DAVID P. FOLEY
PATRICK W. SERRUYS

Introduction: What Do We Mean by Restenosis?

THE most important step in discussing any topic, particularly a controversial one such as restenosis after percutaneous transluminal coronary angioplasty (PTCA), is to clearly describe what exactly we mean by restenosis. This ten letter word is proving extremely challenging to researchers and clinicians in the quest for a definition acceptable to everybody and ultimately a "cure."

We believe that restenosis describes the process by which the blood vessel renarrows following a mechanical injury exerted by a procedure or a device. This process of response has been best described after the injury of balloon dilatation, and in this circumstance consists of three components:

1. **Elastic recoil,** a natural property of intact vessels in response to stretch, is an immediate phenomenon observed with angiography (1,2) and endoluminal ultrasound (3); it has a doubtful contribution to the process of late restenosis
2. **Fibrocellular neointimal hyperplasia** is widely regarded as the

169

main pathologic process by which progressive luminal renarrowing develops in the months following PTCA (4–7)

3. **Reaccumulation of "classic" atherosclerotic plaque** (7).

It is evident that this description differs from "loss of greater than 50% of the gain" or "greater than 50% diameter stenosis at 6 or 12 months follow up," which are two of the most frequently used definitions in daily clinical practice as well as in restenosis trials.

Our intention is not to dismiss conventional methodology but to point out the fallibility of simplistic definitions in trying to describe a complicated process. As long as our understanding of the restenosis process is fragmented, we must be extremely careful not to blindly accept one definition to the exclusion of all others. However, in the meantime it is necessary to make sensible use of the most objective methodological approaches available, particularly in the field of clinical research. In the following sections we will address this evolving concept by discussing the clinical and functional aspects as well as the contribution of available imaging technology, concluding with recommendations for clinical restenosis trials.

Symptoms, Function, or Anatomy as Criteria of Restenosis?

The incidence of late restenosis has remained much the same since the introduction of coronary angioplasty 13 years ago, and a preventive treatment against restenosis must still be developed (8). Primary success and restenosis after PTCA may be defined by symptomatic criteria, such as severity of angina pectoris; by functional criteria, such as various exercise tests; or by anatomic criteria using histology, angiography, or intravascular ultrasound. These three sets of criteria may be considered separately or may be interrelated.

Symptomatic Criteria

Although the subjective improvement of symptoms after PTCA is probably the most desirable end point, it is also the least objective evaluation (9). The frequency of symptomatic improvement appears to be lower than that of angiographic success; only 70% of the patients with a satisfactory angiographic result immediately post-PTCA exhibit such an improvement (10). Furthermore, the reappearance of angina as a criterion of restenosis underestimates the angiographic rate of restenosis because the reported incidence of silent restenosis may be as high as 31% (11).

In a recent review, Califf and colleagues (12) described that in studies with a high rate of angiographic follow-up, the probability that patients with symptoms had restenosis (i.e., the positive predictive value of symptoms) ranged from 48% to 92%, whereas the probability that patients without symptoms were free of restenosis (i.e., the negative predictive value of symptoms) ranged from 70% to 98%. The low positive predictive value found in many of these studies may be explained by the presence of other mechanisms for angina, such as incomplete revascularization or progression of disease in other vessels. In view of the above considerations, the usefulness of symptomatic criteria for the detection of restenosis is at best limited.

Functional Criteria

Exercise Testing: Several studies have examined the ability of the exercise treadmill test to detect restenosis after PTCA. These studies have generally found that the presence of exercise-induced angina, ST segment depression, or both will not predict restenosis whether the test is performed early or late after angioplasty. The positive predictive values of early exercise testing range from 29% to 60%, and the corresponding values for late exercise testing range from 39% to 64% (12, 13). The low positive predictive value is most likely a consequence of incomplete revascularization, that is, either a totally occluded vessel or a significant stenosis at a site other than that dilated by angioplasty. It is also possible that the noninvasive test is accurately demonstrating a functionally inadequate dilatation, despite the appearance of angiographic success.

Thallium Scintigraphy: The positive predictive value of thallium scintigraphy for detecting of restenosis in series with a variable angiographic follow-up ranged from 37% to 100%. Because coronary angiography remains the "gold" standard for detecting restenosis, the reported value of a noninvasive test is determined not only by the actual accuracy of the test but also by the completeness of angiographic follow-up (14). In studies with a high rate of angiographic follow-up, the negative predictive value of thallium scintigraphy varies between 42% and 100%. Potentially, tomographic imaging of nuclear scintigrams may prove superior to planar imaging for detecting restenosis (15).

Anatomic Criteria

Intravascular Ultrasound: Intravascular ultrasound has yielded detailed cross-sectional images of the arterial wall and has the potential for new insight into the mechanisms, complications, and long-term results of coronary interventions. Before it can be accepted as an alternative to arteriography, several significant limitations must be surmounted. In particular, the bulk and relative inflexibility of current devices prevent their routine use. In addition, safety and accuracy have yet to be demonstrated in clinical studies. When these technical obstacles have been overcome and the clinical efficacy of this exciting new imaging modality has been established, its contribution to our understanding of the restenosis process will be invaluable.

Histology: In vivo histologic examination (biopsies of coronary lesions) is currently the only approach that can discriminate between classic atherosclerosis and fibrocellular hyperplasia. However, to what extent single biopsy samples represent the lesion as a whole is undetermined. Furthermore, this technique is probably applicable to a subset of patients, especially when used as both a diagnostic and therapeutic procedure in restenotic lesions or bypass grafts. Some authors have suggested that a relationship exists between the cellular density of the atherectomy specimen (16) or the growth rate and migratory rate of these cells in culture (17–20), and the later development of restenosis. Unfortunately, this approach is inherently limited by sampling bias.

Coronary Angiography: In view of the above, coronary angiography remains the most objective and reliable means of assessing the long-term outcome of interventions. The numerous studies already available on coronary restenosis using angiography lack consistency in their methods and the definition of restenosis used. Figure 6.1 illustrates this point. On the vertical axis of this "nonscientific" figure are the names of investigators who have studied the restenosis problem. On the horizontal axis are the restenosis rates observed in their studies. A restenosis rate ranging between 25% and 35% emerges. However, we must emphasize that the angiographic follow-up in these patients ranged from 57% to 100%, the time to follow-up was between 1 and 9 months, 11 different criteria of restenosis were applied, and finally, visual assessment of the coronary angiogram was used in the majority of these studies.

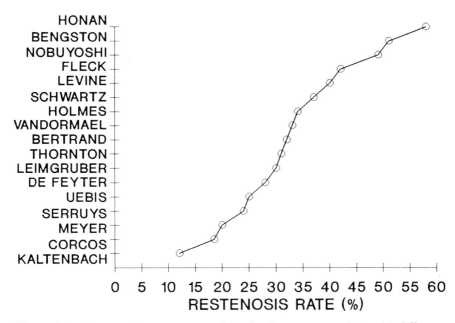

Figure 6.1. Restenosis rates reported in the literature, applying 11 different restenosis criteria, different angiographic follow-up periods (1–9 months), and varying percentages of patients undergoing repeat angiography (57%–100%). In addition, different angiographic analysis techniques (visual or quantitative) were used.

Table 6.1 shows the variety of restenosis criteria in current use. Most are entirely arbitrary, some are based on doubtful logic, and some, although relevant for visual estimation of percent diameter stenosis, are unrealistic when applied to the most accurate values obtained from quantitative angiography. Thus, most of the discrepancies between these studies can be attributed to the selection of patients, the method of analysis, and the definition of restenosis used. To improve the situation three factors must be addressed:

1. **Angiography.** To objectively assess the long-term outcome it is necessary for all patients to be angiographically followed at a predetermined time interval. This will avoid a selection bias in favor of symptomatic patients. The sample size of any clinical trial must be adequate to avoid a type II error.
2. **Analysis.** A well-validated system of analysis with known accuracy and variability must be used. A visual percent diameter ste-

Table 6.1. Criteria for Restenosis in Current Use

1. Loss of at least 50% of the initial gain (NHLBI 4)
2. A return to within 10% of the pre-PTCA diameter stenosis (NHLBI 3)
3. An immediate post-PTCA < 50% diameter stenosis that increases to ≥ 50% at follow-up
4. As for 3, but for a diameter stenosis ≥ 70% at follow-up (NHLBI 2)
5. Reduction ≥ 20% in diameter stenosis
6. Reduction ≥ 30% in diameter stenosis (NHLBI 1)
7. A diameter stenosis ≥ 50% at follow-up
8. A diameter stenosis ≥ 70% at follow-up
9. Area stenosis ≥ 85%
10. Loss ≥ 1 mm^2 in stenosis area
11. Deterioration of ≥ 0.72 mm in MLD from post-PTCA to follow-up
12. Deterioration of ≥ 0.5 mm in MLD from post-PTCA to follow-up

NHLBI = National Heart, Lung and Blood Institute; MLD = minimal lumen diameter

nosis measurement with its inherent interobserver and intraobserver variability (21,22) precludes meaningful results, and edge-detection tracing by hand or other techniques that produce values not physiologically possible are also unacceptable (23,24). Videodensitometry may eventually provide the best measurement because the technique estimates the volume of the lumen independent of geometric assumptions, but for technical reasons this method has not (yet) proven practical (25).

3. **Variables.** The measured variables must be chosen to reflect the restenosis proliferative process and distinguish between the acute results of angioplasty (good or poor) and this proliferative process. We believe that the conventional assessment of percent diameter stenosis is not sufficiently discriminating to achieve this goal and that definitions based on percent diameter stenosis measurement fail to identify lesions undergoing significant deterioration (26, 27). Although this method may be relevant in determining significant stenoses in human atherosclerotic vessels (28), it tells us nothing about the behavior of the lesion following the angioplasty procedure. Percent diameter stenosis criteria are chosen to reflect the change in minimal luminal diameter (MLD) relative to the so-called "normal" diameter of the vessel in the immediate vicinity of the obstruction. This criterion assumes that there is a "nor-

mal" diameter, but diffuse intimal or subintimal thickening is frequently present in arteries with discrete stenoses (particularly in multivessel disease). A coronary angiogram is unable to detect diffuse wall thickening. In addition, this "normal" area almost certainly is diffusely affected by barotrauma of the balloon resulting in a reactive hyperplasia and ultimately luminal narrowing (i.e., the reference area becomes part of the restenosis process; 26). This seriously questions the use of percent diameter stenosis as an index of restenosis.

If we accept the above reasoning, seven of the restenosis criteria summarized in Table 6.1 (criteria 2–8) are disqualified.

Restenosis Definition: Evolving Concept

The choice of restenosis definition has been the subject of much debate, because none currently takes account of both the functional and angiographic outcome after PTCA. A single "stenosis" measurement should not be confused with and cannot replace a measurement of "restenosis" that should represent the change in stenosis severity.

Clinical Observations

In 1988 two studies performing follow-up angiography at different, pre-selected follow-up intervals yielded similar results and showed precisely how lesions behave after angioplasty (29,30). In the study carried out at the Thoraxcenter, the average MLD after PTCA increased slightly from 2.06 mm to 2.11 mm at 30 days and then decreased to 1.93 mm, 1.77 mm, and 1.69 mm after 2, 3, and 4 months (Figure 6.2). An additional important finding following the analysis of the individual data is that almost all lesions deteriorate to some extent. This last observation is crucial in understanding restenosis because it implies that categorical definitions will not reliably describe restenosis. A significant deterioration is also seen in the reference diameter that minimizes the change in the calculated percentage diameter stenosis. A third important finding is that significant lesion progression after 6 months is unusual (29).

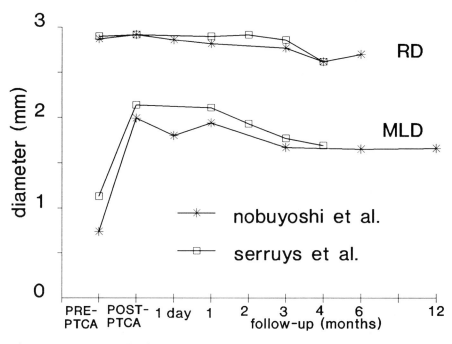

Figure 6.2. MLD and reference diameter values as reported for the studies by Nobuyoshi and colleagues (29) and Serruys and colleagues (30). MLD = minimal luminal diameter; RD = reference diameter.

Different Criteria Identify Different Patients

Although accurate (quantitative) assessment indicates that most lesions tend to restenose, the determination of a cut-off point for restenosis is more difficult. Indeed, the factor that most influences the restenosis rate is the definition of restenosis applied. Figure 6.3 shows the incidence of restenosis according to three criteria taken from a group of 490 lesions analyzed in the first 150 days after angioplasty (27). Two conclusions may be drawn from this figure. First, the incidence of restenosis varies according to the criterion applied, and second, the incidence of restenosis is progressive to at least the third month. At 5 months, the incidence of restenosis as defined by the three separate criteria is similar and ranges from 21% to 34%. However, even a similar incidence of restenosis using different criteria defines different patients. This is illustrated by Figure 6.4, which shows a Venn diagram of the number of lesions fulfilling three different restenosis criteria, taken

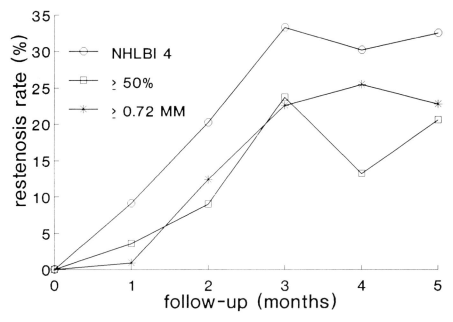

Figure 6.3. Cumulative incidence of restenosis as defined by three different restenosis criteria (NHLBI 4, > 50%, > 0.72 mm) during follow-up of 490 patients. (Reproduced with permission of the American College of Cardiology from ref. 27.)

from the same group of 490 lesions (27). Although the number of lesions fulfilling the three criteria for restenosis were similar, each of the three criteria identified unique lesions that were not identified by the other two. This point has particular relevance when determining the risk factors for restenosis: if restenosis cannot be unequivocally determined, then it is unlikely that the associated risk factors will be identified.

Absolute Change in Angiographically Measured Diameter

As a result of quantitative angiographic studies, a new concept for measuring restenosis has been introduced. The changes in MLD from post-PTCA to follow-up gives a reliable quantitative measurement of restenosis. The restenosis criterion or the cut-off point separating restenosis patients from nonrestenosis patients is then derived from the variability of measurements of the same lesion from different catheterization sessions. Twice the variability defines with reasonable certainty

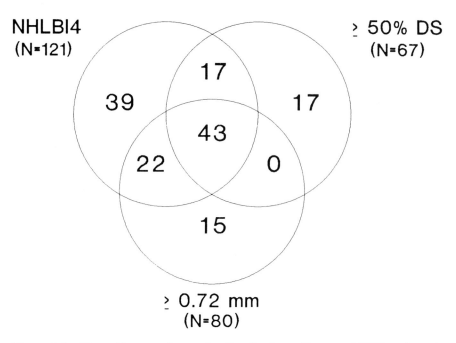

Figure 6.4. Venn diagram shows the distribution of lesions fulfilling the criteria of three different restenosis definitions. (Reproduced with permission of the American College of Cardiology from ref. 27.)

those lesions that have undergone significant deterioration from those that have not. We found this value to be 0.72 mm based on angiograms taken 90 days apart (31), whereas Nobuyoshi and colleagues, using a different measurement system, found 0.5 mm based on angiograms taken 7 to 10 days apart.

Criteria based on the absolute change in MLD are nevertheless limited because they make no attempt to relate the extent of the restenosis process to the size of the vessel. Work is currently in progress to create "sliding-scale" criteria that adjust for vessel size.

Practical Implications for Clinical Trials

Because progression of a stenosis following intervention reflects the process of interest (restenosis) whether or not an arbitrarily defined threshold of obstruction is reached, a continuous measure of luminal reobstruction is preferable for the purposes of clinical trials. When the main concern is clinical decision-making, however, a binary or categorical measure of restenosis provides clinicians with more relevant information. Keeping in mind that an angiographic restenosis study assesses only the anatomic component of the restenosis problem, the threshold above which a loss of luminal diameter would have clinically significant functional or symptomatic consequences is not known. Why then would one bother to try to define a threshold above which "significant" restenosis occurs? To define the threshold by using the reproducibility of the measurement in individual patients is also questionable. The possible benefit of a treatment (pharmacologic or interventional) can be measured with much greater precision by using the change in lumen diameter for the group. For example, if treatment reduces the loss of luminal diameter from 0.4 mm under placebo (27) to 0.25 mm under active medication, to detect a statistically significant difference (probability < 5%) with a power of 90%, it can be calculated that 233 patients will be required per treatment group. The above treatment effect corresponds to restenosis rates (defined as a loss of MLD of ≥ 0.72 mm) of 25% and 17.5%, respectively. Alternatively when a categorical restenosis definition is used (restenosis yes/no) to demonstrate the same difference (with the same power) between the groups, 620 patients per treatment group will be required because the categorical end points do not take full advantage of the available information.

Is a Noncategorical Definition of Restenosis Justified?

To determine the distribution of changes in the angiographically measured MLDs for a large population undergoing PTCA, we constructed a frequency histogram (Figure 6.5). The results indicate that the change in MLD approximately follows a Gaussian distribution. Conventional restenosis can thus be viewed as the tail end of an approximately Gaussian distributed phenomenon with some lesions crossing a more or less arbitrary cut-off point. Results of restenosis prevention trials can be much more elegantly presented as cumulative distribution curves of the individual changes in MLD (Figure 6.6; 32) rather than listing two or more arbitrary restenosis rates that might or might not be significantly different.

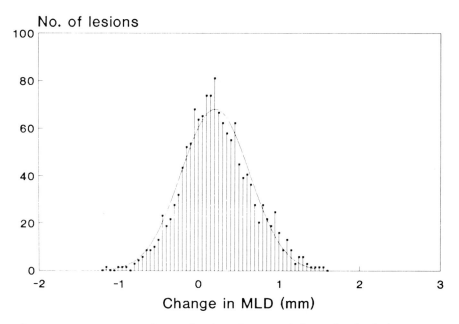

Figure 6.5. Histogram shows the distribution of the individual changes in MLD between the angiogram immediately after angioplasty and that after 6 months of follow-up in 1375 lesions. Lesions that had progressed to total occlusion were excluded. The curve superimposed on the distribution depicts the theoretical Gaussian distribution derived from the mean and standard deviation of the population. A positive value corresponds with a decrease in MLD.

Experiences of a Core Laboratory for Quantitative Coronary Angiography in Restenosis Prevention Trials

Despite the widespread and long-standing use of coronary angiography in clinical practice, the interpretation of an angiogram has changed little and is still visual. However, visual assessment is subjective with a large interobserver and intraobserver variability and, therefore, cannot be used in restenosis prevention trials (21–24). Quantitative coronary angiography has the advantage of being more accurate and reproducible in the assessment of lesion severity than visual and hand-held caliper assessments. At the Thoraxcenter, we have been involved in the development and validation of the computer-assisted Cardiovascular Angiography Analysis System (CAAS) (24,31). A typical example of the quantitative analysis of a coronary obstruction is presented in Figure

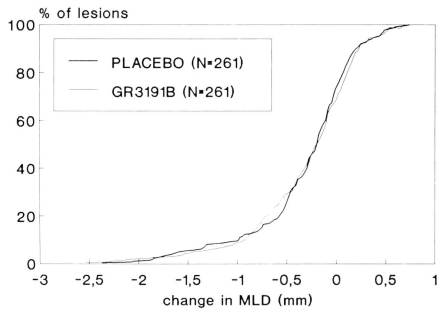

Figure 6.6. Cumulative distribution curves of the individual changes in MLD between postangioplasty angiogram and follow-up angiography for the placebo and the treatment group in a restenosis prevention trial. The practically overlapping curves demonstrate that the active treatment did not differ from placebo in prevention of angiographic luminal narrowing after balloon angioplasty.

6.7. Over the last 3 years, we have functioned as the angiographic core laboratory for four restenosis prevention trials with recruitment of patients in Europe, the United States, and Canada (Table 6.2). If one is to obtain reliable and reproducible quantitative measurements over time from coronary cineangiograms, variations in data acquisition and analysis should be minimized. Table 6.3 summarizes the potential problems in angiographic data acquisition and analysis. An angiographic core laboratory can minimize these problems.

Pincushion Distortion

Pincushion distortion of the image intensifier introduces selective magnification of an object near the edges of the image as compared with its size in the center. A centimeter grid should be filmed in all modes of the image intensifiers in each catheterization suite. CAAS calculates a cor-

A

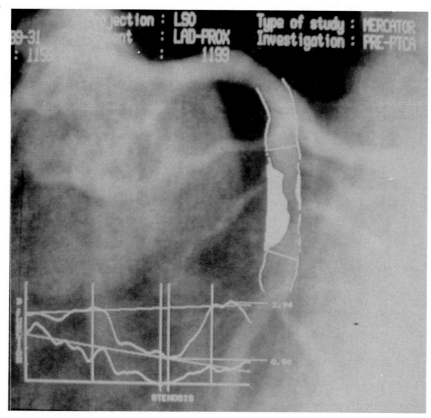

Figure 6.7. (A) Cine frame shows a discrete lesion in the proximal left anterior descending coronary artery (LAD) before PTCA. The diameter function curves of the edge-detection analysis show that the MLD of the lesion is 0.9 mm and the interpolated reference diameter at that site is 2.94 mm.

rection factor for pincushion distortion of each mode. At the present time our database has pincushion correction factors of 557 different modes of magnification (82 clinics and 207 angiographic suites) from Europe, the United States, and Canada.

Differences in Angles and Height Levels of the X-ray Gantry

It is mandatory to repeat the same baseline views. We have thus developed a technician's worksheet (to be completed during the PTCA proce-

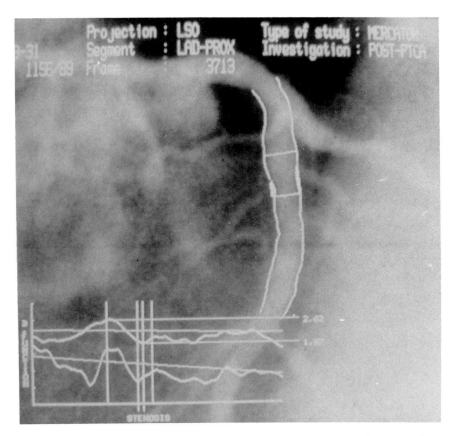

Figure 6.7 *(cont.)* *(B)* Immediately post-PTCA angiographic cine frame in identical mode. The MLD has increased to 1.87 mm.

dure) with detailed information of the procedure: view, catheter type, catheter size, balloon type, balloon size, balloon pressure, kV, mA, and medication given. In this way minimization of differences in x-ray settings at follow-up angiography can be achieved. Furthermore each participating center is requested to send two test films in order to check whether that center is able to comply with these standards.

Differences in Vasomotor Tone of the Coronary Arteries

As the vasomotor tone may differ even during consecutive coronary angiographic studies, it should be controlled at all times of the investigation. An optimal vasodilating drug should produce a quick and maximal

Table 6.2. Angiographic Core Laboratory in Four Restenosis Prevention Trials (1988–1991)

CARPORT:	Coronary Artery Restenosis Prevention on Repeated Thromboxane antagonism Intake and analysis complete, 707 patients.
MERCATOR:	Multicenter European Research Trial with Cilazapril after Angioplasty to prevent Transluminal coronary Obstruction and Restenosis Intake and analysis complete, 735 patients.
MARCATOR:	Multicenter American Research Trial with Cilazapril after Angioplasty to prevent Transluminal coronary Obstruction and Restenosis Intake complete, follow-up analysis pending, 1436 patients
PARK:	Post Angioplasty Restenosis Ketanserin trial Intake complete, follow-up analysis pending, 704 patients.

Table 6.3. Potential Problems with Angiographic Data Acquisition and Analysis

1. Pincushion distortion of image intensifier
2. Differences in angles and height levels of x-ray system settings
3. Differences in vasomotor tone
4. Variation in quality of mixing of contrast agent with blood
5. Catheter used as scaling device (angiographic quality, influence of contrast in catheter tip on the calibration factor, size of catheter)
6. Deviations in size of catheter as listed by manufacturer from its actual size
7. Variation in data analysis

response without influencing the hemodynamic state of the patient. Only nitrates and calcium antagonists satisfy these requirements. Calcium antagonists are more vasoactive on isolated human coronary arteries but they act more slowly; in vivo, however, nitrates are more vasoactive than calcium antagonists (33–35). Therefore, we strongly advocate the use of 0.1 to 0.3 mg nitroglycerin or 1 to 3 mg isosorbide dinitrate (ISDN) pre-PTCA, after the last balloon inflation before repeating the views used pre-PTCA and at follow-up angiography.

Influence of Contrast Agent on Vasomotor Tone of Epicardial Coronary Arteries: Jost and colleagues clearly demonstrated that changes in vessel dimensions due to contrast medium administration are significantly smaller with use of a non-ionic contrast medium than with the use of an ionic contrast medium (36). Therefore, in quantitative coronary angiographic studies, non-ionic contrast media with iso-osmolality should be used.

Catheter Used as Scaling Device for Measurements of Absolute Diameters

Angiographic Versus Microcaliper Measured Size of Catheter: The image quality of the x-ray radiated catheter depends on the catheter material, concentration of the contrast agent in the catheter, and the kV setting of the x-ray source. Studies from Reiber and coworkers in 1985 (37) showed that there was a difference of +9.8% in angiographic-measured size as compared with the true size for catheters made from nylon. Small differences were measured for catheters made from woven dacron (+0.2%), polyvinylchloride (−3.2%) and polyurethane (−3.5%). They concluded that nylon catheters could not be used for quantitative studies.

Influence of Variation in Contrast Filling of the Catheter on Calibration: Catheters made from woven dacron, polyvinylchloride, and polyurethane and flushed with saline possess identical image contrast qualities. After filling with various concentrations of contrast material (Urografin-76, Schering AG, Berlin, Germany; 100%–50%–25%) or air, however, differences among the individual catheters were observed (37). Therefore, we strongly advise flushing catheters before each cine run to prevent this calibration error.

Size of the Catheter: Until recently only 7F and 8F catheters were available and from earlier studies it is known which of the catheters can be used the best (37,38). Currently 5F and 6F catheters are increasingly used during follow-up angiography. Koning and colleagues have shown (Table 6.4) that none of these catheters satisfy earlier established criteria that the average difference of the angiographic and true diameter is lower than 3.5% and that the standard deviation of the measured diameters is smaller then 0.05 mm under the following conditions: filled with 100% contrast concentration, filled with water, acquired at 60 kV and 90 kV. Therefore, 5F or 6F catheters should not be used for quantitative coronary angiography (QCA) studies using CAAS at the present time.

Table 6.4. Mean Values of Angiographically Measured Catheter Dimensions During Three Different Fillings* and Two Kilovoltages[†]

	TRUE SIZE (MM)	ANGIOGRAPHICALLY MEASURED SIZE (MM)	AVG DIF (%)
5F CATHETERS			
Argon	1.66	1.85 ± 0.09	11.3
Cordis	1.73	1.79 ± 0.15	3.2
Edwards	1.66	1.80 ± 0.08	8.5
Mallinckrodt	1.73	1.72 ± 0.14*	−0.8
Schneider	1.69	1.79 ± 0.07	6.1
USCI	1.61	1.75 ± 0.14	8.5
6F CATHETERS			
Argon	1.98	2.14 ± 0.07	8.1
Cordis	2.01	2.03 ± 0.11	1.1
Edwards	1.96	2.10 ± 0.07	7.1
Medicorp (left)	1.97	2.07 ± 0.04	5.1
Medicorp (right)	1.99	2.02 ± 0.10	1.6
Mallinckrodt	1.97	1.91 ± 0.15	−2.9
Schneider	1.94	2.00 ± 0.09	3.0
USCI	1.99	2.06 ± 0.08	3.4

Water, contrast medium at 185 and 370 mg I/cc.
[†] *60 and 90 kV.*

Deviations in the Size of the Catheter as Listed by the Manufacturer

The size of the catheter (especially disposable varieties) as specified by the manufacturer often deviates from its actual size. If a manufacturer cannot guarantee narrow ranges for catheter size, all catheters should be measured by a micrometer. Therefore, during clinical studies we collect all catheters used during angioplasty and follow-up for actual measurement.

Variation in Data Analysis

Reference Diameter: Selection of the reference diameter is hampered by individual variation. In arteries with a focal obstructive lesion and a clearly normal proximal arterial segment, the choice of the reference diameter is straightforward and simple. However, in cases in which the proximal part of the arterial segment shows both stenotic and ectatic areas, the choice may be difficult. To minimize these variations, CAAS is using an interpolated or computer-defined reference technique.

Length of Analyzed Segment: Anatomic landmarks such as bifurcations are used for the manual definition of starting and end points of arterial segments to minimize the problem of variation in analysis. For that purpose, drawings are made by the investigator of all different views suitable for quantitative analysis, pre-PTCA, post-PTCA, and at follow-up.

Frame Selection: Usually, an end-diastolic cine frame is selected for quantitative analysis of a coronary obstruction to avoid the blurring effect of motion. If the obstruction is not optimally visible in a particular frame (e.g., by overlap by another vessel), a neighboring frame in the sequence is selected (39).

Conclusion

Although there is currently no universal agreement regarding the assessment of the restenosis process, we believe it is possible using existing methodology (quantitative coronary angiography) to derive more meaningful information from clinical studies using a noncategorical analytical approach to results obtained.

Acknowledgment: We gratefully acknowledge the skillful secretarial assistance of Hanneke Roerade and Marjo van Ee. Technical assistance of Marie-Angèle Morel in the preparation of this manuscript is gratefully acknowledged.

References

1. Rensing BJ, Hermans WRM, Beatt KJ, et al. Quantitative angiographic assessment of elastic recoil after percutaneous transluminal coronary angioplasty. Am J Cardiol 1990;66:1039–1044.
2. Hjemdahl-Monsen CE, Ambrose JA, Borrico S, et al. Angiographic patterns of balloon inflation during percutaneous transluminal coronary angioplasty: role of pressure-diameter curves in studying distensibility

and elasticity of the stenotic lesion and the mechanism of dilation. J Am Coll Cardiol 1990;16:569–575.

3. Isner JM, Rosenfield K, Losordo DW, et al. Combination balloon-ultrasound imaging catheter for percutaneous transluminal angioplasty. Validation of imaging, analysis of recoil, and identification of plaque fracture. Circulation 1991;84:739–754.

4. Essed CE, van den Brand M, Becker AE. Transluminal coronary angioplasty and early restenosis: fibrocellular occlusion after wall laceration. Br Heart J 1983;49:393–396.

5. Austin GE, Ratliff NB, Hollman J, Tabei S, Phillips DF. Intimal proliferation of smooth muscle cells as an explanation for recurrent coronary artery stenosis after percutaneous transluminal coronary angioplasty. J Am Coll Cardiol 1985;6:369–375.

6. Waller BF. Pathology of transluminal balloon angioplasty used in the treatment of coronary heart disease. Human Pathol 1987;5:476–484.

7. Waller BF, Orr CM, Pinkerton CA, Van Tassel JW, Pinto RP. Morphologic observations late after coronary balloon angioplasty: mechanisms of acute injury and relationship to restenosis. Radiology 1990;174:961–967.

8. Gruentzig AR, Senning A, Siegenthaler WE. Nonoperative dilatation of coronary-artery stenosis. Percutaneous transluminal coronary angioplasty. N Engl J Med 1979;301:61–68.

9. Holmes DR Jr, Schwartz RS, Webster MWI. Coronary restenosis: What have we learned from angiography? J Am Coll Cardiol 1991;17 (suppl B):14B–22B.

10. Kent KM, Bonow RO, Rosing DR, et al. Improved myocardial function during exercise after successful percutaneous transluminal coronary angioplasty. N Engl J Med 1982:306:441–446.

11. Califf RM, Fortin DF, Frid DJ, et al. Restenosis after coronary angioplasty: an overview. J Am Coll Cardiol 1991;17 (suppl B):2B–13B.

12. Califf RM, Ohman EM, Frid DJ, et al. Restenosis: the clinical issues. In: Topol EJ, ed. Textbook of interventional cardiology. Philadelphia: WB Saunders, 1990:363–394.

13. Laarman GJ, Luijten HE, van Zeyl LGPM, et al. Assessment of "silent" restenosis and long-term follow-up after successful angioplasty in single vessel coronary artery disease: the value of quantitative exercise electrocardiography and quantitative coronary angiography. J Am Coll Cardiol 1990;16:578–585.

14. Nelson CL, Tcheng JE, Frid DJ, et al. Incomplete angiographic follow up results in significant underestimation of true restenosis rates after PTCA. Circulation 1990;82 (suppl III):312.

15. Jain A, Mahmarian JJ, Borges-Neto S, et al. Clinical significance of perfusion defects by thallium-201 single photon emission tomography following oral dipyridamole early after coronary angioplasty. J Am Coll Cardiol 1988;11:970–976.

16. Johnson D, Hinohara T, Selmon M, Robertson G, Braden L, Simpson J. Histologic predictors of restenosis after directed coronary atherectomy. J Am Coll Cardiol (abstr) 1991;17(2):53A.

17. Dartsch PC, Voisard R, Betz E. In vitro growth characteristics of human atherosclerotic plaque cells: comparison of cells from primary stenosing and restenosing lesions of peripheral and coronary arteries. Res Exp Med 1990;190:77–87.

18. Voisard R, Dartsch PD, Seitzer U, Hannekum A, Kochs M, Hombach V. The effect of cytostatic agents on proliferative activity and cytoskeletal components of plaque cells from human coronary arteries. Eur Heart J 1991;12 (abstr suppl):385.

19. Strauss BH, Verkerk A, Van Suylen RJ, et al. Smooth muscle cell culture from human coronary lesions. Circulation 1990;82 (suppl III):496.

20. Bauriedel G, Windstetter U, Kandolf R, Höfling B. Increased migratory activity of human smooth muscle cells cultured from peripheral and coronary restenosis plaques. Eur Heart J 1991;12 (abstract suppl): 291.

21. Beaumann GJ, Vogel RA. Accuracy of individual and panel visual interpretation of coronary arteriograms: implications for clinical decisions. J Am Coll Cardiol 1990;16:108–113.

22. Goldberg RK, Kleiman NS, Minor ST, Abukhalil J, Raizner AE. Comparison of quantitative coronary angiography to visual estimates of lesion severity pre- and post-PTCA. Am Heart J 1990;119:178–184.

23. Mancini GBJ. Quantitative coronary arteriographic methods in the interventional catheterization laboratory: an update and perspective. J Am Coll Cardiol 1991;17:23B–33B.

24. Reiber JHC, Serruys PW. Quantitative angiography. In: Marcus ML, Schelbert HR, Skorton DJ, Wolf GL, eds. Cardiac imaging, a companion to Braunwalds heart disease. New York: WB Saunders, 1991:211–280.

25. Reiber JHC. Morphologic and densitometric quantitation of coronary stenoses; an overview of existing quantitation techniques. In: Reiber JHC, Serruys PW, eds. New developments in quantitative coronary angiography. Dordrecht: Kluwer Academic Publishers, 1990:34.

26. Beatt KJ, Luijten HE, De Feyter PJ, Van den Brand M, Reiber JHC, Serruys PW. Change in diameter of coronary artery segments adjacent to stenosis after percutaneous transluminal coronary angioplasty: failure of percent diameter stenosis measurement to reflect morphologic changes induced by balloon dilatation. J Am Coll Cardiol 1988;12:315–323.

27. Beatt KJ, Serruys PW, Hugenholtz PG. Restenosis after coronary angioplasty: new standards for clinical studies. J Am Coll Cardiol 1990;15:491–498.

28. Gould KL, Lipscomb K, Hamilton GW. Physiologic basis for assessing critical stenoses: instantaneous flow response and regional distribution during coronary hyperemia as measures of coronary flow reserve. Am J Cardiol 1974;33:87–94.

29. Nobuyoshi M, Kimura T, Nosaka H, et al. Restenosis after successful percutaneous transluminal coronary angioplasty: serial angiographic follow-up of 299 patients. J Am Coll Cardiol 1988;12:616–623.

30. Serruys PW, Luijten HE, Beatt KJ, et al. Incidence of restenosis after successful coronary angioplasty: a time related phenomenon. A quantitative angiographic study in 342 consecutive patients at 1, 2, 3 and 4 months. Circulation 1988;77:361–371.

31. Reiber JHC, Serruys PW, Kooyman CJ, et al. Assessment of short, medium and long term variations in arterial dimensions from computer assisted quantification of coronary cineangiograms. Circulation 1985; 71:280–288.

32. Serruys PW, Rutsch W, Heyndrickx G, et al. Thromboxane A_2 receptor blockade does not prevent restenosis, despite near complete platelet inhibition. A multicenter randomized clinical trial. Eur Heart J 1991;12 (abstr suppl):386.

33. Feldman RL, Marx JD, Pepine CJ, Conti CR. Analysis of coronary responses to various doses of intracoronary nitroglycerin. Circulation 1982;66:321–327.

34. Lablanche JM, Delforge MR, Tilmant PY, et al. Effects hemodynamiques et coronaries du dinitrate d'isosorbide: Comparison entre les voies d'injection intracoronary et intraveineuse. Arch Mal Coeur 1982;75:303–316.

35. Rafflenbeul W, Lichtlen PR. Release of residual vascular tone in coronary artery stenoses with nifedipine and glyceryl trinitrate. In: Kaltenbach M, Neufeld HN, eds. New therapy of ischemic heart disease and hypertension. Proceedings of the 5th International Adalat Symposium. Amsterdam: Exerpta Medica, 1983:300–308.

36. Jost S, Rafflenbeul W, Gerhardt U, et al. Influence of ionic and non-ionic radiographic contrast media on the vasomotor tone of epicardial coronary arteries. Eur Heart J 1989;10 (suppl F):60–65.

37. Reiber JHC, Kooijman CJ, den Boer A, Serruys PW. Assessment of dimensions and image quality of coronary contrast catheters from cineangiograms. Cath Cardiovasc Diagn 1985;11:521–531.

38. Leung W, Demopulos PA, Alderman EL, Sanders W, Stadius ML. Evalu-

ation of catheters and metallic catheter markers as calibration standard for measurement of coronary dimensions. Cath Cardiovasc Diagn 1990; 21:148–153.

39. Reiber JHC, van Eldik-Helleman P, Kooijman CJ, Tijssen JGP, Serruys PW. How critical is frame selection in quantitative coronary angiographic studies? Eur Heart J 1989;10 (suppl F):54–59.

· ·

CHAPTER 7

Pathology of Postinterventional Coronary Restenosis

——

KENNETH C. HUBER
KIRK N. GARRATT
ROBERT S. SCHWARTZ
WILLIAM D. EDWARDS

FOR the past 150 years, examination of postmortem specimens has been an important tool for investigating disease processes. The evaluation of restenosis following percutaneous coronary revascularization techniques is no exception. Indeed, despite numerous animal models of restenosis, as well as technological advances in coronary artery imaging using quantitative angiography, angioscopy, and intracoronary ultrasound, most of what we know about the mechanisms of percutaneous transluminal coronary angioplasty (PTCA) and restenosis comes from analysis of human specimens obtained at autopsy. Examination of tissues removed from living patients by directional atherectomy has also added substantially to an understanding of restenosis after PTCA.

Following an initially successful interventional procedure, three major clinical (angiographic) scenarios may occur (Figure 7.1; 1). Although many patients achieve long-term success, a significant number do not (2–4). Between 5% and 10% of patients experience immediate or "early" recurrence of stenosis. This abrupt closure typically results from thrombotic occlusion, obstruction by intimal or medial flaps, or medial recoil. Another 30% to 40% of patients will develop "late" recurrence of stenosis (restenosis), usually within 2 to 3 months after the

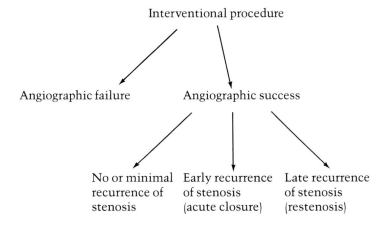

Figure 7.1. Possible clinical/angiographic scenarios following a coronary interventional procedure.

initial procedure (5–6). The major causes of late closure are thought to be medial recoil in overstretched portions of the artery, the development of obstructive fibrocellular proliferation, or a combination of both. It is the latter group, presenting with the clinical phenomenon of restenosis, that will be the focus of this chapter.

Histopathologic Features of PTCA and Restenosis

Before focusing specifically on the histopathologic features of the restenotic neointima, it is worthwhile to review some aspects of the underlying atherosclerotic plaque and currently proposed mechanisms of PTCA. This will provide the framework and context necessary for a discussion of the mechanisms and pathology of restenosis.

Nature of the Underlying Atherosclerotic Plaque

The histopathology of atheromatous coronary plaques has been described in detail (7–9). Certain anatomic features of the underlying plaque have been shown to influence both early and late procedural success (1,10–12). Fibrous and calcific plaques are more likely to have a lower success rate with coronary intervention than soft plaques without angiographic evidence of calcium (12–14). Furthermore, severe concentric stenoses may be more prone to injury than vessels with less extensive lesions (15). Eccentricity of the plaque may influence both the outcome and the nature of the injury produced by PTCA (10). Numerous lesion characteristics, particularly lesion length, have been shown to be important in regard to the incidence of restenosis (16). Intracoronary ultrasound and angioscopy, as well as histopathologic studies, may provide additional information concerning the relationship between plaque characteristics and the likelihood of a successful interventional procedure (17–19).

PTCA-Related Injury

Histopathologic studies indicate that vessel injury, in addition to stretching and dilatation, is the prominent mechanism of most successful PTCA procedures (12,20–27). The initially postulated mechanism of plaque compression has not been substantiated by morphologic studies (21–22). Instead, the most commonly observed lesion following PTCA is plaque fracture, also known as plaque rupture, cracking, breaking, or intimal splitting (12,22–26). In one of the largest studies addressing the effect of PTCA on atherosclerotic plaques, Potkin and colleagues reported plaque rupture following angioplasty in 95% of their cases (12). It is of interest that this was the major mechanism of successful angioplasty described in early animal and human cadaveric heart studies (27).

The *site* of fracture is highly variable and appears to depend largely on the nature of the underlying plaque (Plates I through III). For eccentric plaques, the most common rupture site is at the junction between the atheroma and the disease-free portion of the arterial wall. This was observed in seven of nine cases with eccentric plaques reported by Gravanis and Roubin (28).

The *extent or depth* of injury is also highly variable and can range from shallow intimal tears to deep lacerations that rupture the internal elastic lamina and extend into the media, or rarely the adventitia. The media was involved in 70% to 80% of PTCA cases evaluated at autopsy (28–31).

Damage to disease-free wall has also been reported with eccentric lesions (26,28,32). Gravanis and colleagues described some degree of aneurysmal dilatation in the arterial wall of all patients with eccentric lesions (28). This appears to be due to stretching and thinning of the uninvolved wall, which presumably is more compliant than the atherosclerotic plaque. The initial stretch, however, may be quickly overcome by elastic recoil or more gradually overcome by vasospasm after balloon angioplasty (33). Because postmortem contraction of the stretched segment may occur, it is difficult to know exactly how frequent or permanent the dilatation may be (20). Saffitz reported an extreme case of expansion of the disease-free wall in which vascular rupture caused hemopericardium and tamponade (32).

In some instances there may be no histopathologic evidence of injury at sites of clinically successful PTCA procedures. This was reported by Waller and colleagues in three patients 80, 90, and 150 days after PTCA (34). The most likely explanation was initial distention of the disease-free wall, with no disruption of the internal elastic lamina or media. If recoil causes the lesion to revert back to its original size, the patient may present with signs and symptoms of restenosis. Although the magnitude and frequency of recoil after PTCA is unknown, it is thought to play a role in late restenosis in up to 40% of cases (35).

PTCA-Related Response to Injury

Following a clinically successful PTCA procedure, it is the arterial response to injury (i.e., healing) that in large part determines the long-term success rate. In contrast, acute or subacute thrombosis is the primary cause of early post-PTCA obstruction (Plates IV and V). Healing is accomplished by intimal proliferation and reendothelialization. The extent to which proliferation occurs is thought to be the major factor that determines the severity of restenosis. If intimal hyperplasia is minimal, the arterial lumen will remain functionally unobstructed. Exuberant proliferation, on the other hand, may narrow the lumen to its preprocedural size or may produce even more stenosis than was present before PTCA. Thus, a discussion of the histopathology of restenosis will center on a detailed investigation of neointimal proliferation (synonyms include intimal hyperplasia, intimal fibrous proliferation, fibrocellular tissue, and restenosis tissue).

Historical Perspective: In 1983, Essed and colleagues first reported "fibrocellular occlusion" in a patient who underwent PTCA 5 months prior to death (36). At autopsy, the preexistent atherosclerotic plaque was split, with extension of the fracture into the media. Filling the intramedial false channel and extending into and nearly obliterating the true lumen was a proliferation of fibrocellular tissue.

In 1985, Austin and colleagues reported three patients who died 5, 17, and 62 days following PTCA (37). In the patient who died 62 days after PTCA, an obstructing stenosis consisted of mature atherosclerotic plaque and a sharply demarcated "circumferential inner layer" of intimal proliferation ranging from 0.3 to 0.7 mm in thickness. Immunoperoxidase techniques detected apolipoprotein within the outer layer but not the inner layer of proliferating cells.

Since 1985, several investigators have described the histopathologic features of post-PTCA restenosis (20,24,25,28–31,34,35,38). Although most have been based on observations of tissue acquired at autopsy, some have used specimens removed by coronary atherectomy or surgical excision (39–42).

Frequency of Intimal Hyperplasia: In an analysis of 34 lesions in 20 patients at variable intervals following angioplasty, Nobuyoshi and colleagues detected neointimal proliferation in 83% to 100% of patients between 11 days and 2 years following PTCA (29). It was not detected in lesions less than 10 days or more than 2 years following angioplasty. Gravanis and Roubin reported intimal myoproliferative lesions at 7 of 9 dilatation sites in which the interval from PTCA to death was greater than 30 days (28). Similarly, Morimoto and colleagues reported intimal hyperplasia at 9 of 13 PTCA sites 2 weeks to 2 years and 11 months after the procedure (30).

The frequency of intimal proliferation is similar whether or not there is clinical or angiographic evidence of restenosis (29). This indicates that fibrocellular proliferation represents a general healing response to arterial injury and likely occurs to *some* extent in every patient in whom plaque rupture or other forms of vessel injury have occurred.

Location of Intimal Hyperplasia: Neointimal proliferation generally occurs adjacent to sites of injury. When proliferation is extensive, however, it may form circumferentially around the entire lumen. In nearly every case with plaque rupture or intramedial dissection, the neointima "fills in" the tears and also extends to various degrees over the adjacent underlying wall. In eccentric lesions the proliferative response tends to be most extensive over the nonatheromatous segment of the arterial wall (28). Morimoto and coworkers reported 9 of 13 arteries in which the restenotic proliferative tissue was mainly at the site of internal elastic lamina rupture (30). They suggested that the internal elastic lamina may function as a barrier to prevent smooth muscle cell migration from the media to the intima.

Extent of Intimal Hyperplasia: For cases in which recoil is minimal and neointimal hyperplasia is prominent, the extent of proliferation will determine whether or not restenosis occurs (Plates VI and VII). It is unclear which patient, plaque, or procedural factors are most likely to result in excessive intimal hyperplasia.

Using morphometric analysis techniques, Nobuyoshi and colleagues have measured the area of intimal proliferation and area of lumen and correlated this with the severity of arterial injury as defined by depth of tear into the intima, media, or adventitia (29). They reported a direct correlation between the severity of injury and the extent of intimal proliferation. In another study, Garratt and coworkers found that deep arterial resection (and hence, greater injury) following directional coronary atherectomy was associated with increased angiographic restenosis rates compared to vessels with more shallow injury (41). These two studies, along with Morimoto's observations that the largest amounts of proliferative tissue are found adjacent to the sites of greatest internal elastic lamina fragmentation, support the hypothesis that the severity of arterial injury may be related to the extent of subsequent neointimal proliferation (30). Other factors may be important as well.

Composition of Intimal Hyperplasia: The major cellular component of the fibrocellular proliferative response has been characterized and appears to be a smooth muscle cell or myofibroblast. Nobuyoshi and colleagues reported that the phenotypic characteristics of these cells may change with time (29). In lesions less than 6 months after angioplasty, the neointimal cells were polyhedral in shape with large oval nuclei and abundant cytoplasm. Cases more than 6 months following PTCA revealed cells that were more spindle-shaped with elongated nuclei and less cytoplasm than cells from the younger cases. These two different microscopic appearances were thought to represent "synthetic" and "contractile" phenotypes, respectively (43). Some lesions contained a mixture of both phenotypes. Ultrastructural studies of restenotic tissue have shown abundant cytoplasmic myofibrils and scanty organelles (28, 44).

Restenotic tissue has special staining characteristics typical for smooth muscle cells (Plates VIII and IX; 28–30,38,40,41). Ueda and colleagues showed that the fibrocellular tissue from restenotic lesions stained positively for a monoclonal antiactin antibody against muscle-specific antigen (HHF-35), α and γ actin isotopes specific to smooth muscle cells (GGA-7), and vimentin (38). Interestingly, there was a gradient of GGA-7 antibody reactivity depending on the interval following angioplasty, suggesting that time-dependent changes occur not only in phenotypic appearance but also in expression of different actin isotypes.

Although the origin of neointimal smooth muscle cells is unproven, the subjacent media is generally considered the most likely source.

The extracellular matrix surrounding the proliferating cells can be abundant and in some cases contribute appreciably to the volume of the lesion. Recent evidence also indicates that the composition of the extracellular matrix changes with time. It is composed primarily of proteoglycans (typically chondroitan and dermatan sulfate) initially, but later the extracellular matrix becomes less abundant and is composed chiefly of collagen.

Little human data exist regarding reendothelialization following PTCA regarding its timing and role in the restenotic process. Gravanis and Roubin used a combination of factor VIII-related antigen and *Ulex europeus* immunohistochemical stains to show that reendothelialization was present only in lesions older than 30 days (28). Dartsch and coworkers were unable to demonstrate endothelial cells immunohistochemically in atheromatous specimens obtained by directional atherectomy (42). It is possible that endothelial cells were present but not functioning normally or that they had been damaged or lost by the procedure itself.

Implications from Histopathologic Studies

There are distinct differences between the restenotic neointima and the underlying atherosclerotic plaque. This is true both in regard to cellular and extracellular components, as well as the nature of temporal changes. This observation suggests that the mechanisms involved in the development of restenotic lesions are different from those involved in the development of primary atheromatous lesions and, therefore, implies that extrapolations from the atherosclerotic literature in regard to treatment strategies should be interpreted with caution.

The development of intimal fibrocellular proliferation following PTCA probably represents a general biologic response to vascular injury. This interpretation carries implications for future strategies aimed at reducing the rate of restenosis. Modulation of normal healing responses, rather than elimination of these events, may be effective in controlling restenosis and may be more realistically attained. Interpretation of the restenotic process as a form of wound healing may lead to utilization of current concepts of wound healing to direct therapeutic approaches (45).

The amount of proliferative tissue that develops following angioplasty appears related, in part, to the extent of arterial injury. This implies that less injury is better. Unfortunately, this creates a dilemma since the principal mechanism of successful angioplasty involves injury to the vessel wall. Although injury could be limited by striving for a less ideal result with PTCA, evidence suggests that a small residual luminal diameter is associated with a less satisfactory immediate and long-term outcome. In fact, some investigators have reported that balloon angioplasty procedures that are not associated with sufficient injury to disrupt the intima correlate with more clinical ischemic events afterward than those with intimal disruption (46).

This appears to be true not only for PTCA, but also for newer devices (including laser angioplasty, thermal angioplasty, and atherectomy) that have rates of restenosis similar to those reported for conventional balloon angioplasty. Improved lesion assessment may be important since it does appear that lesion characteristics, and not patient characteristics, are the most important features in predicting acute and long-term outcome after coronary intervention (47,48).

Because arterial injury is required and cannot be easily controlled with current technology, it is unlikely that reduction in restenosis will occur solely with the development of new devices, but rather may rely more on modulating the vascular response to injury.

Limitations of Histopathology Studies of Restenosis

Although much has been learned regarding the morphologic and histopathologic features of human restenotic lesions, important limitations must be addressed.

Temporal Development of Restenotic Lesions

The time course for the clinical and angiographic presentation of restenosis has been well studied and confirmed by two large independent studies (5,6). Both have confirmed that most patients present with angiographic evidence of restenosis between the first and third months after successful angioplasty. Little is known, however, about the temporal sequence of events for the development of restenotic lesions on a cellular level. An appreciable gap exists in the literature regarding the histopathologic characteristics of human PTCA sites when initial formation of the neointima takes place (i.e., during the first month when healing should be starting).

Typically, lesions are segregated into two groups: those less than 30 days and those greater than 30 days following angioplasty (so-called early and late lesions). The vast majority of patients dying early following PTCA do so within hours or a few days following PTCA—too early for the cellular characteristics of wound healing to have begun. On the other hand, most patients dying late after angioplasty do so months to years following PTCA, when the healing process has been completed for quite some time. This arbitrary temporal distinction has led to the characterization of two separate histopathologic populations: those with early restenosis after PTCA, in whom thrombus or vasospasm are often responsible for lumen occlusion and those with late restenosis after PTCA in whom the response to injury is described as neointimal proliferation.

Virtually no information describes what occurs between the first and third weeks following angioplasty. Characterization of healing of PTCA-induced injury during this elusive window of time would potentially offer new insight into effective methods for controlling intimal proliferation. For example, although inflammation is an important part of the general response to injury, its presence (or absence) has never been documented in the literature on post-PTCA restenosis in patients.

Literature Bias

Apart from the inherent bias in the autopsy literature toward a "worst-case scenario," other limitations make the restenosis literature difficult to interpret. First, the indications for intervention vary, with some procedures performed in the setting of stable angina and others in cases of unstable angina or acute myocardial infarction, where the underlying pathology is expected to be different. Second, it is often unclear whether patients had clinical evidence of functional late restenosis. Finally, many reports describe a mixture of patients who died either of cardiac or noncardiac causes. Clearly, this interpretation of the "natural history" of restenotic neointimal proliferation should be interpreted with caution.

References

1. Ellis SG. Elective coronary angioplasty: Technique and complications. In: Topol E, ed. Textbook of Interventional Cardiology. Philadelphia: WB Saunders, 1990:199–222.

2. Holmes DR Jr, Vlietstra RE, Smith HC, et al. Restenosis after percutaneous transluminal coronary angioplasty (PTCA): a report from the PTCA Registry of the National Heart, Lung and Blood Institute. Am J Cardiol 1984;53:77C–81C.

3. Levine S, Ewels CJ, Rosing DR, et al. Coronary angioplasty: clinical and angiographic follow-up. Am J Cardiol 1985;55:673–676.

4. Leimgruber PP, Roubin GS, Hollman J, et al. Restenosis after successful coronary angioplasty in patients with single vessel disease. Circulation 1986;73:710–717.

5. Nobuyoshi M, Kimura T, Nosaka H, et al. Restenosis after successful percutaneous coronary angioplasty: serial angiographic follow-up of 229 patients. J Am Coll Cardiol 1988;12:616–623.

6. Serruys PW, Luijten HE, Beatt J, et al. Incidence of restenosis after successful coronary angioplasty: a time related phenomenon. A quantitative angiographic study in 324 consecutive patients at 1, 2, 3 and 4 months. Circulation 1988;77:361–377.

7. Ross R, Glomset JA. The pathogenesis of atherosclerosis. N Engl J Med 1976;295:369–420.

8. Ross R. The pathogenesis of atherosclerosis. An update. N Engl J Med 1986,314:488.

9. Baroldi G. Diseases of extramural coronary arteries. In Silver MD, ed. Cardiovascular Pathology, 2nd ed. New York: Churchill-Livingstone, 1991:487–563.

10. Ellis SG, Roubin GS, King SB, et al. Angiographic and clinical predictors of acute closure after native vessel angioplasty. Circulation 1988; 77:372–379.

11. Ellis SG, Vandormael MG, Cowley MJ, et al. Coronary morphologic and clinical determinants of procedural outcome of angioplasty for multivessel coronary disease. Implications for patient selection. Circulation 1990;82:1193–1202.

12. Potkin BN, Roberts WC. Effects of coronary angioplasty on atheroscle-

rotic plaques and relation of plaque composition and arterial size to outcome. Am J Cardiol 1988;62:41–50.

13. Savage M, Goldberg S, Hirshfield J, et al. Clinical and angiographic determinants of primary coronary angioplasty success: M-HEART investigators. J Am Coll Cardiol 1991;17:22–28.

14. Ellis SG, DeCesare NB, Popma JJ, et al. Quantitative core lab analysis of directional coronary atherectomy results: relation to lesion morphology and operator experience (abstr). Circulation 1990;82:312.

15. Cowley MJ, Dorros G, Kelsey SF, et al. Acute coronary events associated with percutaneous transluminal coronary angioplasty. Am J Cardiol 1983;53:12C–16C.

16. Hirshfeld JW, Schwartz JS, Jugo R, et al. Restenosis after coronary angioplasty: a multivariate statistical model to relate lesion and procedure variables to restenosis. The M-HEART Investigators. J Am Coll Cardiol 1991;18:647–656.

17. Lyon RT, Zarins CK, Lu CT, et al. Vessel plaque and lumen morphology after transluminal balloon angioplasty: quantitative study in distended human arteries. Arteriosclerosis 1987;7:306–314.

18. Nishimura RA, Edwards WD, Warnes CA, et al. Intravascular ultrasound imaging: in vitro validation and pathologic correlation. J Am Coll Cardiol 1990;16:145–154.

19. Uchida Y, Hasegawa K, Kawamura K, Shibuya I. Angioscopic observations of the coronary luminal changes induced by coronary angioplasty. Am Heart J 1989;117:769–776.

20. Waller BF. "Crackers, breakers, stretchers, drillers, scrapers, shavers, burners, welders and melters"—The future treatment of atherosclerotic coronary artery disease? A clinical-morphologic assessment. J Am Coll Cardiol 1989;13:969–987.

21. Dotter CT, Judkins MP. Transluminal treatment of atherosclerotic obstructions: descriptions of new technique and a preliminary report of its application. Circulation 1964;30:654–670.

22. Block PC, Myler RK, Stertzer S, Fallon JT. Morphology after transluminal angioplasty in humans. N Eng J Med 1981;305:382.

23. Waller BF. Pathology of transluminal balloon angioplasty used in the treatment of coronary heart disease. Hum Pathol 1987;18:476–484.

24. Kohchi K, Takebayashi S, Block PC, et al. Arterial changes after percutaneous transluminal coronary angioplasty: results at autopsy. J Am Coll Cardiol 1987;10:592–599.

25. Mizuno K, Kurita A, Imazeki N. Pathologic findings after percutaneous transluminal coronary angioplasty. Br Heart J 1984;52:588–590.

26. Sanborn TA, Faxon DP, Haudenshild C, et al. The mechanism of trans-

luminal angioplasty: evidence for formation of aneurysms in experimental atherosclerosis. Circulation 1983;68:1136–1140.

27. Lee G, Ikeda RM, Joye JA, et al. Evaluation of transluminal angioplasty of chronic coronary artery stenosis: value and limitations assessed in fresh human cadaver hearts. Circulation 1980;61:77–83.

28. Gravanis MB, Roubin GS. Histopathologic phenomena at the site of percutaneous transluminal coronary angioplasty: the problem of restenosis. Hum Pathol 1989;20:477–485.

29. Nobuyoshi M, Kimura T, Ohishi H, et al. Restenosis after percutaneous coronary angioplasty: pathologic observations in 20 patients. J Am Coll Cardiol 1991;17:433–439.

30. Morimoto S, Mizuno Y, Hiramitsu, et al. Restenosis after percutaneous transluminal coronary angioplasty: a histopathologic study using autopsied hearts. Jap Circ J 1990;54:43–56.

31. Waller BF. Morphologic correlates of coronary angiographic patterns at the site of percutaneous transluminal coronary angioplasty. Clin Cardiol 1988;11:817–822.

32. Saffitz JE, Rose TE, Oaks JB, Roberts WC. Coronary arterial rupture during coronary angioplasty. Am J Cardiol 1983;51:902.

33. Bertrand ME, LaBlanche JM, Fourrier JL, et al. Relationship of restenosis after percutaneous transluminal coronary angioplasty to vasomotion of the dilated coronary arterial segment. Am J Cardiol 1989;63:277–281.

34. Waller BF, Garfinkel HJ, Rogers FJ, et al. Early and late morphologic changes in major epicardial coronary arteries after percutaneous transluminal coronary angioplasty. Am J Cardiol 1987;53:42C–47C.

35. Waller BF, Pinkerton CA. Coronary balloon angioplasty restenosis: Pathogenesis and treatment strategies from a morphologic perspective. J Intervent Cardiol 1989;2:167–178.

36. Essed CE, VanDenbrand M, Becker AE. Transluminal coronary angioplasty and early restenosis. Fibrocellular occlusion after wall laceration. Br Heart J 1983;49:393–396.

37. Austin GE, Ratliff NB, Hollman J, Tabei S, Phillips DF. Intimal proliferation of smooth muscle cells as an explanation for recurrent coronary artery stenosis after percutaneous transluminal coronary angioplasty. J Am Coll Cardiol 1985;6:369–375.

38. Ueda M, Becker AE, Tsukada T, et al. Fibrocellular tissue response after percutaneous transluminal coronary angioplasty: an immunocytochemical analysis of the cellular composition. Circulation 1991;83:1327–1332.

39. Simpson JB, Selmon MR, Robertson GC, et al. Transluminal atherectomy for occlusive peripheral vascular disease. Am J Cardiol 1988;61:96G–101G.

40. Garratt KN, Edwards WD, Kaufman UP, et al. Differential histopathology of primary atherosclerotic and restenotic lesions in coronary arteries and saphenous vein bypass grafts: Analysis of tissue obtained from 73 patients by directional atherectomy. J Am Coll Cardiol 1991;17:442–448.

41. Garratt KN, Holmes DR Jr, Bell MR, et al. Restenosis following directional coronary atherectomy: differences between primary atheromatous and restenosis lesions and influence of subintimal resection. J Am Coll Cardiol 1990;16:1665–1671.

42. Dartsch PC, Bauriel G, Schinko I, et al. Cell constitution and characteristics of human atherosclerotic plaques selectively removed by percutaneous atherectomy. Atherosclerosis 1989;80:149–157.

43. Chamley-Campbell JH, Campbell GR, Ross R. Phenotype- dependent response of cultured aortic smooth muscle to serum mitogens. J Cell Biol 1981;89:379–383.

44. Ohara T, Nanto S, Asada S, et al. Ultrastructural study of proliferating and migrating smooth muscle cells at the site of PTCA as an explanation for restenosis (abstr). Circulation 1988;78(suppl II):290.

45. Forrester JS, Fishbein M, Helfant R, Fogin J. A paradigm for restenosis based on cell biology: clues for the development of new preventive therapies. J Am Coll Cardiol 1991;17:758–769.

46. Black D, Hamay D, Niederman A, et al. Tear or dissection after angioplasty: morphologic correlates of an ischemic complication. Circulation 1989;79:1035–1042.

47. Ellis SG, Cowley MJ, DiSciascio G, et al. Determinants of 2-year outcome after coronary angioplasty in patients with multivessel disease on the basis of comprehensive preprocedural evaluation: implications for patient selection. Circulation 1991;83:1905–1914.

48. Berger PB, Bell MR, Bresee SJ, et al. Is the risk of restenosis after a second PTCA higher among patients with a history of prior restenosis at another site? (abstr). J Am Coll Cardiol 1991;17:267A.

. . . .

CHAPTER 8

Cellular Mechanisms of Restenotic Neointima in a Porcine Coronary Model

—

ROBERT S. SCHWARTZ
WILLIAM D. EDWARDS

CORONARY restenosis remains a major limitation of all interventional coronary revascularization procedures. Many "off-the-shelf" drugs have failed to show benefit in expensive and time-consuming clinical trials (1–12). Early optimism of a "magic bullet" in the form of a simple medication has increasingly turned to skepticism and resulted in a search for more exotic therapies (13–18).

Therapeutic trials have failed for various reasons, including the possibility that an effective agent has not yet been tested, one or more effective agents have been tested but at incorrect dosages or administration times, or more than a single agent is needed. Various therapeutic approaches (Table 8.1) have been based on an accepted but unproven paradigm shown in Figure 8.1.

In this sequence, platelet and fibrin deposition follow arterial injury, in turn causing medial smooth muscle cell (SMC) migration and proliferation to form an exuberant, stenosing neointima (19–25). This sequence of cellular events, however, is poorly documented in patients because neither autopsy nor atherectomy tissues are generally available during the formative periods after dilatation.

A better understanding of the restenosis process may result in more

Table 8.1. Current Strategies for Treatment of Restenosis

STRATEGY	EXAMPLES	PROPOSED MECHANISM
Lipid lowering	Lovastatin	Uncertain
Antimitotic	Colchicine	Inhibit SMC proliferation
Antiproliferative	Heparin (LMW)	Inhibit SMC proliferation
	Angiopeptin	
Cytotoxic	Methotrexate	Inhibit SMC proliferation
ACE inhibition	Cilazapril	? Matrix volume inhibition
Gene therapy transfection	Direct gene transfer	Native resistance
Anticoagulant antiplatelet antithrombin	IIb/IIIa receptor Ab Hirudin/analogs	Limit local thrombus
Antigrowth factors	PDGF Ab Antisense nucleotides	Inhibit SMC migration and proliferation

SMC = smooth muscle cell; LMW = low molecular weight; ACE = angiotensin-converting enzyme; PDGF = platelet-derived growth factor

effective therapies. This chapter discusses the development of restenotic neointima in an animal model. If applicable to human beings, these results provide evidence that the cellular causes of restenosis may differ from currently accepted hypotheses.

Figure 8.1.   Current paradigm for neointimal formation. According to the current hypothesis of restenosis, smooth muscle cells at the site of medial injury migrate into the intima, proliferate, and synthesize extracellular matrix to form a lesion encroaching on the lumen.

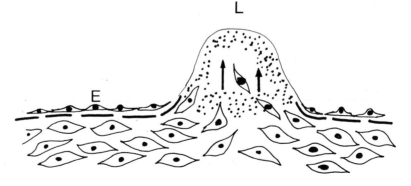

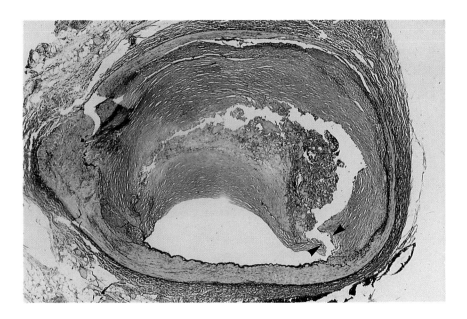

Plate I. Arterial injury following PTCA. Rupture of eccentric plaque at junction with disease-free portion of wall, resulting in focal intraplaque dissection (arrow; elastin-van Gieson; 32 ×).

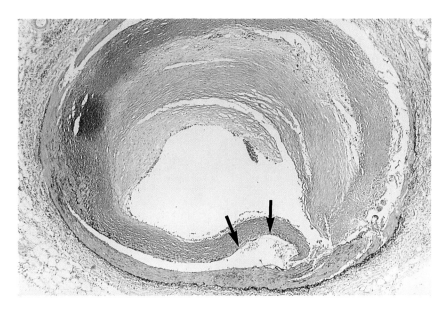

Plate II. Rupture of eccentric plaque at junction with disease-free portion of wall, resulting in focal intramedial dissection (arrows; elastin-van Gieson; 48.5 ×).

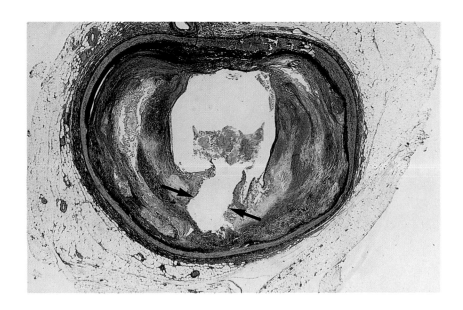

Plate III.   Rupture within body of atheromatous plaque (arrows; elastin-van Gieson; 24.5 ×).

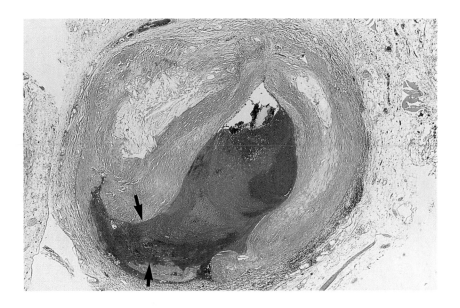

Plate IV.   Post-PTCA restenosis lesion. Acute thrombotic occlusion, with evidence of PTCA-related intramedial dissection (arrows; hematoxylin-eosin; 24.5 ×).

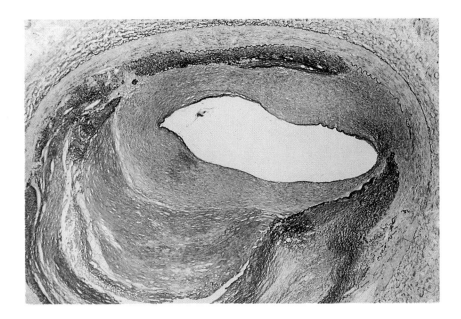

Plate V. Luminal obstruction by excessive intimal hyperplasia (elastin-van Gieson; 48.5 ×).

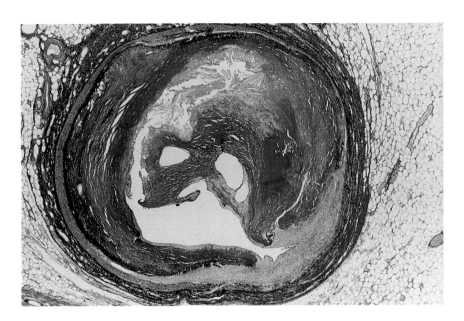

Plate VI. Variable extent of neointimal proliferation. Mild intimal hyperplasia, with filling in of PTCA-related fracture (elastin-van Gieson; 32 ×).

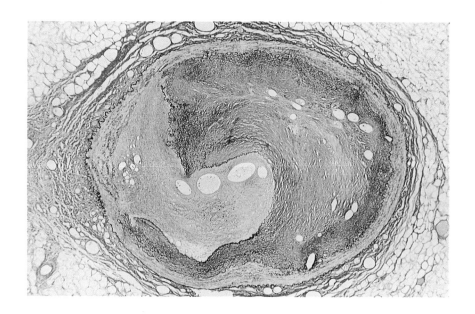

Plate VII. Extensive intimal hyperplasia, with severe luminal restenosis (elastin-van Gieson; 24.5 ×).

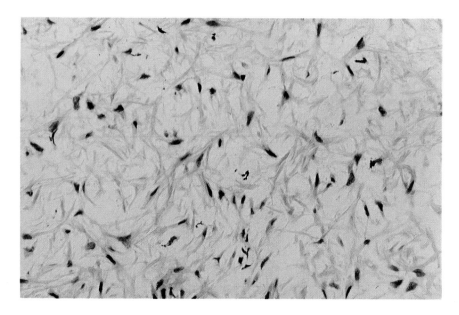

Plate VIII. Cellular composition of post-PTCA restenotic lesion. Cells have typical smooth muscle appearance (hematoxylin- eosin; 485 ×).

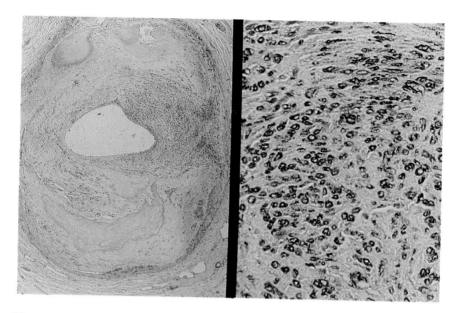

Plate IX. Immunohistochemical stain for actin indicates smooth muscle population (actin stain; left 42.5×; right 485×).

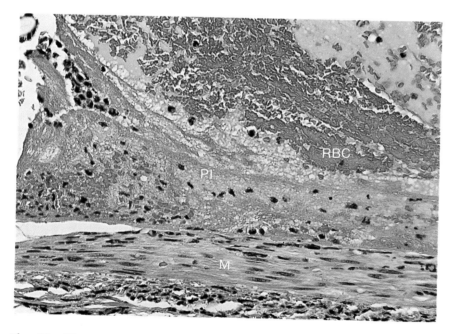

Plate X. Time course of restenotic neointimal formation. **Stage I. Thrombosis:** Fresh thrombus early (6 h) after vessel injury, consisting of platelets, fibrin, and erythrocytes. M = media, Pl = aggregated platelets and fibrin, RBC = erythrocytes and fibrin (hematoxylin-eosin; 750×).

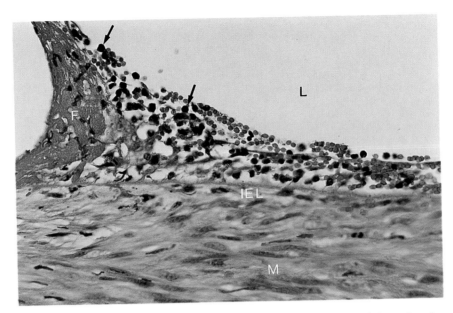

Plate XI. Stage II. Recruitment: Complete reendothelialization of thrombus has occurred within 4 days following injury. Monocytes and lymphocytes (arrows) line both sides of endothelium, with degenerating thrombus below. L = lumen, M = media, F = degenerating fibrin/thrombus, IEL = internal elastic lamina (hematoxylin-eosin; 500×). See Plate X for additional abbreviations.

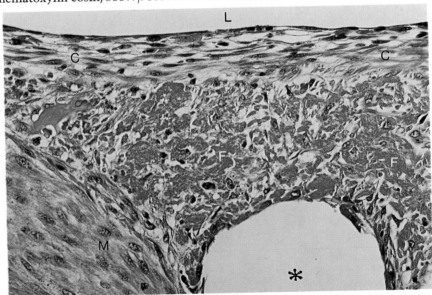

Plate XII. Stage III. Proliferation: A "cap" of smooth muscle cells is seen along the *luminal* surface of degenerating thrombus, 13 days after injury. The cap will progressively increase in thickness downward toward media as thrombus is resorbed, leaving a healed vessel. L = lumen, M = media, F = fibrin/degenerating thrombus, * = hole from wire, C = cap (hematoxylin-eosin; 125×).

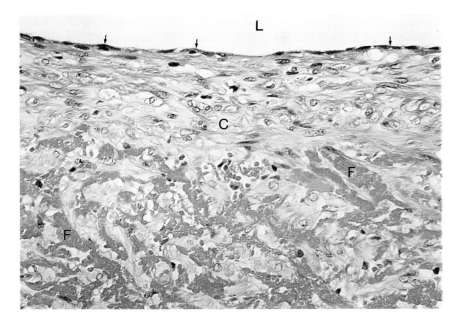

Plate XIII. Smooth muscle cell cap from a different animal shows resorbing thrombus below. Endothelium is shown by small arrows. L = lumen, F = fibrin/degenerating thrombus, * = hole from wire, C = cap (hematoxylin-eosin; 500×).

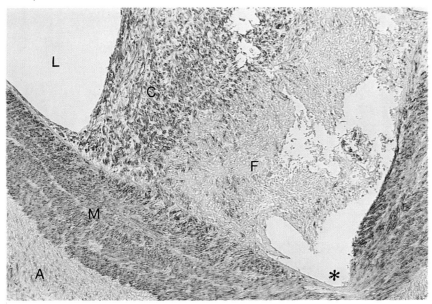

Plate XIV. Actin stain shows smooth muscle cells (brown) not only in media (M) but also in neointimal cap (arrows), most densely along luminal aspect rather than medial aspect of injury site. A = adventitia, L = lumen, F = fibrin/degenerating thrombus, M = media, * = hole from wire, C = cap (actin stain; 250×).

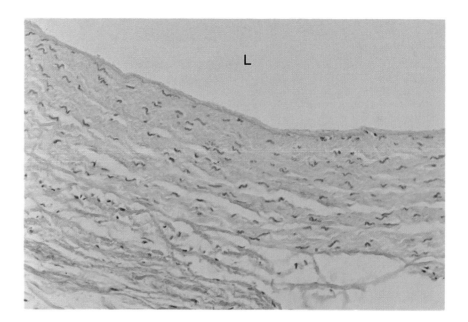

Plate XV. Neointimal growth following acute medial necrosis. Acute, severe medial cell injury. Corkscrew and pyknotic nuclei are prominent, and the media is edematous. This injury was caused by microwave energy delivered 24 hours earlier. Heat was delivered at 80°C for 30 seconds. L = lumen (hematoxylin-eosin; 500×).

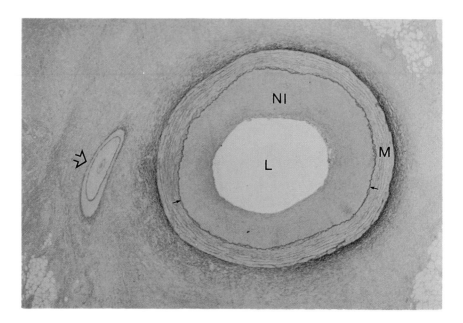

Plate XVI. Neointimal formation is seen 28 days following heat injury, despite an intact internal elastic lamina (small arrows). Prominent neointimal concentric hyperplasia is seen in the larger artery, as well as in the smaller vessel (open arrow). L = lumen, M = media (elastin-van Gieson; 500×).

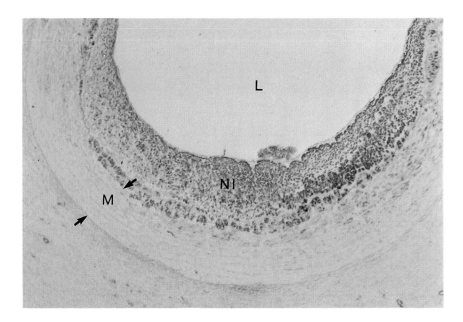

Plate XVII. Neointima stains prominently for α actin, whereas media does not, indicating extensive medial cell death 28 days following heat injury. M = media, NI = neointima, L = lumen (actin stain; 250×).

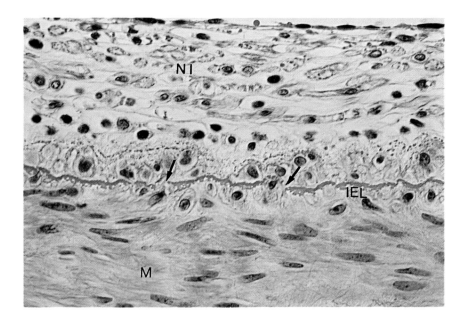

Plate XVIII. Cellular activity at a site *distant* from coronary injury. Note the normal thin endothelialized neointima. Along the internal elastic lamina, medial cells seem to be transforming to a more rounded shape and migrating through breaks in the internal elastic lamina (arrows). The arterial lumen is at the top of the picture. E = endothelium, IEL = internal elastic lamina, M = media, NI = neointima (hematoxylin-eosin; 750×).

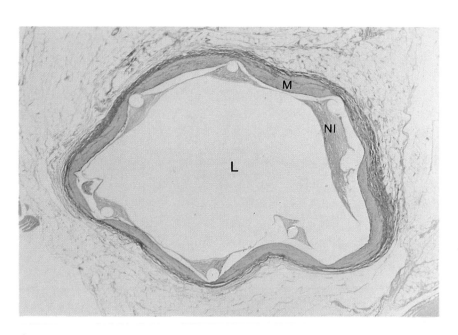

Plate XIX. Histopathologic cross-section of a canine coronary artery that underwent oversized coil injury. Little neointimal proliferation is evident in comparison to that expected for a pig with similar vessel injury. L = lumen, NI = neointima, M = media (elastin-van Gieson 100×).

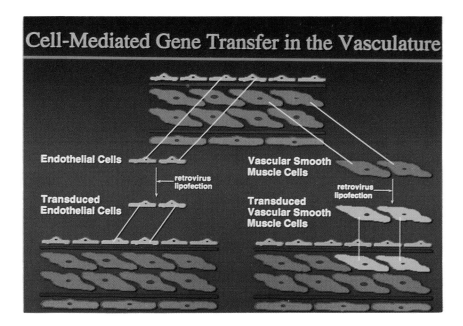

Plate XX. Cell-mediated gene transfer is performed in vascular cells by removing endothelial or vascular smooth muscle cells from an animal and genetically modifying them in tissue culture by use of a retroviral vector or a DNA liposome complex.

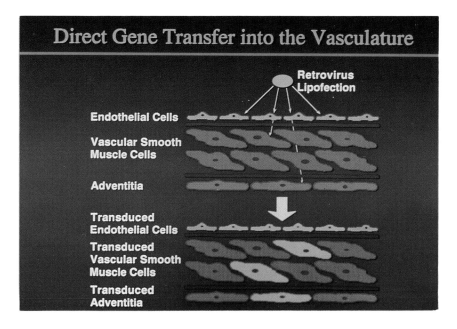

Plate XXI. Direct gene transfer allows the introduction of the recombinant gene directly into vascular cells by infection with a retrovirus or transfection with DNA/liposome complexes in vivo.

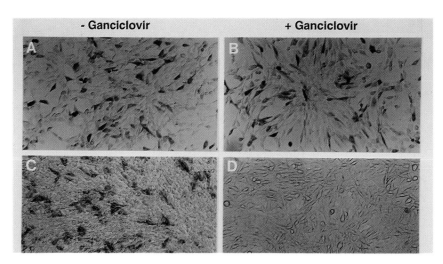

Plate XXII. Expression of β-galactosidase and herpesvirus TK in cells transduced by the suicide retroviral vector. NIH-3T3 cells were analyzed by histochemical staining for β-galactosidase activity after infection with the retroviral vector transducing β-galactosidase and neomycin resistance and after incubation in (A) media only or (B) media with ganciclovir, or after infection with the suicide retroviral vector and cultured for 4 days in (C) media only or (D) media with ganciclovir. Following infection with a suicide vector and treatment with ganciclovir, NIH-3T3 cells lost β-galactosidase expression and cell death occurred (200×). (Reprinted from Plautz G, Nabel EG, Nabel GJ. Selective elimination of recombinant genes in vivo with a suicide retroviral vector. The New Biologist 1991;3:709–715.)

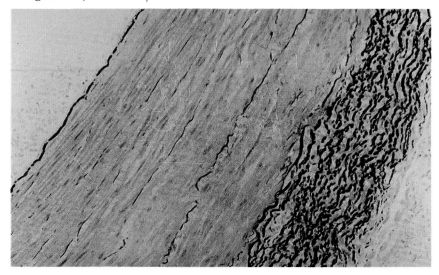

Plate XXIII. A section of a pig femoral artery following an injection of heparin through the local delivery catheter. The heparin is detectable by a dark stain with toluidine blue. There is a thin line of heparin deposition on the intimal surface, scattered heparin throughout the media, and a substantial collection of heparin in the adventitia.

Although excessive neointimal proliferation is the major cause of late coronary restenosis, other causes include arterial spasm, vessel recoil, and thrombus formation (26). This discussion will deal only with the genesis of neointima and will be limited to a review of observations from the porcine coronary injury model.

The Porcine Coronary Injury Model

The coronary arteries of juvenile domestic crossbred swine are focally injured using excessive balloon dilatation and implantation of metallic tantalum coils, as described previously (27–29). Restenotic neointima forms within 1 month in prolific amounts (Figure 8.2) and has a histopathologic appearance similar to human restenosis. Limitations of this model will be discussed later.

Figure 8.2. Macroscopic appearance of porcine neointima. Prolific neointima routinely develops with enough volume to cause luminal stenosis (right). A normal segment of artery proximal to the lesion is shown for comparison (left). Residual wire fragments are visible (arrows).

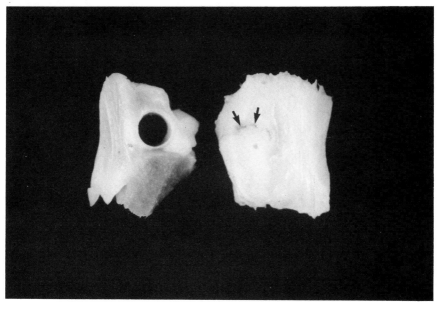

Neointimal Volume Development Over Time

To understand the mechanisms by which neointima develops over time, experiments have been performed in which pigs were killed at intervals varying from 6 hours to 28 days after coronary artery injury (30). Histopathologic tissue examination revealed three distinct stages in the genesis of neointima, summarized in Table 8.2.

Stage I: Thrombosis

The earliest response to arterial injury is the formation of thrombus at the injury site similar to coronary thrombi described in patients. It is typically pale tan grossly and platelet-rich microscopically. Red thrombus is found on top of the platelets and consists primarily of fibrin and erythrocytes (Plate X). Fibrin and platelets often deposit concurrently and produce a heterogeneous microscopic appearance. Thrombus literally develops within minutes after arterial injury. By 24 hours the thrombus becomes more dense and homogeneous as platelets, and later erythrocytes, lyse and agglutinate. Platelet lysis results in discharge of granules and release of many bioactive substances within the thrombus including platelet-derived growth factor (PDGF; 31,32).

Stage II: Cellular Recruitment

The next morphologic stage begins 3 to 4 days after injury. In this stage the thrombus itself becomes covered by endothelium. The functionality of this endothelium has not yet been assessed, but it may limit further deposition of thrombus. Following reendothelialization, monocytes and lymphocytes are attracted from the flowing blood to the newly formed endothelial surface, at about 4 to 8 days. Both cell types

Table 8.2. Stages of Neointimal Development

STAGE	NAME	CELLULAR EVENTS
I	Thrombosis	Plaelet-rich thrombus Fibrin-rich thrombus
II	Cellular recruitment	Endothelialization of mural thrombus Recruitment of lymphocytes and monoocytes
III	Cellular proliferation	Smooth muscle cell migration, proliferation and matrix synthesis

appear in large quantities and frequently are found on both the luminal and the thrombotic side of the endothelium (Plate XI).

These cells may be attracted by endothelial cells or by thrombus itself. Lymphocytes and monocytes pass through the endothelium into the degenerating fibrin thrombus. The monocytes become macrophages. Both macrophages and lymphocytes release a variety of growth factors and cytokines that affect SMCs (33–37). Chemoattractants are presumably involved in SMC migration and proliferation as described in other animal arterial injury models.

Macrophages and monocytes also elaborate fibrinolytic enzymes (38,39). Over time these cells are found at progressively deeper levels within the degenerating thrombus and are surrounded by clear regions, suggesting focal thrombolysis is occurring. Importantly, this process occurs from the luminal (endothelial) direction *toward* the medial injury site rather than vice versa.

Stage III: Cellular Proliferation

In the next stage, cells staining positively for actin form an intimal "cap" on the *luminal* side of the healing mass (Plates XII through XIV). The proliferative tissue is thought to be SMC in origin. The plump appearance of the cells presumably represents a phenotypic transformation from contractile spindle cells. The thickness of the cap is proportional to lesion age, suggesting that cap growth also occurs in a luminal-to-adventitial direction. Residual thrombus is gradually resorbed and replaced by neointima until healing is complete.

A prominent extracellular matrix is presumably secreted by the SMCs and consists of collagen and glycosaminoglycans. The role of this matrix in the final volume of neointima is unclear but under investigation.

Smooth Muscle Cells: Site of Origin

The neointimal SMCs do not necessarily originate from the site of medial injury. This may be inferred from the cap noted in stage III, which forms along the luminal surface and thickens over time toward the media and adventitia. These cells may thus arise from uninjured media in nearby portions of the artery, or they may arise from other sites such as intima, adventitia, or even macrophages.

In an early experiment, it was reasoned that elimination of SMCs from media might prevent restenosis because no cells would be available to migrate and proliferate. Therefore, normal pig coronary arteries were exposed to localized, intraluminal microwave heat energy sufficient to cause medial necrosis. This energy was delivered by an angioplasty balloon that raised local surface temperatures to 80°C for 30 seconds. The balloon itself was sized so that mechanical damage to the artery was minimal (Plate XV).

At 28 days, a large volume of neointima was consistently observed at burn sites (Plate XVI). Secondary medial atrophy and fibrosis were also noted, with little actin uptake (Plate XVII). The greatest volume of neointima formed at sites of maximal medial injury. Yet because medial SMCs had been killed early at the burn site, it is difficult to hypothesize that SMC migration occurred from the medial injury site when these cells died at an early stage. It seems likely that migration into the neointima occurred from a distant uninjured medial site.

Smooth Muscle Cells in Restenosis

The delineation of three stages in neointimal development implies that the cellular basis of restenosis is complex. In the current popular hypothesis, SMCs migrate, proliferate, and synthesize extracellular matrix in response to vessel injury to generate a stenotic lesion. If the stages of neointimal formation in human beings are similar to the pig, then medial SMCs may have a more passive role in restenosis than previously thought. Rather than proliferating uncontrollably, they may only proliferate to fill an existing thrombotic mass to complete a normal arterial healing process. Matrix synthesis may stabilize the mass and contribute additional volume to the lesion.

Neointimal formation as described above is consistent with current ideas of SMC migration and proliferation. It differs only in the location of origin and direction of proliferation. Migration seems to occur from more distant sites; proliferation occurs into a degenerating bioabsorbable matrix. This is confirmed by examination of injury sites on the border of injury, away from maximal neointimal growth. At these sites there is much cellular activity in the subintimal space. Cells in these areas stain strongly for α actin, and regions are found where SMCs seem to be migrating through the internal elastic lamina into the subintimal space, presumably to form the cap across the endothelialized thrombus (Plate XVIII). These findings enhance rather than contradict current hypotheses of neointimal formation. To summarize these observations:

1. SMCs forming neointima do not necessarily originate at the site of medial injury.
2. Endothelialized and degenerating thrombus, colonized by monocytes and lymphocytes, provides a bioabsorbable matrix into which the SMC migrates and proliferates and synthesizes extracellular matrix.
3. The "thrombus burden" that accumulates at the arterial injury site over time may directly determine the volume of eventual neointimal tissue.

The Proportional Response of Neointima to Arterial Injury

In the pig model neointimal thickness is directly proportional to the depth of arterial injury (29). An ordinal injury score (Table 8.3) was prospectively developed and tested to quantitate injury. Linear regression analysis of mean arterial injury score and mean neointimal thickness indicated a strongly proportional relationship (Figure 8.3A). Accordingly, more injury causes more neointimal proliferation. A similar relationship has also been inferred for human beings (Figure 8.3B; 40). Deeper injury causes thicker neointimal proliferation and thus more stenosis. These findings may have important implications for restenosis research: injury extent may be a strong covariate and should be included when histologically comparing therapies. Although depth of injury cannot be measured from angiographic data in human studies, it

Table 8.3. Values Used for Vessel Injury Score

SCORE	DESCRIPTION OF INJURY
0	Internal elastic lamina intact; endothelium typically denuded; media compressed but not lacerated
1	Internal elastic lamina lacerated; media typically compressed but not lacerated
2	Internal elastic lamina lacerated; media visibly lacerated or crushed; external elastic lamina intact
3	Large lacerations of media extending through the external elastic lamina; coil wires sometimes residing in adventitia

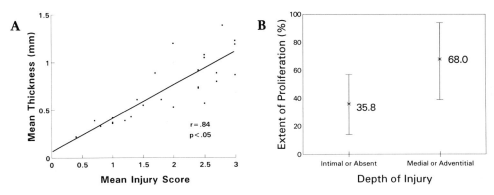

Figure 8.3. (A) Mean neointimal thickness is proportional to mean injury score in 26 porcine coronary arterial segments (p < 0.05). The slope appears relatively constant across experiments. (B) Data from human beings suggests depth of injury is related to neointimal proliferation. When no medial or adventitial injury was present, the extent of proliferation was significantly less (adapted from Nobuyoshi et al, 1991).

can be assessed histopathologically and may be essential in future animal trials.

Application of the Proportional Injury–Response Relationship

The injury–response relationship is described by a linear function and is characterized by a slope and intercept. These two parameters provide a powerful method for testing potential restenosis therapies in animal models where histopathology is used as an end point.

The **slope** of the injury–neointimal thickness line relates differential injury to the resulting neointimal thickness, that is, the **incremental** increase in neointimal volume for an incremental change in depth of injury. The **intercept** of the regression line measures differences in neointima for any degree of injury. In an experiment testing a treatment for inhibition of neointima, these two parameters are calculated for the treated and control groups. Different slopes, intercepts, or both may result (Figure 8.4). The regression lines are compared for statistically significant differences.

To illustrate this method, consider a hypothetical treatment that is highly effective against neointimal formation. It will generate an injury–response regression line with a much lower slope, intercept, or

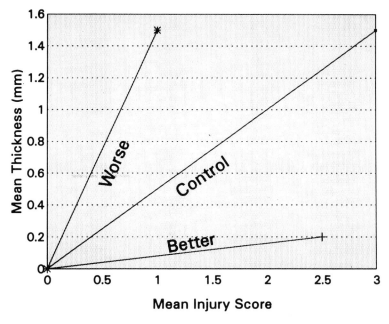

Figure 8.4. Different slopes, intercepts, or both may result when comparing two regression lines in neointimal response studies. This figure illustrates the appearance of different slopes. Effective treatments lower slope, intercept, or both in injury response regression lines. Treatments that cause more neointima cause higher slope, intercept, or both.

both. This successful treatment causes less incremental neointimal formation from injury. Conversely, a treatment that worsened neointimal formation would have a larger slope, intercept, or both.

Variability in the Proportional Neointimal Response to Injury

Early results using injury–response regression in pigs indicate that it is the intercept that varies across treatment groups; slopes are similar. This interesting finding suggests that the **differential** arterial injury response is constant: differences in neointimal thickness because of treatment are constant and independent of injury depth. For pigs, the slope typically ranges from 0.35 mm/injury unit to 0.45 mm/injury unit.

Early studies in dogs using coronary stents showed less neointima than is found in pigs (Plate XIX). An intriguing possibility is that the arteries of different species may respond with variable amounts of neointima for a given amount of injury. Interspecies variability may occur in the injury–response relationship, with each having a characteristic injury–neointimal response slope or intercept. A preliminary study is underway to test this hypothesis. If true, some animal models may be more appropriate than others for the study of restenotic neointima. The cause of this species difference might be investigated in order to develop therapeutic strategies.

Restenosis Treatments: Planning an Approach

Simple description of neointimal development following injury does not imply an understanding of the process. The major question to be answered in solving the restenosis problem is which factor or factors (recoil, thrombus, and the like) are most important in determining neointimal volume because it is this volume that impinges on the arterial lumen. Which stage or stages in neointimal development determine this volume?

If each stage identified above could be separately blocked or severely reduced, the effects on eventual neointimal volume could be carefully studied. If blocking single stages does not prove effective, multiple stages could be simultaneously blocked and the effects observed.

A rational strategy might consist of severely limiting platelet deposition (stage I); severely limiting fibrin deposition (stage I); limiting monocyte and lymphocyte recruitment or blocking their secretory products (stage II); or limiting SMC migration, proliferation, and matrix synthesis in the degenerating fibrin thrombus (stage III). The effect of each intervention alone and in combination should be studied.

Limitations

The observations described in this chapter should be interpreted in the context of the animal model in which they were found. Do the same stages hold true for development of human neointima? The answer is unknown but relates to the larger question of appropriate animal restenosis models in general. Other models are discussed in Chapter 13.

Although neointimal formation in the porcine model resembles human neointima, a wire coil is responsible for producing it. This has raised questions about the role played by the wire itself. There is little indication of either foreign body response or ongoing injury in the majority of arteries examined. Inflammatory responses occur when arterial injury is most severe, when wires are found within the adventitia. The proportional response of neointima and injury suggests that the injury done by the wire rather than the wire itself is responsible for neointimal proliferation. A "properly" placed stent caused little neointima. Oversized balloon inflation also results in neointimal proliferation in the pig when no metal coil is present.

Another concern is the possibility that the wire injury model generates more thrombus than found in patients following angioplasty. This possibility cannot be easily assessed. The evidence suggests that thrombus is an important part of neointimal volume in the pig model. Until the evolution of neointimal formation can be assessed in patients, the question will remain unanswered.

Summary

Significant reduction in coronary restenosis remains a major priority in interventional cardiology. Large amounts of time, money, and emotional resources have produced no solutions. The time and expense of clinical trials increasingly mandate a better understanding of animal models so that preliminary treatments may be assessed rapidly and inexpensively.

References

1. Bowles MH, Klonis D, Plavac TG, et al. EPA in the prevention of restenosis post PTCA. Angiology 1991;42:187–194.
2. Corcos T, David PR, Bal PG, et al. Failure of diltiazem to prevent restenosis after percutaneous transluminal coronary angioplasty. Am Heart J 1985;109:926–931.
3. Ellis SG, Roubin GS, Wilentz J, Douglas JSJ, King SB III. Effect of 18- to 24-hour heparin administration for prevention of restenosis after uncomplicated coronary angioplasty. Am Heart J 1989;117:777–782.
4. Hill JA, Macdonald RG, Jugo R, et al. Multi-Hospital Eastern Atlantic

Restenosis Trial: design, recruitment, and feasibility. M-HEART Investigators. Cathet Cardiovasc Diagn 1990;20:227–237.

5. Pepine CJ, Hirshfeld JW, Macdonald RG, et al. A controlled trial of corticosteroids to prevent restenosis after coronary angioplasty. M-HEART Group. Circulation 1990;81:1753–1761.

6. Reis GJ, Boucher TM, Sipperly ME, et al. Randomized trial of fish oil for prevention of restenosis after coronary angioplasty. Lancet 1989;2:177–181.

7. Schwartz L, Bourassa MG, Lesperance J, et al. Aspirin and dipyridamole in the prevention of restenosis after percutaneous transluminal coronary angioplasty. N Engl J Med 1988;318:1714–1719.

8. Stone GW, Rutherford BD, McConahay DR, et al. A randomized trial of corticosteroids for the prevention of restenosis in 102 patients undergoing repeat coronary angioplasty. Cathet Cardiovasc Diagn 1989;18:227–231.

9. Taylor R, Gibbons F, Cope G, et al. Effects of low dose aspirin on restenosis after coronary angioplasty. Am J Cardiol 1991;68:874–878.

10. Thornton MA, Gruentzig AR, Hollman J, King SB III, Douglas JS Jr. Coumadin and aspirin in prevention of recurrence after transluminal coronary angioplasty: a randomized study. Circulation 1984;69:721–727.

11. Whitworth HB, Roubin GS, Hollman J, et al. Effect of nifedipine on recurrent stenosis after percutaneous transluminal coronary angioplasty. J Am Coll Cardiol 1986;8:1271–1276.

12. Dehmer G, Popma J, van den Berg E, et al. Reduction in the rate of early restenosis after coronary angioplasty by a diet supplemented with n-3 fatty acids. N Engl J Med 1988;319:733–740.

13. Epstein S, Siegall C, Biro S, Fu Y, Fitzgerald D, Pastan I. Cytotoxic effects of a recombinant chimeric toxin on rapidly proliferating vascular smooth muscle cells. Circulation 1991;84:778–787.

14. Lundergan C, Foegh ML, Vargas R, et al. Inhibition of myointimal proliferation of the rat carotid artery by the peptides, angiopeptin and BIM 23034. Atherosclerosis 1989;80:49–55.

15. Jenkins RD, Sinclair IN, Leonard BM, Sandor T, Schoen FJ, Spears JR. Laser balloon angioplasty versus balloon angioplasty in normal rabbit iliac arteries. Lasers Surg Med 1989;9:237–247.

16. Finci L, Hofling B, Ludwig B, et al. Sulotroban during and after coronary angioplasty. A double-blind, placebo controlled study. Z Kardiol 1989;3:50–54.

17. Calcagno D, Conte JV, Howell MH, Foegh ML. Peptide inhibition of neointimal hyperplasia in vein grafts. J Vasc Surg 1991;13:475–479.

18. Powell J, Clozel J, Muller R, et al. Inhibitors of angiotensin-converting enzyme prevent myointimal proliferation after vascular injury. Science 1989;245:186–188.

19. Clowes A, Reidy M, Clowes M. Kinetics of cellular proliferation after arterial injury: I. Smooth muscle growth in absence of endothelium. Lab Invest 1983;49:327–332.

20. Fingerle J, Johnson R, Clowes A, Majesky M, Reidy M. Role of platelets in smooth muscle cell proliferation and migration after vascular injury in the rat carotid artery. Proc Natl Acad Sci USA 1989;86:8412–8416.

21. Reidy M, Clowes A, Schwartz S. Endothelial regeneration: V. Inhibition of endothelial regrowth in arteries of rat and rabbit. Lab Invest 1983;49:569–575.

22. Adams PC, Badimon JJ, Badimon L, Chesebro JH, Fuster V. Role of platelets in atherogenesis: relevance to coronary arterial restenosis after angioplasty. Cardiovasc Clin 1987;18:49–71.

23. Harker LA. Role of platelets and thrombosis in mechanisms of acute occlusion and restenosis after angioplasty. Am J Cardiol 1987;60:21B–28B.

24. Ip JH, Fuster V, Israel D, Badimon L, Badimon J, Chesebro JH. The role of platelets, thrombin and hyperplasia in restenosis after coronary angioplasty. J Am Coll Cardiol 1991;17(suppl B):77B–88B.

25. Minar E, Ehringer H, Ahmadi R, Dudczak R, Porenta G. Platelet deposition at angioplasty sites and platelet survival time after PTA in iliac and femoral arteries: investigations with indium-111 oxine labelled platelets in patients with ASA (1.0 g/day) therapy. Thromb Haemost 1987; 58:718–723.

26. Bertrand ME, Lablanche JM, Fourrier JL, Gommeaux A, Ruel M. Relation to restenosis after percutaneous transluminal coronary angioplasty to vasomotion of the dilated coronary arterial segment. Am J Cardiol 1989;63:277–281.

27. Schwartz RS, Murphy JG, Edwards WD, Camrud AR, Vlietstra RE, Holmes DR. Restenosis after balloon angioplasty: A practical proliferative model in porcine coronary arteries. Circulation 1990;82:2190–2200.

28. Schwartz RS, Murphy JG, Edwards WD, Camrud AR, Vlietstra RE, Holmes DR. Restenosis occurs with internal elastic lamina laceration and is proportional to severity of vessel injury in a porcine coronary artery model. Circulation 1990;4(suppl III):656.

29. Schwartz RS, Murphy JG, Edwards WD, Camrud AR, Vlietstra RE, Holmes DR Jr. Restenosis and the proportional neointimal response to coronary artery injury: results in a porcine model. J Am Coll Cardiol 1992;19:267–274.

30. Schwartz RS, Edwards WD, Murphy JG, Camrud AR, Holmes DR Jr.

Restenosis develops in four stages: serial histologic studies in a coronary injury model. J Am Coll Cardiol 1991;17:52A.

31. Ross R, Raines E, Bowen-Pope D. The biology of platelet-derived growth factor. Cell 1986;46:155–169.

32. Williams L. Signal transduction by the platelet-derived growth factor receptor. Science 1989;243:1564–1570.

33. Krane SM, Goldring MB, Goldring SR. Cytokines. Ciba Found Symp 1988;136:239–256.

34. Martin CA, Dorf ME. Differential regulation of interleukin-6, macrophage inflammatory protein-1, and JE/MCP-1 cytokine expression in macrophage cell lines. Cell Immunol 1991;135:245–258.

35. McKay IA, Leigh IM. Epidermal cytokines and their roles in cutaneous wound healing. Br J Dermatol 1991;124:513–518.

36. Schaefer RM, Paczek L, Heidland A. Cytokine production by monocytes during haemodialysis. Nephrol Dial Transplant 1991;2:14–17.

37. Yamada Y, Kimball K, Okusawa S, et al. Cytokines, acute phase proteins, and tissue injury. C-reactive protein opsonizes dead cells for debridement and stimulates cytokine production. Ann NY Acad Sci 1990;587:351–361.

38. Bevilacqua M, Pober J, Wheeler M, Cotran R, Gimbrone M. Interleukin-1 acts on cultured human vascular endothelium to increase adhesion of polymorphonuclear leukocytes, monocytes, and related leukocyte cell lines. J Clin Invest 1985;76:2003–2011.

39. Davies MJ, Woolf N, Rowles PM, Pepper J. Morphology of the endothelium over atherosclerotic plaques in human coronary arteries. Br Heart J 1988;60:459–464.

40. Nobuyoshi M, Kimura T, Osishi H, et al. Restenosis after percutaneous transluminal coronary angioplasty: pathologic observations in 20 patients. J Am Coll Cardiol 1991;17:433–439.

CHAPTER 9

Thrombosis and Restenosis After Angioplasty

J. H. Chesebro
M. W. I. Webster
P. Zoldhelyi
J. J. Badimon
L. Badimon
V. Fuster

ANGIOPLASTY by balloon, atherectomy catheter, or laser may improve the minimal lumen diameter (MLD) of the coronary artery (measured by quantitative angiography) from 0.8 mm to 1.5 to 2.5 mm immediately after the procedure. However, after 3 to 6 months more than 40% of patients may have more than 50% loss of the measured gain to an MLD of 1.3 to 1.4 mm (1,2). New methods of maintaining this acute improvement are needed. Because portions of the arterial circumference may be normal in the presence of eccentric plaque, indiscriminate injury of the entire artery would ideally be avoided with targeted removal of the obstructing plaque in the future.

Mechanisms that may contribute to restenosis include accelerated progression of atherosclerosis, mural thrombus and its organization, proliferation of smooth muscle cells (SMC) and fibroblasts, production of connective tissue matrix by these cells, vasoconstriction, and recoil following dilatation and stretch (3).

This chapter discusses the role of thrombus, platelets, thrombin, and cellular proliferation in restenosis and includes the pathology of restenosis, risk factors for thrombosis and restenosis, SMC proliferation, migration and thrombus, mechanisms of mural thrombus and the role of thrombin, reasons for the high risk of preexisting thrombus, and future directions.

Pathology of Restenosis

Coronary angioscopy, tissue specimens from atherectomy, and postmortem examination have provided valuable information about the nature of the arterial injury and the morphologic sequelae. Coronary angioscopy immediately after the angioplasty procedure has documented plaque fissures and tears with mural thrombus in 70% to 80% of arteries despite the usual doses of heparin and antiplatelet therapies (4–6). Thus, current therapies are not preventing mural thrombus in most patients.

Postmortem examination after balloon angioplasty documents the incomplete displacement or dissolution of atherosclerotic plaque; tears, fissures, and dissections into or around the plaque; eccentric and serpigeonous residual lumens; and residual thrombus within and extruding from the breaks in the arterial wall. Furthermore, injury and tears through the internal elastic lamina into the media with associated mural thrombus may also occur in normal portions of the arterial circumference opposite an eccentric plaque (7–16). Turbulent flow and stasis of blood flow within the same artery are inevitable within such lumens; future antithrombotic therapies should thus be effective at both high and low shear forces.

Arterial tissue from atherectomy confirms the presence of mural thrombus, and intimal SMC and fibroblast proliferation within the first 15 to 30 days after the angioplasty procedure in a high proportion of cases. Thereafter, collagen and extracellular matrix, which are likely synthesized by the SMCs and fibroblasts, are more abundant. Some cells are primitive with positive vimentin immunohistochemical staining and are not yet declared to be an SMC or fibroblast. Atherectomy specimens from peripheral arteries of patients with restenosis showed intimal SMC cell hyperplasia in 75%, some thrombus in 65%, and a large amount of thrombus (> 20% of the specimen) in 25%. The presence of thrombus was unrelated to the type of antithrombotic therapy (17). Experimental studies in pigs also suggest that all current therapies are inadequate for preventing thrombus (18,19).

Risk Factors for Thrombosis and Restenosis

Restenosis is more likely in those with risk factors for thrombosis. These include diabetes, smoking, angina at rest, eccentric plaque, and arterial dissection. Other risk factors associated with restenosis also increase arterial thrombosis via the rheology of blood flow and include significant residual stenosis immediately after percutaneous transluminal coronary angioplasty (PTCA; most platelets within MLD), proximal lesions of the left anterior descending coronary artery (high flow and thus high shear rate), and long lesions greater than 10 mm (more platelet deposition within stenosis; 20–29; see the section on mechanisms of mural thrombosis). In addition, exercise tests were positive 3 days after angioplasty in 79% of patients who restenose later compared to 18% positive tests in those who do not restenose (30). This suggests that the restenosis process starts early and may be due to acute mural thrombus, which also forms quite early.

Smooth Muscle Cell Proliferation, Migration, and Thrombus

Proliferation and migration of SMCs, which follow acute arterial injury, are independent processes. The proliferative response can be divided into three phases based on experimental data. Phase I or the first wave of proliferation and hypertrophy peaks at 48 hours in medial SMCs. Phase II or the intermediate phase of SMC proliferation involves migration of SMCs from media to intima and proliferation within the intima from approximately 4 to 14 days. In phase III or later, SMC proliferation, hypertrophy and production of extracellular matrix predominate (31–33).

Phase I

In phase I the medial SMC proliferation appears related to arterial injury or stretch of the media and not to the presence or absence (severely decreased by antiplatelet antibody) of platelets. In gentle denudation without medial injury and no significant stretch, only small increases in proliferation occurred despite generation of some large platelet thrombi (31,34–37). In pigs the degree of stretch by number of atmospheres of balloon inflation (probably influencing medial SMC injury and necrosis) correlated with the proportion of medial SMCs proliferating at 48 hours after injury. The presence or absence of deep or mild injury or the severity of ^{111}In-labeled platelet deposition did not correlate with the degree of medial SMC proliferation (38). Thus, the first wave of SMC proliferation after injury appears to correlate with arterial stretch and probably cellular injury but not platelet deposition.

Phase I medial proliferation appears to be stimulated by basic fibroblast growth factor (bFGF). Rat SMCs express mRNA for bFGF, and bFGF protein was found by immunoblot analysis. Minimal injury denuded endothelium and when followed by intravenous bFGF infusion increased medial proliferation. Infusion of anti-bFGF-antibody decreased medial SMC proliferation. Uninjured arteries without endothelial denudation were not responsive to an intravenous infusion of bFGF (34–37).

Additional stimuli or helper functions in phase I may come from other growth factors (GF) such as platelet-derived growth factor (PDGF) or thrombin. Thrombin appears to be mitogenic in neonatal rat SMCs but in the adult rat stimulates protein synthesis but not DNA synthesis (hypertrophic but not mitogenic). Thrombin also activates a number of transmembrane signaling pathways common to PDGF; these may also induce chemotactic activity (39–41). Thus, thrombin, PDGF, or both may have a helper function in conjunction with bFGF. Proliferation in phase I may influence phase II, especially in the presence of cellular migration from media to intima.

Phase II

In phase II or the intermediate phase, intimal thickening depends on the separable phenomena of SMC proliferation and migration from media to intima (42–48). The SMCs show chemotaxis in response to PDGF but proliferate in response to several GFs including bFGF, PDGF, epidermal GF, insulin GF, and transforming GF-β (45–47,49). These mitogens may be released from or regulated by platelets, endothelial cells, monocytes, macrophages, SMCs, or thrombus (49–51). SMC migration does not depend on proliferation (52,53). Nonproliferating SMCs can migrate and contribute to intimal cells; approximately 50% of intimal SMCs do not divide (54). Peak SMC proliferation in the intima occurs at 96 hours in the rat (31). In pigs intimal SMCs are evident by 4 to 7 days after injury with 48% proliferating by 1 week after injury by 6 atm of balloon dilation (55). In the presence of a macroscopic mural thrombus after deep injury, a cap of SMCs forms just below the endothelium by 2 weeks after injury and is associated with significant intimal cellular proliferation (55). This subpopulation of neointimal SMCs may also be present in the rat and has a different pattern of gene expression (strongly positive for PDGF-A and PDGF-B receptor transcripts) (32).

Mural thrombi have been qualitatively related to SMC proliferation along with platelet antigens and bands of fibrin in experimental and human plaques (50,56–62). Fibromuscular plaque formation can result from distal propagation of thrombus to a distal uninjured segment, and pulmonary embolization of platelet-rich thrombi can result in fibromuscular plaquelike lesions rich in lipids and connective tissue, in the absence of lipid feeding (56). Intimal proliferation in the rabbit aorta induced by an indwelling polyethylene cannula or after balloon injury is considerably reduced by antiplatelet sera, which drastically lowered the platelet count to less than 10,000 (50,62). Thrombocytopenia in rats prevented intimal lesions at 7 days following balloon injury (34). Because neointimal SMCs in the rat contain abundant PDGF β-receptor messenger RNA, the effect of thrombocytopenia suggests that PDGF-BB from platelets plays a significant role in neointimal formation. Deep arterial injury results in macroscopic, platelet- rich, mural thrombus (63) with increased delivery of GFs from platelets to the arterial wall compared with mild injury, which results in only a single layer of platelets and markedly decreased fibrin, thrombin, and delivery of GFs to the arterial wall. These facts may account for the increased proliferative response after deep compared to mild arterial injury (55,63). As will be discussed under mural thrombus, increased thrombin is associated with deep arterial injury. In addition, a close correlation also exists between the number of thrombin molecules and the extent of GF secretion by platelets (64). Thus, thrombus, platelets, and their secretory products appear to play a significant role in phase II or the intermediate phase of SMC proliferation (Figure 9.1).

Phase III

In phase III SMC proliferation slows, but intimal cellular hypertrophy and extracellular matrix production from SMCs may continue and appear to be influenced by factors that affect SMCs (33). Intimal thickening progressively increases in chronically denuded areas (by both continued proliferation and matrix formation) but not in reendothelialized areas where proliferative activity usually returns to baseline in about 4 weeks (65). Species differences and lipids may alter this (66,67). With

PROPOSED MECHANISMS

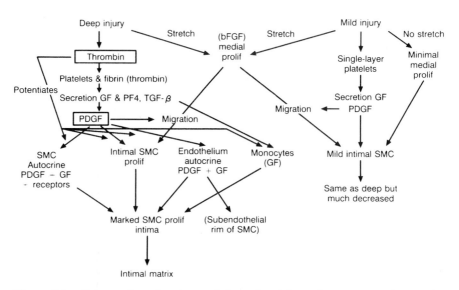

Figure 9.1. Proposed mechanisms of the role of thrombus in smooth muscle cell (SMC) proliferation. Phase I or the first wave of proliferation due to arterial stretch or direct injury peaks at 48 hours, appears directly related to basic fibroblast growth factor (bFGF, center), and is independent of platelet deposition. Lack of stretch results in minimal phase I proliferation (right). Similar mechanisms are present after deep (into plaque or through internal elastic lamina) injury (left) or mild (endothelial denudation only) injury (right). The degree of phase II intimal proliferation of SMC at 1 to 2 weeks after arterial injury is considerably greater after deep injury. The reasons for this are presumably due to increased amounts of thrombin, which stimulates platelet and fibrin deposition, platelet secretion of platelet-derived growth factor (PDGF) and other growth factors (GF), oncogene activation, and potentiation of other GFs, which may originate from platelets, monocytes, macrophages, endothelium, or SMCs. PDGF appears to play a pivotal role in migration of SMC from media to intima and presumably is also an important GF in the phase II intimal proliferation (see text). Other secretory products from platelets such as platelet factor 4 (PF4) may be chemotactic to monocytes or transforming growth factor-β (TGF-β) may contribute to proliferation of SMC. Similar mechanisms are present after mild injury (right) but occur to a lesser degree.

complete endothelial denudation, only partial ingrowth from healthy endothelial borders is possible (65).

Endothelial Cells

Endothelial cells may regulate SMC proliferation. Synthesis and secretion of $PDGF_C$ are increased in injured endothelial cells (68). Several agonists may stimulate production and release of $PDGF_C$ by endothelial cells and include tumor necrosis factor, TGF-β (present in large quantities in platelets), thrombin (induces dose-dependent $PDGF_C$ secretion), factor Xa, and agents that injure endothelial cells such as bacterial endotoxin phorbol esters (68–73). Because thrombin is adsorbed to fibrin within thrombi and intimal lesions and appears active from histochemical demonstration using fluorogenic substrate (74–82), thrombin within intimal lesions might stimulate production and release of $PDGF_C$ by endothelial cells. In the pig, endothelial cells are regrown by 1 week after balloon injury at which time they are also functional (63, 83). Thus, in vivo production of GFs or inhibitors may be closely regulated by endothelial cells.

Endothelium may also release other factors that stimulate SMC proliferation (84). Endothelium is a rich source of bFGF, a cell-associated mitogen released by agents that injure endothelial cells and appears important in the maintenance of endothelial cells, but also stimulates proliferation of SMCs and fibroblasts (37). Porcine vascular cells produce a PDGF-like mitogen, and porcine SMCs respond to purified porcine PDGF with a proliferative response (85). Many other factors may also play a role in cellular proliferation after arterial injury. These may act alone or synergistically with PDGF and include interleukin-1, angiotensin-converting enzyme (which may induce PDGF-A expression in SMCs), and insulin-like GF (86–89).

Mechanisms of Mural Thrombosis: The Role of Thrombin

Arterial mural thrombosis with severe platelet and fibrinogen deposition is thrombin dependent, occurs within minutes of type III or deep arterial injury, tracks along the region of deep injury, and appears related to the surface area of deep injury after balloon dilation. Mural thrombosis may lead to acute occlusion, even in previously normal arteries, or subsequent organization of mural thrombus with fibromuscular proliferation and arterial stenosis within a month of injury (55,63, 90–94). Major factors contributing to thrombosis are the rheology of blood flow and arterial wall substrates for thrombosis. These are modified by less potent systemic factors such as the blood lipids, catecholamines, lipoprotein-associated coagulation inhibitor (LACI), factor VII, fibrinogen levels, and modifiers of thrombolysis such as plasminogen activator inhibitor (PAI-1).

Arterial substrates for thrombosis are similar whether type III or deep injury is into the normal media or intimal plaque. These substrates include collagen types I and III, tissue thromboplastin, decreased prostacyclin, phospholipid in cell membranes for formation of activator complexes within the coagulation cascade, and loss of endothelium and its antithrombotic protection (1,3). Macroscopic mural thrombus is strongly anchored to the deeply injured arterial wall. Mild injury or endothelial denudation exposes less thrombogenic collagen types IV and V to flowing blood and results in only a single layer of platelet deposition.

The *rheology of blood flow* may be aggravated by vasoconstriction. Shear force is directly related to blood flow and inversely to the third power of the lumen diameter. Higher shear forces cause red blood cells to force platelets to the periphery and increase cell membrane adenosine diphosphate (ADP). Platelet deposition is maximal within the MLD of the stenosis and becomes red and more fibrin-rich distal to the stenosis (1,3,95–97). These factors increase the risk of occlusion and restenosis in inadequately dilated arteries after PTCA (22–29).

Thrombogenic Risk of Mural Thrombus

Residual mural thrombus is a more thrombogenic substrate than the deeply injured arterial wall (98). This results in increased risk of acute occlusion (6%–68% incidence) and restenosis after PTCA in patients with unstable angina or after thrombolysis (26,98–102). The increased thrombogenicity of mural thrombus also accounts for the increased risk of myocardial infarction, refractory angina, and death in patients with unstable angina (102,103). This increased thrombogenicity relates to the substrate of mural thrombus, which contains active thrombin adsorbed to fibrin by a site on thrombin near the C-terminal end and separate from its catalytic site (75–81). Thrombin adsorbed to fibrin becomes internalized as the thrombus grows and is freshly exposed to flowing blood by catheter dislodgment, partial embolization, or lysis.

This stimulates more platelets to deposit because platelets are exquisitely sensitive to activation by thrombin (64, 92, 93).

Role of Thrombin

Although in vitro activation and aggregation of platelets can be stimulated by a variety of substances including thromboxane A_2, serotonin, ADP, collagen, and thrombin, inhibition of in vitro aggregation does not predict the in vivo response to inhibitors of these substances. Blockade of thromboxane A_2, serotonin, or both receptors did not significantly decrease platelet deposition after deep arterial injury, but did decrease injury-associated vasoconstriction (104).

Heparin has both antithrombin and antifactor Xa effects. To test the possible effectiveness of antithrombin or antifactor Xa effects in vivo, we administered increasing doses of unfractionated heparin immediately before balloon angioplasty. Increasing doses of unfractionated heparin significantly reduced quantitative platelet and fibrinogen deposition but did not completely eliminate mural thrombus after deep injury (92). Administration of low molecular weight heparin (CY216), which has a greater antifactor Xa effect, was not significantly different than unfractionated heparin for the reduction of mural thrombosis, platelet deposition, or fibrinogen deposition. Reduction in arterial thrombosis was most closely correlated with the antithrombin rather than the anti-Xa effect (105). Additional in vivo studies defined the importance of thrombin in deep arterial injury. Specific thrombin inhibition with hirudin, the anticoagulant of the European leech, inhibits platelet aggregation to thrombin but not to thromboxane A_2, serotonin, ADP, or collagen. However, recombinant hirudin (CGP 39393) reduces fibrinogen deposition at lower doses (mean activated partial thromboplastin time, aPTT 1.7 × control) and at higher doses (aPTT 2 to 3 × control) totally eliminates mural thrombosis and reduces platelet deposition to a single layer or less in vivo after deep arterial injury by angioplasty (93). Combining heparin with low-dose aspirin (1 mg/kg/per day) or aspirin plus dipyridamole was better than placebo in reducing mural thrombosis but did not eliminate mural thrombus as did specific and potent (K_A 10^{-14}) thrombin inhibition with hirudin (19). Thus, specific thrombin inhibition with hirudin sets a new treatment standard and therapeutic goal for the total elimination of mural thrombus after deep arterial injury by angioplasty.

Different blood levels of thrombin inhibition are required depending on the pathogenesis of thrombosis and which action of thrombin is being inhibited. Hirudin forms a 1:1 stoichiometric complex with thrombin. The blood level of hirudin required to totally inhibit thrombosis in vivo appears to be a measure of the thrombin content of the pathologic condition or lesion. In the absence of any arterial injury fives times the blood level of hirudin is required to inhibit platelet thrombi compared to fibrin thrombi in the pulmonary circulation during disseminated intravascular coagulation (106). This illustrates the exquisite sensitivity of platelets to thrombin. Studies in pigs and rats suggest that the thrombin content of deeply injured arteries appears to be eight to ten times greater than that of mildly injured (type II injury) or deendothelialized arteries (93,106,107). Immunohistochemical staining for thrombin within thrombus overlying a total occlusion with adjacent deep arterial injury compared to adjacent mild injury shows positive staining for thrombin adjacent to deep injury but not adjacent to mild injury; this is a second method of demonstrating the increased thrombin content and thus increased thrombogenicity of deeply injured artery (108).

The addition of an arterial *metallic stent* to deeply injured artery appears to further increase the thrombin content of the pathologic condition because the dose of hirudin that totally inhibited mural thrombus will no longer totally prevent mural thrombus when the metallic stent is placed in the deeply injured artery (109). However, high-dose thrombin inhibition can prevent thrombosis within a metallic stent under other circumstances (metallic stent placed within a Gortex graft; 110).

Thrombin also binds to arterial subendothelial matrix and remains active (111). We are currently studying whether additional thrombin is present (bound or generated) in the matrix of deeply injured artery.

Future Directions

The first step and probably the cornerstone of reducing the incidence of restenosis appears to be total prevention of mural thrombosis after deep arterial injury by angioplasty. Without prevention of thrombus, a large bulk of intraluminal material and a huge supply of GFs will not be eliminated.

Other mechanisms of blocking arterial thrombosis may be examined. The blocking of glycoprotein platelet–membrane receptors such as against glycoprotein IIb/IIIa do not appear as promising because antibodies to glycoprotein IIb/IIIa do not appear to be effective at low shear (112) where total prevention of mural thrombus after successful dilation would appear to be desirable. In addition, hirudin (but not heparin) completely blocks growth of mural thrombus at high and low shear (113).

Blocking thrombin generation at a more proximal level in the coagulation cascade may be effective and perhaps safer than direct inhibition of thrombin because systemic anticoagulation may be avoided. This is currently being explored.

Intravenous specific thrombin inhibition can totally prevent intraluminal mural thrombus (92,93). However, our preliminary observations suggest that it does not prevent intramural thrombus within the tears and fissures of the arterial wall. Because tears and fissures are a normal occurrence with balloon angioplasty (7–16), new approaches are needed. This may involve local delivery of antithrombotic therapy in high concentrations into the arterial wall, newer methods of lasing or cutting to prevent tears and fissures, or both. Both approaches are being studied and show promise.

The duration of antithrombotic therapy after angioplasty is under study in animals and also requires definition in patients. The dosage of antithrombin therapy for total prevention of intraluminal mural thrombus requires definition in human beings and is under study.

Inhibitors of specific GFs require study in a large animal model such as the pig or baboon under balloon angioplasty conditions that produce deep arterial injury as in patients. Only after successful completion of such animal studies should human studies be considered. In this way unnecessary, expensive, time-consuming, and possibly risky human studies may be avoided.

References

1. Chesebro JH, Webster MWI, Reeder GS, et al. Coronary angioplasty: antiplatelet therapy reduces acute complications but not restenosis (abstr). Circulation 1989;80(suppl II):64.
2. Rogers J, Garratt KN, Kaufmann UP, Vlietstra RE, Bailey KR, Holmes DR. Restenosis after atherectomy vs PTCA: initial experience (abstr). J Am Coll Cardiol 1990;15:197A.
3. Ip JH, Fuster V, Israel D, Badimon L, Badimon J, Chesebro JH. The role of platelets, thrombin and hyperplasia in restenosis after coronary angioplasty. J Am Coll Cardiol 1991;17(suppl):77B–88B.

4. Uchida Y, Hasegawa K, Kawamura K, Shibuya I. Angioscopic observation of the coronary luminal changes induced by percutaneous transluminal coronary angioplasty. Am Heart J 1989;117:769–776.

5. Mizuno K, Miyamoto A, Sakurada M, et al. Evaluation of coronary thrombi after PTCA by angioscopy (abstr). Circulation 1989;80(suppl II):523.

6. Yanagida S, Mizuno K, Miyamoto A, et al. Comparison of findings between coronary angiography and angioscopy (abstr). Circulation 1989;80(suppl II):376.

7. Kohchi K, Takebayashi S, Block PC, Hiroki T, Nobuyoshi M. Arterial changes after percutaneous coronary angioplasty: results at autopsy. J Am Coll Cardiol 1987;10:592–599.

8. Ueda M, Becker AE, Fujimoto T. Pathological changes induced by repeated percutaneous transluminal coronary angioplasty. Br Heart J 1987;58:635–643.

9. Block PC, Myler RK, Stertzer S, Fallen JT. Morphology after PTCA in human beings. N Engl J Med 1981;305:382–385.

10. Farb A, Virmani R, Atkinson JB, Kolodgie FD. Plaque morphology and pathologic changes in arteries from patients dying after coronary balloon angioplasty. J Am Coll Cardiol 1990;16:1421–1429.

11. Essed CE, van den Brand M, Becker AE. Transluminal coronary angioplasty and early restenosis: fibrocellular occlusion after wall laceration. Br Heart J 1983;49:393–396.

12. Austin GE, Ratliff NB, Hollman J, Tabei S, Phillips DF. Intimal proliferation of smooth muscle cells as an explanation for recurrent coronary artery stenosis after percutaneous transluminal coronary angioplasty. J Am Coll Cardiol 1985;6:369–375.

13. Colavita PG, Ideker RE, Reimer KA, Hackel DB, Stack RS. The spectrum of pathology associated with percutaneous transluminal coronary angioplasty during acute myocardial infarction. J Am Coll Cardiol 1986;8:855–860.

14. Solymoss BC, Gote G, Leung TK, et al. Pathology of percutaneous transluminal coronary angioplasty complications (abstr). Circulation 1988;78(suppl II):445.

15. O'Hara T, Nanto S, Asada S, Konamura K, Wang DY. Ultrastructural study of proliferating and migrating smooth muscle cells at the site of percutaneous transluminal coronary angioplasty as an explanation for restenosis (abstr). Circulation 1988;78(suppl II):290.

16. Potkin BN, Roberts WC. Effects of percutaneous transluminal coronary angioplasty on atherosclerotic plaques and relation of plaque composition and arterial size to outcome. Am J Cardiol 1988;62:41–50.

17. Johnson DE, Hinohara T, Selmon MR, Braden LJ, Simpson JB. Primary peripheral arterial stenoses and restenoses excised by transluminal atherectomy: a histopathologic study. J Am Coll Cardiol 1990;15:419–425.

18. Heras M, Chesebro JH, Penny WJ, Bailey KR, Badimon L, Fuster V. Effects of thrombin inhibition on the development of acute platelet-thrombus deposition during angioplasty in pigs: heparin versus recombinant hirudin, a specific thrombin inhibitor. Circulation 1989;79: 657–665.

19. Lam JYT, Chesebro JH, Steele PM, Heras M, Badimon L, Fuster V. Antithrombotic therapy for arterial injury by angioplasty: Efficacy of common platelet-inhibitors versus thrombin inhibition in pigs. Circulation 1991;84:814–820.

20. Schwartz L, Bourassa MG, Lesperance J, et al. Aspirin and dipyridamole in the prevention of restenosis after percutaneous transluminal coronary angioplasty. N Engl J Med 1988;318:1714–1719.

21. Dehmer GJ, Popma JJ, van den Berg EK, et al. Reduction in the rate of early restenosis after coronary angioplasty by a diet supplemented with n-3 fatty acids. N Engl J Med 1988;319:733–740.

22. Guiteras VP, Bourassa MG, David PR, et al. Restenosis after successful percutaneous transluminal coronary angioplasty: the Montreal Heart Institute experience. Am J Cardiol 1987;60(suppl B):50B–55B.

23. Kaltenbach M, Kober G, Scherer D, Vallbaracht C. Recurrence rate after successful coronary angioplasty. Eur Heart J 1985;6:276–281.

24. Levine S, Ewels CJ, Rosing DR, Kent KM. Coronary angioplasty: Clinical and angiographic follow-up. Am J Cardiol 1985;55:673–676.

25. Mata LA, Bosch X, David PR, Rapold HJ, Corcos T, Bourassa MG. Clinical and angiographic assessment 6 months after double vessel percutaneous transluminal coronary angioplasty. J Am Coll Cardiol 1985; 6:1239–1244.

26. Leimgruber PP, Roubin GS, Hollman J, et al. Restenosis after successful coronary angioplasty in patients with single-vessel disease. Circulation 1986;73:710–717.

27. Wijns W, Serruys PW, Reiber JHC. Early detection of restenosis after successful percutaneous transluminal coronary angioplasty by exercise redistribution. Am J Cardiol 1985;55:357–361.

28. Holmes DR Jr, Vlietstra RE, Smith HC, et al. Restenosis after percutaneous transluminal coronary angioplasty (PTCA): a report from the PTCA registry of the National Heart, Lung, and Blood Institute. Am J Cardiol 1984;53:77C–81C.

29. Chesebro JH, Webster MWI, Reeder GS, et al. Coronary angioplasty:

antiplatelet therapy reduces acute complications but not restenosis. Circulation 1989;80(suppl II):64.

30. El-Tamimi H, Davies GJ, Hackett D, Fragasso G, Crea F, Maseri A. Very early prediction of restenosis after successful coronary angioplasty: anatomic and functional assessment. J Am Coll Cardiol 1990;15:259–264.

31. Clowes AW, Reidy MA, Clowes MM. Kinetics of cellular proliferation after arterial injury. I. Smooth muscle growth in the absence of endothelium. Lab Invest 1983;49:327–333.

32. Majesky MW, Reidy MA, Bowen-Pope DF, Hart CE, Wilcox JN, Schwartz JM. PDGF ligand and receptor gene expression during repair of arterial injury. J Cell Biol 1990;111:2149–2158.

33. Snow AD, Bolender RP, Wright TN, Clowes AW. Heparin modulates the composition of the extracellular matrix domain surrounding arterial smooth muscle cells. Am J Pathol 1990;137:313–330.

34. Fingerle J, Johnson R, Clowes AW, Majesky MW, Reidy MA. Role of platelets in smooth muscle cell proliferation and migration after vascular injury in rat carotid artery. Proc Natl Acad Sci USA 1989;86:8412–8416.

35. Fingerle J, Au WPT, Clowes AW, Reidy MA. Intimal lesion formation in rat carotid arteries after endothelial denudation in absence of medial injury. Arteriosclerosis 1990;10:1082–1087.

36. Capron L, Bruneval P. Influence of applied stress on mitotic response of arteries to injury with a balloon catheter: quantitative study in rat thoracic aorta. Cardiovasc Res 1989;23:941–948.

37. Lindner V, Lappi DA, Baird D, Majack RA, Reidy MA. Role of basic fibroblast growth factor in vascular lesion formation. Circ Res 1991;68:106–113.

38. Webster MWI, Chesebro JH, Heras M. Mruk JS, Grill DE, Fuster V. Effect of balloon inflation on smooth muscle cell proliferation in the porcine carotid artery. J Am Coll Cardiol 1990;15:188A.

39. Huang C-L, Ives HE. Growth inhibition by protein kinease C late in mitogenesis. Nature 1987;329:849–850.

40. Berk BC, Taubman MB, Gragoe EJ, Fenton JW, Griendling KK. Thrombin signal transduction of mechanisms in rat vascular smooth muscle cells. J Cell Biol 1990;265:17334–17340.

41. Berk BC, Taubman MB, Griendling KK, et al. Thrombin-stimulated events in cultured vascular smooth muscle cells. Biochem J 1991;274:799–805.

42. Hassler O. The origin of the cells constituting arterial intima thickening: an experimental autoradiographic study with the use of H3-thymidine. Lab Invest 1970;22:286–293.

43. Webster WS, Bishop SP, Geer JC. Experimental aortic intimal thickening. Am J Pathol 1974;76:245–260.

44. Thorgeirsson G, Robertson AL, Cohen DH. Migration of human vascular endothelial and smooth muscle cells. Lab Invest 1979;41:51–62.

45. Grotendorst GR, Seppa HEJ, Kleinman HK, et al. Attachment of smooth muscle cells of collagen and their migration toward platelet-derived growth factor. Proc Natl Acad Sci USA 1981;78:3669–3672.

46. Ihnatowycz IO, Winocour PD, Moore S. A platelet-derived factor chemotactic for rabbit arterial smooth muscle cells in culture. Artery 1981;9:316–317.

47. Battegay EJ, Raines EW, Seifert RA, Bowen-Pope DF, Ross R. TGF-Beta induces biomodal proliferation of connective tissue cells via complex control of an autocrine PDGF loop. Cell 1990;63(3):515–524.

48. Nakao J, Ooyama T, Chang WC, et al. Platelets stimulate aortic smooth muscle cell migration in vitro. Atherosclerosis 1982;43:143–150.

49. Ferns GA, Raines EW, Sprugel KH, Montani AS, Reidy MA, Ross R. Inhibition of neointimal smooth muscle accumulation after angioplasty by an antibody to PDGF. Science 1991;253:1129–1132.

50. Moore S, Friedman RJ, Singal DP, et al. Inhibition of injury induced thromboatherosclerotic lesions by anti-platelet serum in rabbits. Thromb Haemost 1976;35:70–81.

51. Libby P, Warner SJC, Salomon RN, Birinyi LK. Production of platelet-derived growth factor-like mitogen by smooth-muscle cells from human atheroma. N Engl J Med 1988;318:1493.

52. Bernstein LR, Antantoniades H, Zetter BR. Migration of cultured vascular cells in response to plasma and platelet-derived factors. J Cell Sci 1982;56:71–82.

53. Weinstein R, Stemerman MB, Maciag T. Hormonal requirements for growth of arterial smooth muscle cells in vitro: an endocrine approach to atherosclerosis. Science 1981;212:818–820.

54. Clowes AW, Schwartz SM. Significance of quiescent smooth muscle migration in the injured rat carotid artery. Circ Res 1985;56:139–145.

55. Webster MWI, Chesebro JH, Grill DE, Badimon JJ, Badimon L. Influence of deep and mild injury on smooth muscle cell proliferation after angioplasty. Circulation 1991;84(suppl II):296.

56. Woolf N. Interaction between mural thrombi and underlying artery wall. Haemostasis 1979;8:127–141.

57. Woolf N, Carstairs KC. Infiltration and thrombosis in atherogenesis: a study using immunofluorescent techniques. Am J Path 1967;51:373–386.

58. Woolf N, Carstairs KC. The survival time of platelets in experimental mural thrombi. J Path 1969;97:595–601.

59. Woolf N, Bradley JWP, Crawford T, et al. Experimental mural thrombi in the pig aorta. The early natural history. Br J Exp Path 1968;49:257–264.

60. Woolf N, Davies MJ, Bradley JPW. Medial changes following thrombosis in the pig aorta. J Path 1971;105:205–209.

61. Woolf N, Crawford T. Fatty streaks in the aortic intima studied by an immuno-histochemical technique. J Path Bact 1960;80:405–408.

62. Friedman RJ, Stemerman MB, Wenz B, et al. The effect of thrombocytopenia on experimental atherosclerotic lesion formation in rabbits. J Clin Invest 1977;60:1191–1201.

63. Steele PM, Chesebro JH, Stanson AW, et al. Balloon angioplasty: natural history of the pathophysiologic response to injury in a pig model. Circ Res 1985;57:105–112.

64. Shuman MA. Thrombin-cellular interactions. Ann NY Acad Sci 1986;485:228–239.

65. Clowes AW, Clowes MM, Reidy MA. Kinetics of cellular proliferation after arterial injury. III. Endothelial and smooth muscle growth in chronically denuded vessels. Lab Invest 1986:54:295–303.

66. Clowes AW, Reidy MA, Cloes MM. Mechanisms of stenosis after arterial injury. Lab Invest 1983;49:208–215.

67. Minick CR, Stemerman MB, Insull W Jr. Role of endothelial and hypercholesterolemia in intimal thickening and lipid accumulation. Am J Pathol 1979;95:131–158.

68. Fox PL, DiCorleto PE. Regulation of production of a platelet-derived growth factor-like protein by cultured bovine aortic endothelial cells. J Cell Physiol 1984;121:298–308.

69. Hajjarka KA, Hajjarka DP, Silverstein RL, et al. Tumor necrosis factor-mediated release of platelet-derived growth factor from cultured endothelial cells. J Exp Med 1987;166:235–245.

70. Daniel TO, Gibbs VC, Milfay DF, et al. Agents that increase cAMP accumulation block endothelial c-SIS induction by thrombin and transforming growth factor-beta. J Biol Chem 1987;262:11893–11896.

71. Daniel TO, Gibbs VC, Milfay DF, et al. Thrombin stimulates c-SIS gene expression in microvascular endothelial cells. J Biol Chem 1986;261:9579–9582.

72. Gajdusek C, Carbon S, Ross R, et al. Activation of coagulation releases endothelial cell mitogens. J Cell Biol 1986;103:419–428.

73. Harlan JM, Thompson PJ, Ross RR, et al. Alpha-thrombin induces re-

lease of platelet-derived growth factor-like molecule(s) by cultured human endothelial cells. J Cell Biol 1986;103:1129–1133.

74. Oka K, Tanaka K. Histochemical demonstration of thrombin using fluourogenic substrate. Thrombos Res 1980;19:125–128.

75. Seegers WH, Nieft M, Loomis EC. Note of the absorption of thrombin on fibrin. Science 1945;101:520–521.

76. Liu CY, Nossel HL, Kaplan KL. The binding of thrombin by fibrin. J Biol Chem 1979;254:10421–10425.

77. Francis CW, Markham RE Jr, Barlow GH. Thrombin activity of fibrin thrombi and soluble plasmic derivatives. J Lab Clin Med 1983; 102:220–230.

78. Kaminski M, McDonagh J. Studies on the mechanism of thrombin: Interaction with fibrin. J Biol Chem 1983;258:10530–10535.

79. Berliner LJ, Sugawara Y. Human α-thrombin binding to nonpolymerized fibrin-sepharose: evidence for an anionic binding region. Biochemistry 1985;24:7005–7009.

80. Kaminski M, McDonagh J. Inhibited thrombins: Interactions with fibrinogen and fibrin. Biochem J 1987;242:881–887.

81. Vali Z, Scheraga HA. Localization of the binding site on fibrin for the secondary binding site of thrombin. Biochemistry 1988;27:1956–1963.

82. Tam WS, Fenton JW, Detwiler TC. Dissociation of thrombin from platelets by hirudin. J Biol Chem 1979;254:8723–8725.

83. Webster MWI, Chesebro JH, Heras M, Mruk JS, Grill DE. Acetylcholine infusion identifies regrowth after porcine coronary endothelial denudation. Circulation 1989;80(suppl II):648.

84. Koo EWY, Gottlieb AI. Endothelial stimulation of intimal cell proliferation in a porcine aortic organ culture. Am J Path 1989;134:497–503.

85. Johnson CM, Hanson MN, Helgeson SC, et al. Porcine cardiac valvular subendothelial cells in culture: cell isolation and growth characteristics. J Mol Cell Cardiol 1987;19:1185–1193.

86. Clinton SK, Dinarello CA, Cannon JG, Shaw AR, Libby P. Induction in vivo of interleukin-1 (IL-1) gene expression in rabbit aortic tissue. Circulation 1988;78(suppl II):65.

87. Powell JS, Clozel JP, Muller RKM, et al. Inhibitors of angiotensin-converting enzyme prevent myointimal proliferation after vascular injury. Science 1989;245:186.

88. Naftilan AJ, Pratt RE, Dzau VJ. Induction of platelet-derived growth factor A-chain and c-myc gene expression by angiotensin II in cultured rat vascular smooth muscle cells. J Clin Invest 1989;83:1419.

89. Ross R, Raines EW, Bowen-Pope DF. The biology of platelet-derived growth factor. Cell 1986;46:155.

90. Ip JH, Fuster V, Badimon L, Badimon JJ, Taubman MB, Chesebro JH. Syndromes of accelerated atherosclerosis: role of vascular injury and smooth muscle cell proliferation. J Am Coll Cardiol 1990;15:1667–1687.

91. Heras M, Chesebro JH, Penny WJ, Bailey KR, et al. Importance of adequate heparin dosage in arterial angioplasty in a porcine model. Circulation 1988;78:654–660.

92. Heras M, Chesebro JH, Penny WJ, Bailey KR, Badimon L, Fuster V. Effects of thrombin inhibition on the development of acute platelet-thrombus deposition during angioplasty in pigs: heparin versus recombinant hirudin, a specific thrombin inhibitor. Circulation 1989; 79:657–665.

93. Heras M, Chesebro JH, Webster MWI, et al. Hirudin, heparin and placebo during deep arterial injury in the pig: the in vivo role of thrombin in platelet-mediated thrombosis. Circulation 1990;82:1476–1484.

94. Lam JYT, Chesebro JH, Steele PM, Badimon L, Fuster V. Is vasospasm related to platelet deposition? Relationship in a porcine preparation of arterial injury in vivo. Circulation 1987;75:243–248.

95. Lam JYT, Chesebro JH, Fuster V. Platelets, vasoconstriction, and nitroglycerin during arterial wall injury: a new antithrombotic role for an old drug. Circulation 1988;78:712–716.

96. Badimon L, Badimon JJ, Galvez A, Chesebro JH, Fuster V. Influence of arterial damage and wall shear rate on platelet deposition. Ex vivo study in a swine model. Arteriosclerosis 1986;6:312–320.

97. Badimon L, Badimon JJ. Mechanism of arterial thrombosis in non-parallel streamlines: platelet growth at the apex of stenotic severely injured vessel wall. Experimental study in the pig model. J Clin Invest 1989;84:1134–1144.

98. Badimon L, Lassila R, Badimon J, Vallabhajosula S, Chesebro JH, Fuster V. Residual thrombus is more thrombogenic than severely damaged vessel wall (abstr). Circulation 1988;78(suppl II):119.

99. Califf RM, Topol EJ, George BS. Characteristics and outcome of patients in whom reperfusion with intravenous tissue- type plasminogen activator fails. Circulation 1988;77:1090–1099.

100. Baim DS, Diver DJ, Knatterud GL. PTCA "salvage" for thrombolytic failures—implications from TIMI II-A. Circulation 1988;78(suppl II):112.

101. Mabin TA, Holmes DR Jr, Smith HC, et al. Intracoronary thrombus: role in coronary occlusion complicating percutaneous transluminal coronary angioplasty. J Am Coll Cardiol 1985;5:198–202.

102. Chesebro JH, Lam JYT, Badimon L, Fuster V. Restenosis after arterial angioplasty: a hemorrhagic response. Am J Cardiol 1987;60:10B–16B.

103. Theroux P, Ouimet H, McCans J, et al. Aspirin, heparin, or both to treat acute unstable angina. N Engl J Med 1988;319:1105–1111.
104. Lam JYT, Chesebro JH, Badimon L, Fuster V. Serotonin and thromboxane A_2 receptor blockade decrease vasoconstriction but not platelet deposition after deep arterial injury. Circulation 1986;74(suppl II):97.
105. Heras M, Chesebro JH, Webster MWI, et al. Antithrombotic efficacy of low molecular weight heparin after arterial injury in the pig (abstr). Arteriosclerosis and Thrombosis 1992;12:250–255.
106. Markwardt F, Kaiser B, Novak G. Studies on antithrombotic effects of recombinant hirudin. Throm Res 1989;54:377–388.
107. Ambler J, Butler KD, Kerry R, et al. Comparative effects of selective thrombin inhibition by hirudin on coagulation and thrombosis. Circulation 1989;80(suppl II):316.
108. Chesebro JH, Webster MWI, Zoldhelyi P, Roche PC, Badimon L, Badimon JJ. Antithrombotic therapy in the progression of coronary artery disease. Circulation 1992 (in press).
109. Garratt KN, Heras M, Holmes DR Jr, Roubin GS, Chesebro JH. Platelet deposition and thrombosis in arterial stents: effect of hirudin compared with heparin plus antiplatelet therapy. J Am Coll Cardiol 1990;15(suppl):209A.
110. Krupski WC, Bass A, Kelly AB, et al. Heparin-resistant thrombus formation by endovascular stents in baboons: interruption by a synthetic antithrombin. Circulation 1990;82:570–577.
111. Bar-Shavit R, Eldora A, Vlodavsky I. Binding of thrombin to subendothelial extracellular matrix. J Clin Invest 1989;84:1096–1104.
112. Badimon L, Badimon JJ, Cohen M, Chesebro JH, Fuster V. Thrombus formation in stenotic and laminar flow conditions: effect of an antiplatelet GPIIb/IIIa monoclonal antibody fragment. Circulation 1989;80(suppl II):422.
113. Badimon L, Badimon J, Lassila R, Heras M, Chesebro JH, Fuster V. Thrombin inhibition by hirudin decreases platelet thrombus growth on areas of severe vessel wall injury. J Am Coll Cardiol 1989;13:145A.

· ·

CHAPTER 10

Restenosis: Cellular Mechanisms

——

JAMES A. FAGIN
BOJAN CERCEK
JAMES S. FORRESTER

RESTENOSIS, currently estimated to occur in 40% to 50% of the dilated lesions, continues to be a major limitation to the success of transluminal angioplasty (1). No established therapy prevents or ameliorates this complication. Most vessel dilatation achieved by balloon inflation is due to stretching of the normal arterial wall. The atheromatous plaque is largely nondistensible and may fissure or crack, but does not significantly contribute to luminal enlargement. The endothelial layer, in turn, is stripped away from the balloon-treated surface, exposing the underlying media. These immediate effects of endoluminal angioplasty on the vessel wall trigger a series of events destined to repair the injury. Restenosis can be considered an undesirable consequence of this repair process (2).

In previous chapters, the role of the platelets and arterial thrombosis in the genesis of restenosis have been discussed in detail. In this review, we focus on the influence of growth factors (GF) in the vascular repair process that occurs after arterial injury. Vascular smooth muscle cells (SMCs) provide structure and elasticity to the vessel wall and are therefore primarily involved in the control of blood pressure and flow. In their differentiated, "contractile" state, they lie embedded in the medial layer of the vessel, where they constitute the only cell type. Medial SMCs are normally in a near-quiescent state, with a replication rate of approximately 0.02%. Each cell is surrounded by a basement membrane composed of collagen type IV, laminin, entactin (nidogen), and heparin sulphate proteoglycans. This macromolecular network plays an important role in regulating homeostasis of the cells and in establishing a link with surrounding extracellular matrix proteins (3). When subjected to appropriate stimuli, a subpopulation of medial SMCs develops the ability to migrate, and also regains the capacity to proliferate. These relatively dedifferentiated, "synthetic" SMCs have additional phenotypic properties that distinguish them from their "contractile" precursors: they develop a fibroblastlike appearance and secrete extracellular matrix proteins such as elastin and collagen type I. This is accompanied by suppression of SMC-specific α-actin and myosin and loss of contractile function (4). Proliferating "synthetic" SMCs are the predominant histologic feature of the neointimal proliferative response occurring after balloon angioplasty. It is important to define the signalling mechanisms that determine the phenotypic transition, because this may provide us with better strategies to modify the biologic response to arterial injury.

As an immediate consequence of balloon dilatation, the endothelial layer is removed from the injured site. At least three major events result from deendothelialization: platelet adhesion, loss of growth inhibitory factors made by endothelial cells, and absence of the normal permeability barrier to compounds present in plasma.

Role of Platelets

Within minutes of endothelial injury, platelets adhere to the denuded surface and rapidly degranulate. A number of platelet factors stored in α granules are released locally into the exposed intimal layer. Prominent among them is platelet-derived growth factor (PDGF), a glycoprotein dimer with powerful mitogenic and chemotactic activity on vascular SMCs. PDGF is a glycoprotein homodimer or heterodimer made of two chains (A and B) linked by disulfide bonds. It has been postulated that this growth factor may be the major initiator of the local vascular response to injury (5). It is noteworthy that adhering platelets largely disappear within hours of injury, yet SMC migration and proliferation occur over a course of days or weeks (6). PDGF can bind to the glycosaminoglycan heparin, which is present in the extracellular milieu of the vascular wall, and could conceivably serve as a reservoir for the GF long after platelets are no longer present in the injured vessel surface. Several lines of evidence indicate, however, that platelets are not an absolute requirement for vascular repair. Inhibition of platelet adhesion with antiplatelet drugs before endothelial denudation results in only partial decrease of neointimal proliferation in New Zealand rabbits (7) and has almost no effect in rats (8). In clinical studies, the incidence of restenosis after coronary angioplasty is not affected by prior therapy with aspirin and dipyridamole (9). These data support the concept that the restenotic process is not entirely dependent on platelet function and that other regulatory pathways must be involved in controlling the response to injury.

Endothelium-Derived Growth Inhibitors

After angioplasty, areas that remain denuded of endothelium for a longer period have greater SMC hyperplasia, whereas reendothelialization is often associated with cessation of SMC growth. Because of this, it has been postulated that endothelial cells may elaborate factors that inhibit SMC proliferation (10). Endothelial cell–conditioned medium blocks vascular SMC replication in vitro, an effect largely abolished by prior digestion with heparanase, suggesting that the inhibitory effect is due to heparinlike products made by endothelial cells. Heparin and heparinlike species are effective antiproliferative agents for vascular SMC. The action of heparin is probably not due to binding and inactivation of mitogens such as PDGF or fibroblast growth factors (FGF), but rather to a specific receptor-mediated inhibition of cell division. Thus, SMC proliferation after injury may be facilitated through loss of the tonic growth inhibition normally exerted by heparinlike species made by endothelial cells.

Loss of Permeability Barrier

Deendothelialization is associated with removal of the normal permeability barrier of the vessel wall, thus allowing unrestricted access of factors present in plasma to the inner layers of the artery. In this manner, plasma-derived mitogens (i.e., insulinlike growth factors [IGF], epidermal growth factor [EGF], serotonin, and many others) may be directly involved in inducing migration or growth of medial SMC. The plasma protein fibronectin has also been shown to have major effects on the phenotypic properties of SMC. Fibronectin promotes the transition of rat aortic SMCs from a contractile to a synthetic phenotype (3). The dedifferentiating effects of fibronectin on SMC are mediated through the cell attachment sequence of the protein (Arg-Gly-Asp-Ser, RGDS). Interestingly, DNA replication and SMC proliferation do not occur in the presence of fibronectin unless serum or PDGF is also present. This suggests that plasma-derived fibronectin may modulate SMC phenotype, rendering the cells competent to divide in response to GFs.

Role of Growth Factors in Restenosis

As discussed above, the histologic hallmark of restenosis is neointimal SMC proliferation. There is considerable information on the potential role played by various polypeptide mitogens and cytokines in this process. We will discuss the significance of some of the candidate GFs of major pathophysiologic significance.

Fibroblast Growth Factors

Injuries that cause little or no trauma to the media elicit only minor SMC hyperplasia (11). It is possible that trauma disrupts the basement membrane or the extracellular matrix network surrounding SMC, therefore allowing free interaction with mitogens or other regulatory proteins. Additionally, SMC death may promote growth of neighboring cells through liberation of stored growth factors or cytokines. Vascular SMC synthesize angiogenic factors such as FGF, with powerful mitogenic activity for SMC and endothelial cells (12). Solid evidence indicates that FGFs remain largely cell associated. Because they lack a signal peptide sequence, they cannot be secreted in a similar fashion as other growth factors such as PDGF and IGF-I. For reasons presently unclear, FGFs are found not only associated with cells, but also stored in the basement membrane and extracellular matrix. After traumatic injury to the arterial media, FGFs could be released from damaged or dying SMC. Furthermore, heparanases and proteases from infiltrating macrophages have the potential to degrade the extracellular matrix and release FGFs stored in the pericellular space. The potential biologic relevance of these observations was recently demonstrated in vivo (13).

Rats treated with a blocking antibody to basic FGF had decreased SMC proliferation after balloon catheter injury, suggesting that this GF may be significant in the process of vessel repair and restenosis.

Platelet-Derived Growth Factors

As mentioned above, a number of powerful mitogens are released by platelets on adhesion to the damaged vessel wall (i.e., PDGF, EGF, transforming GFs). However, the process of restenosis is not adequately prevented by blocking platelet function. Because of this, it has been postulated that GFs or cytokines elaborated within the vessel wall may be involved with the induction or perpetuation of SMC migration and proliferation. Balloon injury induces medial SMC to produce PDGF-AA, an isoform of PDGF that has strong mitogenic activity but is not as effective as PDGF-AB or PDGF-BB in promoting migration (14). Expression of PDGF-AA peaks a few hours after injury and falls to near basal levels within 24 hours (15). Additionally, regenerating endothelial cells and macrophages secrete PDGF-BB, although the production of this PDGF isoform is not significantly modulated during experimental vascular injury. These data are compatible with the following role for PDGF in the first hours after balloon angioplasty: platelets release PDGF-AB and -BB, which serve as an initial stimulus to both SMC migration and proliferation; on activation, SMC produce PDGF-AA, which further induces cellular growth in a paracrine fashion but does not contribute to cell chemotaxis. A recent observation compatible with this hypothesis was made in rats rendered thrombocytopenic with antiplatelet antibodies. In these animals, SMC proliferation after balloon injury was unimpaired, whereas neointimal plaque formation did not take place, demonstrating a platelet-dependent effect on SMC migration (16).

Insulinlike Growth Factors

Platelet-derived growth factor stimulates cell growth through interaction with specific plasma membrane receptors and activation of an intracellular signal cascade, which ultimately leads to DNA synthesis and cell division. However, PDGF requires the presence of additional GFs to maximally stimulate cell replication. PDGF has been termed a "competence factor" in that it enables cells to move from the quiescent (G0) to the G1 phase of the cell cycle. The target cells require a second class of GFs, termed "progression factors," in order for DNA synthesis to take place. One of the best characterized progression factors for PDGF-mediated mesenchymal cell growth is IGF-I (17). IGF-I, also termed somatomedin C, mediates the growth-promoting effects of pituitary growth hormone and is abundantly present in plasma. IGF-I is markedly synergistic with PDGF to induce SMC growth in vitro. Furthermore, there is evidence that SMC can make IGF-I, and that this production is, in turn, stimulated by PDGF (18,19). Thus, PDGF can induce the production of its own progression factor. It is likely that this process may also be occurring in vivo. IGF-I gene expression is markedly increased in rat aorta after balloon angioplasty, with maximal production at 7 days after injury (20). Besides functioning as a progression factor for PDGF-induced growth, local overproduction of IGF-I in the vascular media may serve other important reparative functions. IGF-I is an effective stimulus for tropoelastin biosynthesis (21), and thus may be involved in regenerating the damaged medial elastin layer after balloon trauma. Indeed, vascular IGF-I gene expression after injury is prominent among SMCs in the vascular media, potentially providing a paracrine stimulus to repair the elastin macromolecular network.

The significance of the synergism between PDGF and IGF-I is highlighted by recent studies on another in vivo model of wound healing (22). When applied topically to partial thickness porcine skin wounds, the combination of PDGF and IGF-I was by far the most effective stimulator of healing (compared to nine individual factors and eight other combinations). This synergism was apparent in the promotion of dermal cell proliferation as well as hydroxyproline content of the 7-day-old wounds.

The IGFs circulate in plasma complexed with a number of high affinity-binding proteins. Four IGF-binding proteins have been isolated from human and rat samples and the complete cDNA and amino acid sequences determined: IGFBP-1, IGFBP-2, IGFBP-3, and IGFBP-4. IGFBP-3 is the major IGFBP in serum, is growth hormone dependent, and binds IGF-I and IGF-II with equal affinity. IGFBP-1 has a predicted mass of 25.3 kd; is expressed by multiple cell types including placenta, uterus, and HEP-G2 cells; and binds IGF-I and IGF-II with equally high affinity. IGFBP-2 has been purified from conditioned medium of BRL-3A rat liver cells, has a molecular mass of 31 kd, and has a much higher affinity for IGF-II than IGF-I. Recently an inhibitory IGF-binding protein, IGFBP-4, has been isolated and cloned from a human osteoblastlike osteosarcoma cell line (23). The role of IGFBPs in regulating the function of IGFs is complex and appears to depend on the nature of the IGFBP, the cell type, and culture conditions. In most systems, IGFBPs have been found to antagonize IGF action by interfering with ligand binding to the receptor. Relatively little is known about IGFBPs in vascular SMCs. We have recently observed that IGFBP-4 is abundantly expressed by SMCs, and that PDGF can markedly induce its expression (19). The functional role of tissue IGF-binding proteins in vivo and in vitro is not understood. They may serve as carriers, endogenous agonists or antagonists, or storage sites for the IGFs. It is likely, however, that they modulate the local bioavailability of these growth factors.

Transforming Growth Factor-β

Transforming growth factor-β (TGF-β) is a homodimeric polypeptide ubiquitously expressed by mammalian cells and is released by cells localized at the site of tissue repair, such as activated macrophages, lymphocytes, and possibly vascular SMCs (24). Depending on cell type, and experimental conditions, it has both growth inhibitory and growth stimulatory properties. A latent form of TGF-β is stored in the α granules of platelets, indicating that SMCs may be exposed to this polypeptide after endothelial injury. At low concentrations, TGF-β stimulates SMC growth, probably through autocrine induction of PDGF-AA production. At higher concentrations, TGF-β decreases the expression of the PDGF-α receptor, and thus functions as a growth inhibitor (25). Thus, the ultimate effects of this peptide depend on its bioavailability within the vascular wall. Besides its effects on cell proliferation, TGF-β is a major regulator of extracellular matrix production, as will be discussed below.

Angiotensin II

Recently, angiotensin-converting enzyme (ACE) inhibitors (cilazapril and captopril) inhibited myointimal proliferation after balloon arterial injury in rats (26). These effects were not due to the hypotensive effects of the compounds since calcium channel antagonists such as verapamil did not prevent SMC proliferation despite eliciting an equivalent decrease of mean arterial blood pressure. A preliminary retrospective study suggests that ACE inhibitors may also decrease restenosis in human subjects (27). Angiotensin II alone is not considered a significant mitogen for SMCs, although it does significantly stimulate protein synthesis (28). However, angiotensin II induces the expression of the proto-oncogenes c-fos, c-jun, and c-myc, suggesting that at least part of the subcellular cascade of events necessary for DNA synthesis and cell growth is activated. It is possible that angiotensin II requires one or more cofactors to effectively promote SMC growth. Although angiotensin II probably does not augment PDGF-induced cell proliferation, evidence indicates that it may enhance growth of mouse fibroblast NIH3T3 cells induced by EGF. Recently, the angiotensin II receptor has been identified and cloned. Additionally, competitive and noncompetitive inhibitors of the receptor are now available (29). It is, therefore, possible to effectively block angiotensin II action in vivo, which will allow a better understanding of its potential significance in inducing smooth muscle hyperplasia.

Extracellular Matrix Production

In the clinical setting, restenosis occurs 3 to 6 months following intervention, well beyond the time course of SMC migration and proliferation. The bulk of the increase in plaque size is due to deposition of extracellular matrix proteins by synthetic vascular SMCs. Histologic evaluation of human restenotic lesions reveals that the predominant matrix components are collagen and glycosaminoglycans (GAG). GAG appear to be the more important component of the early restenotic lesions, followed by collagen deposition after 6 months. The two major GAG synthesized by vascular SMCs are dermatan sulphate and chondroitin sulphate. TGF-β is a powerful stimulus to the production of GAG and may be a major factor regulating the early matrix deposition phase of vascular repair. In fibroblasts TGF-β can also activate the expression of other matrix proteins, such as collagen and fibronectin (30). In contrast, the effects of TGF-β on SMC production of collagen subtypes and fibronectin are at best modest. Interestingly, angiotensin II markedly stimulates GAG synthesis, a fact that might explain the beneficial effects of angiotensin II in preventing restenosis (Bailey WL, et al., unpublished observations). Much remains to be learned, however, about the complex control mechanisms for matrix deposition after vascular injury. However, because proteoglycan deposition forms the bulk of the restenotic plaque, this aspect of the process is attractive for targeted therapeutic interventions.

Conclusions

We have discussed the role of GFs in the vascular response to injury and restenosis. It is increasingly apparent that the healing process is subject to multiple redundant and often overlapping control mechanisms. For instance, at least two powerful mitogens, PDGF and FGF, are likely to play a role in inducing SMC proliferation. PDGF derives from a variety of sources (i.e., platelets, SMCs, macrophages), and simply preventing release from one of these (i.e., platelets) provides only a marginal decrease in myointimal proliferation and clinical restenosis. IGF-I may be an "amplifying factor" for SMC growth, a final common pathway for the full-blown mitogenic effects of PDGF and FGF to take place. The potential role of angiotensin II (either derived from plasma or generated locally within the vessel wall) is clearly intriguing and offers opportunities for therapeutic interventions.

References

1. Nobuyoshi M, Kimura T, Noksaka H, et al. Restenosis after successful percutaneous transluminal coronary angioplasty: serial angiographic follow-up of 229 patients. J Am Coll Cardiol 1988;12:616–623.
2. Forrester JS, Fishbein M, Helfant R, Fagin JA. A paradigm for restenosis based on cell biology: clues for the development of new prevention therapies. J Am Coll Cardiol 1990;17:758–769.
3. Thyberg J, Hedin U, Sjolund M, et al. Regulation of differentiated properties and proliferation of arterial smooth muscle cells. Arteriosclerosis 1990;10:966–990.
4. Gabbiani G, Kocher O, Bloom WS, et al. Actin expression in smooth muscle cells of rat aortic intimal thickening, human atheromatous plaque, and cultured rat aortic media. J Clin Invest 1984;73:148–152.
5. Ross R. The pathogenesis of atherosclerosis—an update. N Engl J Med 1986;314:488–500.
6. Wilentz J, Sanborn T, Haudenschild C, Valeri C, Repan T, Faxon D. Platelet accumulation in experimental angioplasty: time course in relation to vascular injury. Circulation 1987;75:636.
7. Faxon DP, Sanborn JA, Haudenschild CC, Ryan TJ. Effect of antiplatelet therapy on restenosis after experimental angioplasty. Am J Cardiol 1984;53:72C–76C.
8. Clowes AW, Karnovsky MJ. Failure of certain antiplatelet drugs to affect

myointimal thickening following arterial endothelial injury in the rat. Lab Invest 1977;36:452–464.

9. Schwartz L, Bourassa MG, Lesperance J, et al. Aspirin and dipyridamole in the prevention of restenosis after percutaneous transluminal coronary angioplasty. N Engl J Med 1988;318:1719–1724.

10. Castellot JJ, Wright TC, Karnovsky MJ. Regulation of vascular smooth muscle cell growth by heparin and heparan sulphates. Semin Thromb Hemost 1987;13:489–503.

11. Fingerle J, Tina Au YP, Clowes AW, Reidy MA. Intimal lesion formation in rat carotid arteries after endothelial denudation in absence of medial injury. Arteriosclerosis 1990;10:1082–1087.

12. Klagsbrun M, Edelman ER. Biological and biochemical properties of fibroblast growth factors. Implications for the pathogenesis of atherosclerosis. Arteriosclerosis 1989;9:269–278.

13. Lindner V, Reidy MA. Proliferation of smooth muscle cells after vascular injury is inhibited by an antibody against basic fibroblast growth factor. Proc Natl Acad Sci USA 1991;88:3739–3743.

14. Siegbahn A, Hammacher A, Westermark B, Heldin C-H. Differential effects of the various isoforms of platelet-derived growth factor on chemotaxis of fibroblasts, monocytes, and granulocytes. J Clin Invest 1990;85:916–920.

15. Majesky MW, Reidy MA, Bowen-Pope DF, Hart CE, Wilcox JN, Schwartz SM. PDGF ligand and receptor gene expression during repair of arterial injury. J Cell Biol 1990;111:2149–2158.

16. Fingerle J, Johnson R, Clowes AW, Majesky MW, Reidy MA. Role of platelets in smooth muscle proliferation and migration after vascular injury in rat carotid artery. Proc Natl Acad Sci USA 1989;86:8412–8416.

17. Stiles CD, Capone GT, Scher CDE, Antoniades HN, Van Wyk JJ, Pledger WJ. Dual control of cell growth by somatomedins and platelet-derived growth factor. Proc Natl Acad Sci USA 1979;76:1279–1282.

18. Clemmons DR. Variables controlling the secretion of a somatomedin-like peptide by cultured porcine smooth muscle cells. Circ Res 1985; 56:418–426.

19. Giannella-Neto D, Kamyar A, Forrester J, Fagin JA. PDGF isoforms induce IGF-I gene expression in rat vascular smooth muscle cells and stimulate the biosynthesis of IGF-binding proteins. Circulation 1990; 82:828A.

20. Cercek B, Fishbein MC, Forrester JS, Helfant RH, Fagin JA. Induction of insulin-like growth factor I messenger RNA in rat aorta after balloon denudation. Circ Res 1990;66:1755–1760.

21. Foster J, Rich CB, Florini J. Insulin-like growth factor I, somatomedin C,

induces the synthesis of tropoelastin in aortic tissue. Coll Relat Res 1987;7:161–169.

22. Lynch SE, Colvin RB, Antoniades HN. Growth factors in wound healing. Single and synergistic effects on partial thickness porcine skin wounds. J Clin Invest 1989;84:640–646.

23. LaTour D, Mohan S, Linkharb TA, et al. Inhibiting insulin-like growth factor-binding protein: cloning, complete sequence, and physiological regulation. Mole Endocrinol 1990;4:1806–1814.

24. Sporn MB, Roberts AB, Wakefield LM, deCrombrugghe B. Some recent advances in the chemistry and biology of transforming growth factor-beta. J Cell Biol 1987;105:1039–1045.

25. Battegay EJ, Raines EW, Seifert RW, et al. TGF-beta induces bimodal proliferation of connective tissue cells via complex control of an autocrine PDGF loop. Cell 1990;63:515–524.

26. Powell JS, Clozel JP, Muller RKM, et al. Inhibitors of angiotensin-converting enzyme prevent myointimal proliferation after vascular injury. Science 1989;245:186–188.

27. Gottlieb NB, Gottlieb RS, Morganroth J, et al. Prevention of restenosis after PTCA by angiotensin converting enzyme inhibitors. J Am Coll Cardiol 1990;17:181A.

28. Berk BC, Vekshtein V, Gordon HM, et al. Angiotensin II- stimulated protein synthesis in cultured vascular smooth muscle cells. Hypertension 1989;13:305–314.

29. Chiu AT, Carini DJ, Duncia JV, et al. DuP 532: a second generation of nonpeptide angiotensin II receptor antagonists. Biochem Biophys Res Commun 1991;177:209–217.

30. Ignotz RA, Massague J. Transforming growth factor-beta stimulates the expression of fibronectin and collagen and their incorporation into the extracellular matrix. J Biol Chem 1986;261:4337–4345.

CHAPTER **11**

. . . .

Lipids and Restenosis

——

JAMES J. FERGUSON
JAMES T. WILLERSON

ATHEROSCLEROTIC coronary vascular disease remains the leading cause of death in the industrialized world, accounting for more than a million deaths per year in the United States alone. The treatment of cardiovascular disease has advanced considerably over the last three decades, with the development of direct coronary angiography by Mason Sones in 1959 (1), the pioneering efforts of Rene Favoloro in developing coronary artery bypass grafting (CABG) surgery in 1968 (2), and the visionary work of Andreas Gruentzig in developing and applying the technique of balloon angioplasty to human coronary vessels in 1977 (3). The therapeutic options of CABG and balloon angioplasty are currently widely applied to the treatment of atherosclerotic coronary vascular disease. In 1987, approximately 332,000 CABG procedures and 184,000 percutaneous transluminal coronary angioplasty (PTCA) procedures were performed (4). Although the volume of CABG has remained relatively constant over recent years, the initial strict indications for PTCA have been expanded, and this technique is applied with increasing frequency. In 1991 an estimated 300,000 PTCA procedures were done.

Both CABG and PTCA are not without limitations. CABG has associated risks, and the grafts have a finite life span. The occlusion rate of saphenous bypass grafts is 15% to 20% in the first year. Between year 1 and year 5, the occlusion rate is approximately 2% per year, which increases to approximately 4% per year in year 6. By 5 to 7 years after bypass surgery, the overall occlusion rate is 25% to 35%; by 10 years, the occlusion rate is 40% to 50% (5).

Balloon angioplasty also has associated procedural risks and, as it is currently applied, has a restenosis rate of somewhere between 20% and 45%, depending on the criteria used for the definition of restenosis. Most restenosis lesions occur in the first 6 months following the procedure. As the application of PTCA has expanded, the incidence of restenosis has become a major limiting factor. It appears that the incidence of restenosis may be even higher following "high-risk" or complex PTCA procedures, and that the currently higher overall incidence of restenosis seen at some centers may be because of the expanding application of PTCA to more complex lesions and multivessel disease. Restenosis is also a problem for the new interventional modalities, such as lasers, atherectomy devices, and stents. Initial hopes that mechanical factors might improve the rate of restenosis have not been borne out, and for the most part, these new techniques appear to have restenosis rates similar to conventional balloon angioplasty.

This chapter focuses on the relationship between serum lipids and restenosis. The issues are complex and require an understanding not only of background issues relating lipids (in the form of cholesterol) to the development of atherosclerosis, but the importance of lipids and lipoproteins to the complex process of restenosis, which involves interactions among the coagulation system, blood elements, and vessel wall. This chapter reviews some of the clinical and experimental work examining the effect of lipid-lowering therapy on atherosclerosis and restenosis, both from an epidemiologic and a preventive standpoint. This chapter also examines the potential relationships between lipoprotein-a (Lp[a]) and the coagulation system, and further discusses the role of agents (such as HMG-CoA reductase inhibitors and fish oils) whose role in the prevention of restenosis may have nothing to do with their lipid-lowering effects. With this background information, clinicians should be able to draw meaningful conclusions about the potential relationships between lipids and restenosis following PTCA and begin to interpret the current contradictory clinical data.

Background Issues

Lipids and Lipoprotein Metabolism

Three types of lipids play a major metabolic role in the body: cholesterol, triglycerides, and phospholipids. It is important to understand some background information about each of the three (Table 11.1). Cholesterol is the most abundant sterol in human plasma; it is both absorbed from dietary intake and synthesized in vivo. In normal people, about one sixth to one third comes from dietary sources and enters the blood indirectly via the thoracic duct in the form of chylomicra. The rest is synthesized by the liver and enters the blood in lipoprotein form. Approximately two thirds of cholesterol is in the form of cholesterol esters rather than free cholesterol. The liver, because it can esterify cholesterol, is the major organ involved in regulating serum cholesterol levels. Regardless of its source, cholesterol is incorporated into plasma lipoproteins and cells throughout the body and serves as a substrate for the synthesis of steroid hormones. Cholesterol is broken down in the

Table 11.1. Blood Lipids

CHOLESTEROL

Absorbed from diet and synthesized (liver)
Dietary cholesterol enters blood as chylomicra
66% in ester form
Broken down in liver

TRIGLYCERIDES

Absorbed from diet and synthesized (throughout body)
Ester of 3 fatty acids with glycerol
Dietary triglycerides hydrolyzed, absorbed, resynthesized, and enter blood as
    chylomicron
Removed and stored by adipose tissue, can be broken down later for use as
    energy source

PHOSPHOLIPIDS

Most abundant lipid in plasma
Widely distributed throughout the body, mostly in form of lecithin
Most synthesized in liver
Play important role in coagulation
May help stabilize cholesterol and triglycerides in plasma

liver; bile acids, the major detergents in bile, are the direct result of cholesterol breakdown.

Triglycerides arise from both dietary intake and in vivo synthesis. Synthesis occurs in almost all tissues of the body, especially in adipose tissues, liver, and intestine. Triglycerides themselves are esters of three fatty acid molecules with glycerol. Dietary triglycerides must first be hydrolyzed to monoglycerides and free fatty acids, which are then absorbed across the intestinal wall, resynthesized into triglycerides by intestinal cells, and released as chylomicra into intestinal lymph. They also enter the blood finally as chylomicra via the thoracic duct. Chylomicra can be used as an energy source by skeletal or cardiac muscle, but are more frequently removed by adipose tissue and stored. When needed, stored triglycerides are broken down to fatty acids and released into the circulation where they can be used as an energy source. Nonused free fatty acids are taken up again by the liver and resynthesized to triglycerides. The liver can also synthesize triglycerides from nonlipid precursors, such as glucose.

Phospholipids are the most abundant lipid in plasma and a major component of plasma lipoproteins. Like cholesterol, they are widely distributed throughout the body, both in cells and in myelinated nerve sheaths. Most ($\sim 70\%$) of plasma phospholipids are in the form of lecithin (phosphatidyl choline). Phospholipids can be synthesized by all cells, but most of the plasma phospholipids are probably synthesized in the liver; they can be broken down by most of the cells in the body. Phospholipids play an important role in the coagulation system; additionally, they may help stabilize the less polar lipids (cholesterol and triglyceride) within the lipoprotein molecules in plasma.

It is also important to understand the metabolic pathways of lipoproteins as they are synthesized in the liver and metabolized in the body (Figure 11.1). The lipoprotein cascade is initiated in the liver, which produces very low-density lipoprotein (VLDL), the first of a series of lipoprotein molecules. Circulating VLDL contains much less cholesterol than triglyceride and is acted on by lipoprotein lipase in the tissue capillaries to remove a large amount of triglyceride (and some protein), producing intermediate-density lipoprotein (IDL) with nearly equal amounts of cholesterol and triglyceride. IDL is further reduced to low-density lipoprotein (LDL) by lipoprotein lipase, with almost all of the triglyceride being removed, leaving cholesterol as the primary lipid component. LDL then serves as the primary vehicle whereby cholesterol is delivered to the tissues.

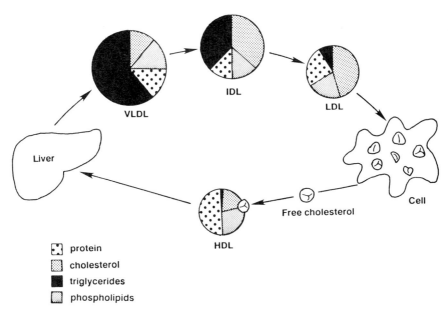

Figure 11.1. The lipoprotein metabolic cycle. The liver produces VLDL, which is converted to IDL, and then LDL by lipoprotein lipase. LDL serves as the primary vehicle for delivery of cholesterol to tissues. HDL acts to remove cholesterol from the peripheral tissues and return it to the liver, where it can be catabolized and excreted.

High-density lipoprotein (HDL) is mostly protein and acts to remove cholesterol from cells and tissues. It picks up cholesterol from peripheral tissues by means of an enzyme (lecithin/cholesterol acyltransferase), which esterifies cholesterol and pulls it into the interior of the HDL molecule. This allows cholesterol to be brought back to the liver, where it can be catabolized and excreted. The specific mechanisms by which HDL removes cholesterol from cells are currently under investigation. Thus, the higher the serum HDL level, the more molecules available to remove the cholesterol deposited in the tissues by LDL (6).

Lipoprotein lipase is the enzyme primarily responsible for the removal of lipoprotein triglycerides from the circulation (7). It is activated on the walls of capillaries in the tissue beds to hydrolyze chylomicrons and lipoproteins, ultimately producing LDL. One interesting aspect of lipoprotein lipase is its relationship to heparin. Hahn originally reported that the administration of heparin totally cleared diet-induced lipemia in dogs (8). The fact that this phenomenon occurred only in vivo suggested that some factor was released from intact tissues into the circulation by heparin. This factor ultimately turned out to be none other than lipoprotein lipase. Furthermore, lipoprotein lipase has an affinity for heparin and binds to it avidly. Lipoprotein lipase also plays a key role in lipid and energy metabolism in the peripheral tissues.

Lipids and Atherosclerosis

An elevated blood cholesterol level appears to be an important clinical risk factor for coronary artery disease. Current theories relating to the pathogenesis of atherosclerosis revolve around the "response-to-injury" hypothesis, proposing that the critical initiating event for the development of atherosclerosis is some form of "injury" to the endothelium (9). Atherosclerotic lesions themselves consist of smooth muscle cells (SMCs) and macrophages, and may represent a continuum that spans the range from a normal defensive response to injury to a clinically significant pathologic response. Recent modifications of the response-to-injury hypothesis (10) suggest that at least two pathways may result in the formation of SMC proliferative lesions. The first pathway (present in hypercholesterolemia) involves an interaction between the vessel wall and monocytes to stimulate the growth of fibrous plaque via the release of growth factors from all four of the principal cells involved in the process of atherosclerosis: endothelium, smooth muscle, platelets, and monocyte/macrophages. The second pathway (possibly important in clinical circumstances associated with increased atherosclerosis, such as diabetes and hypertension) is a direct stimulation of the endothelium, which, in turn, releases growth factors that promote the migration and proliferation of SMCs.

The Framingham group has been studying the relationship of LDLs to coronary artery disease for nearly four decades (11) and a strong relationship between LDL and VLDL and coronary artery disease has become evident over time (Figure 11.2). On the basis of initial data from the Framingham study as well as data from other epidemiologic and experimental studies, additional prevention trials were conducted to determine whether lowering blood cholesterol could significantly reduce the incidence of coronary artery disease (12).

The Wadsworth Veterans' Administration study randomized 800 patients to a usual versus a low-cholesterol diet (13). Over an 8-year period of follow-up, an average difference of 12.7% in the serum cholesterol levels was noted between the two groups. The low-cholesterol diet

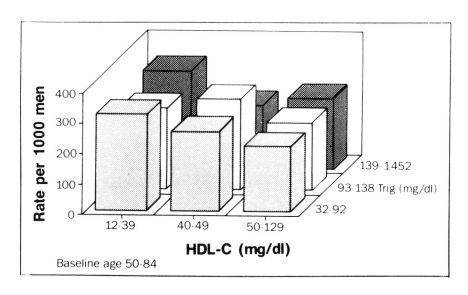

Figure 11.2. The age-adjusted 14-year rates of coronary heart disease (y axis) as a function of serum high-density lipoprotein cholesterol (HDL-C, x axis) and serum triglyceride (Trig, z axis) for men and women. (Reprinted with permission from reference 11.)

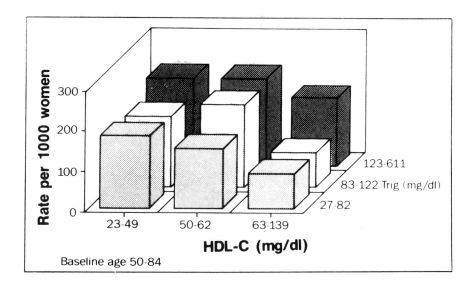

group had significantly fewer cardiovascular end points, although the study end points were mixed and somewhat subjective. Two studies in Oslo provided similar results (14,15), although the number of "hard" end points in these studies was too small to draw broad conclusions.

These preliminary studies provided a background for the large National Heart, Lung, and Blood Institute (NHLBI)-sponsored Lipid Research Clinics coronary primary prevention trial (LRC-CPPT), which involved 3806 middle-aged men with elevated (> 265) serum cholesterol levels, all of whom received dietary therapy (16). Patients with persistently elevated LDL (> 175) were randomized to diet alone versus cholestyramine and followed for 7 to 10 years. Cholestyramine therapy was effective in lowering cholesterol and LDL by 17% and 30%, respectively, and resulted in a 19% reduction in major cardiovascular end points by myocardial infarction and death, a 20% decrease in the need for bypass surgery, and a 25% decrease in the incidence of angina.

The Helsinki Heart Study was a similar primary prevention trial in which 4000 men were randomized to either gemfibrozil or placebo and followed for 5 years (17). Treatment with gemfibrozil resulted in a 30% to 40% decrease in serum triglycerides and a 10% to 11% reduction of both total and LDL cholesterol. Over the first 3 years of the trial, there was relatively little difference between the groups in primary cardiac end points. However, over the next 2 years of the study, there was a 34% decrease in cardiac events in the gemfibrozil-treated group (Figure 11.3).

Carlson and colleagues recently reported the results of a secondary prevention trial of cholesterol-lowering therapy that compared diet alone to diet plus colestipol and clofibrate in men with a recent myocardial infarction (18). After 5 years of follow-up, the treatment group had significantly lower cardiovascular mortality and total mortality.

Additional studies evaluated the effect of lowering serum cholesterol on the actual progression or regression of atherosclerosis (19). Anitschkow was the first to show that atheromatous lesions regress in an animal model of diet-induced atherosclerosis when the cholesterol-rich diet was discontinued (20). These results were confirmed in a number of other animal models of atherosclerosis, but the findings of a specific study often depend on the model chosen, the severity of the initial lesion, the other components of the plaque (calcium, fibrous tissue) as well as the absolute level of serum cholesterol (21–24).

Human studies have shown similar results. Both Vartiainen (25) and Wilens (26) showed that caloric deprivation was associated with a lower incidence of atheromatous lesions at autopsy in early studies before the

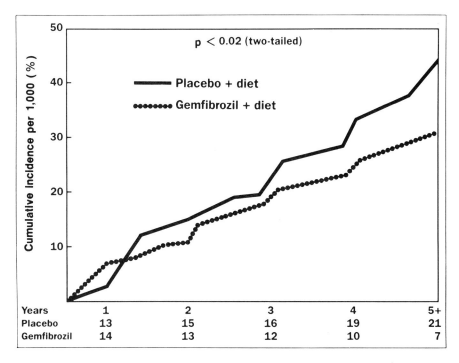

Figure 11.3. The cumulative incidence of death and myocardial infarction in the Helsinki Heart Study. (Reprinted with permission of The New England Journal of Medicine from N Engl J Med 1987;317:1237–1245.)

development of angiography. The development of angiography allowed more quantitative assessment of the extent of atherosclerosis in living human subjects. Other subsequent open-label trials incorporating angiographic assessment of disease severity have suggested that lipid-lowering therapy may result in regression of atherosclerotic lesions (27).

Brensike and colleagues (28) and Levy and coworkers (29) reported the results of the NHLBI type II coronary intervention study, in which 116 patients with type II hyperlipoproteinemia and coronary artery disease were placed on a low-fat, low-cholesterol diet and randomized to either cholestyramine (6 g qid) or placebo for a period of 5 years. Coronary angiography was performed at the end of the study, with visual interpretation of the angiograms. There was progression of coronary artery disease in 28 of 57 (49%) placebo-treated patients versus 19 of 59 (32%) of cholestyramine-treated patients. However, when only definite progression was considered, the difference did not reach statistical significance. Analysis of other end points (percent of baseline lesions with progression, lesions progressing to occlusion, regression of lesions, amount of lesion change, all cardiovascular end points) also favored cholestyramine treatment, but did not achieve statistical significance because of the limited sample size. Changes in the ratio of HDL to total cholesterol or HDL to LDL were the best predictors of change in coronary artery disease, independent of treatment with cholestyramine.

The Cholesterol-Lowering Atherosclerosis Study (CLAS) examined 160 men with established coronary artery disease who underwent coronary artery bypass grafting (30). Subjects were randomized to receive either diet alone or diet plus maximal doses of colestipol and niacin. The severity of vascular lesions in both native arteries and bypass grafts was assessed with quantitative angiography. Lesion severity was significantly reduced in the treatment group (Figure 11.4). The incidence of new lesions significantly decreased, and the old lesions already present grew less rapidly (and in some cases even regressed). This was one of the first trials to show that lipid-lowering therapy can be of significant benefit in patients with already established coronary artery disease.

Brown and coworkers also used quantitative angiography to show the effect of intensive lipid-lowering therapy on coronary atherosclerosis in

Figure 11.4. Progression/regression of vascular lesions in the CLAS study. (Adapted from reference 30.)

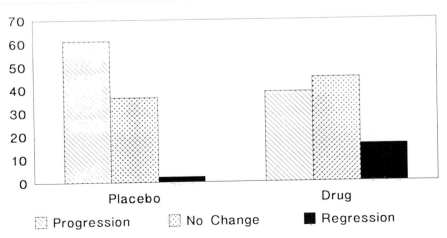

Progression / Regression of Vascular Lesions

(% of Patients)

146 men (62 years of age or younger) with documented coronary artery disease treated with either dietary counseling, diet plus lovastatin and colestipol, or diet plus niacin and colestipol (31). Treatment was maintained for a period of $2\frac{1}{2}$ years with baseline and final angiograms. Forty-six percent of the diet-alone group had angiographic progression compared to 21% of the lovastatin/colestipol group and 25% of the niacin/colestipol group. Regression was more frequent in the lovastatin/colestipol group (32%) and niacin/colestipol group (39%) than in the diet alone group (11%; Figure 11.5). Clinical events (myocardial infarction, death, revascularization) were more frequent in the diet alone group (10/52) than either the lovastatin/colestipol (3/46) or niacin/colestipol (2/48) groups.

Lipids and Restenosis

As previously mentioned, restenosis is a major factor limiting the current application of balloon angioplasty. Restenosis is a more accelerated process (< 6 months) than de novo atherosclerosis, and the role of lipids in the process of restenosis is much less clear than the role of lipids in

Figure 11.5. Progression/regression of vascular lesions in 146 men with documented coronary artery disease treated with either diet, diet plus lovastatin and colestipol, or diet plus niacin and colestipol. (Adapted from reference 31.)

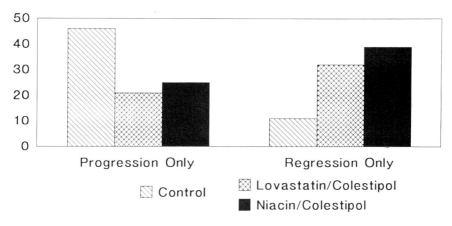

Frequency of Progression / Regression

(> 10% change in diameter stenosis)

Progression Only   Regression Only

⬚ Control   ▧ Lovastatin/Colestipol   ■ Niacin/Colestipol

atherosclerosis. A recent morphologic study by Waller and coworkers examined necropsy specimens from 20 patients with restenosis, a mean of 4.2 months after initially successful PTCA (32). Histologic analysis showed that restenosis was due to intimal proliferation in 12 of 20 (60%) patients. Nine of these 12 patients (75%) had evidence of intimal or medial balloon injury. Atherosclerotic plaque was the cause of restenosis in the eight remaining angioplasty sites, none of which had intimal proliferation. None of these eight lesions showed any evidence of previous angioplasty injury, and none showed evidence of new or accelerated atherosclerotic plaque. Six of the eight were eccentric, with variable amounts of disease-free wall.

Thus, at least two mechanisms may be responsible for restenosis. The first relates to the injury from the angioplasty procedure itself and involves intimal proliferation at the injury site. As discussed elsewhere in this book, the process of intimal proliferation is generally considered a response to damage to the endothelium or media or both, and results from a complex interaction between the coagulation system, blood elements, and the vessel wall. Plaque disruption is followed by local deposition of platelets and initiation of a restenosis "cascade" that involves platelets, SMCs, leukocytes, and the endothelium with potential humoral mediators of thromboxane, serotonin, and a variety of tissue and platelet-derived growth factors. The role of lipids in this cascade is uncertain, except as they relate to interactions with coagulation or fibroproliferative processes. Ross and Harker have shown that hypercholesterolemia promotes intimal proliferation after endothelial injury to normal arteries (33).

The second and presumably less common mechanism for restenosis is atherosclerotic progression. It has been well documented that lipids bear a direct relationship to normal atherosclerotic progression, but it is uncertain whether this mechanism is of real importance for the accelerated process of clinical restenosis. Waller and others have emphasized the importance of gradual elastic recoil as opposed to accelerated atherosclerosis (32), but as yet data are not definitive. The technique of balloon angioplasty does not physically remove any atherosclerotic material, so the progression of disease at the site of severe balloon-induced tissue injury remains a possible (albeit less likely) mechanism for restenosis.

The recent availability of directional coronary atherectomy has provided some preliminary information about the histologic composition of restenosis lesions. Initial reports emphasized the role of intimal proliferation (34,35), but recent reports suggested that it is not always possible to distinguish between restenosis lesions and de novo atherosclerosis (36). The technique of directional atherectomy provides only a focal limited sample of the overall disease process in the vessel wall, and patient selection factors may also play a role in the makeup of atherosclerotic lesions.

Do serum lipids relate to restenosis? Current data are contradictory. Myler and coworkers reported that hypercholesterolemia was an independent risk factor for restenosis following PTCA (37), but other workers found no such association (38–45). A report of pooled data from four studies (46–49) also showed no effect of cholesterol on restenosis (50). Austin and colleagues reported that restenosis developed in 5 of 6 patients in a selected subset of patients with severe (> 350) hypercholesterolemia (46). Bergelson reported a significant relationship between a number of baseline lipid measures (including total cholesterol, HDL, LDL, apolipoprotein A [apo A], apolipoprotein B [apo B], and venous ratios) and the risk of restenosis (51). Hearn and coworkers reported an association between Lp(a) and restenosis but no relationship between total cholesterol and restenosis (52). A number of other studies have not identified any lipid subfractions as predictors of restenosis (53, 54). To date, elevated triglyceride levels have not been associated with restenosis (38,40,41,44).

The sum total of all available data suggest that there *may* be an association between serum lipids and restenosis, but if present, such a relationship does not apply to the population at large, does not necessarily relate only to cholesterol, and may involve complex interactions with other risk factors. Blood lipids and serum cholesterol do not appear to be major risk factors for restenosis in the overall population, but in conjunction with other risk factors, they may have a role in the development of restenosis in selected patients. A recent preliminary study of Schmidt and colleagues also showed that elevated serum cholesterol may also be associated with the development of restenosis following directional coronary atherectomy (55).

Lipoprotein(a) and Restenosis

One intriguing aspect of the relationship of blood lipids and restenosis following PTCA is Lp(a) content (56). This unique lipoprotein combines structural elements of both the coagulation system and the lipoprotein system and is associated with an increased incidence of premature coronary artery disease and stroke. Lp(a) is assembled from LDL and a large glycoprotein called apo A. Structurally, there is striking homology between apo A and plasminogen, which plays a key role as a precursor to plasmin and the regulation of endogenous fibrinolysis. Plasminogen is cleaved by endogenous (and exogenous) plasminogen activators to form plasmin, which lyses fibrin. Lp(a) has a specific binding site for fibrin, which is a "kringle" exactly homologous to the fibrin binding sites of plasmin (Figure 11.6). The binding of Lp(a) to fibrin may be responsible for lipid and lipoprotein accumulation at sites of endothelial damage, and it may competitively interfere with the endogenous activation of plasminogen to plasmin. A number of epidemiologic studies have

Figure 11.6. There is considerable homology between the structure of Lp(a) and the structure of plasminogen. The "kringles" on both molecules act as fibrin binding sites.

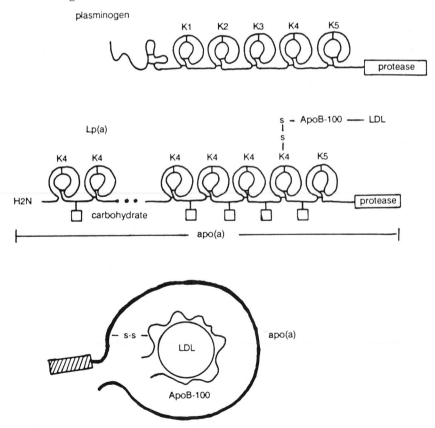

shown a positive relationship between Lp(a) and premature coronary artery disease and myocardial infarction. Lp(a) is generally felt to be an independent genetic risk factor for atherosclerotic vascular disease.

A recent study by Hodenberg and colleagues (57) examined whether a relationship exists between the serum level of Lp(a) and the outcome of thrombolysis. Theoretically, if Lp(a) plays a key role in inhibiting endogenous thrombolysis, it may also affect the therapeutic efficacy of exogenously administered plasminogen activators for the treatment of acute myocardial infarction. This study in 41 patients (30 with successful reperfusion, 11 with unsuccessful reperfusion) showed no relationship between the level of Lp(a) and the outcome of thrombolytic therapy, but this same question is currently under active investigation at other centers.

Other studies have examined possible relationships between lipoproteins and restenosis. The previously cited study by Bergelson and colleagues demonstrated a significant relationship between apo B and apo A-I and restenosis (51). Hearn and coworkers have also shown that Lp(a) and the HDL-cholesterol ratio are independent predictors of restenosis (52). Much work needs to be done to further elucidate how Lp(a) may fit into the restenosis process.

A fundamental question currently unanswered is whether Lp(a) is related to atherogenesis because of its lipoproteinlike qualities or whether it is due to its plasminogenlike structure. A number of potential mechanisms are possible, including competitive inhibition of plasminogen activators, impairment of endogenous thrombolytic activity, or perhaps some manner in which Lp(a) becomes incorporated into a site of endothelial injury and serves as a nidus for the deposition of additional atherosclerotic material. A recent study by Ring and colleagues showed the presence of intracoronary fibrin degradation following routine balloon angioplasty (58), and given the ability of Lp(a) to bind fibrin, Lp(a) may have an important role in influencing the events that occur shortly after balloon angioplasty. Lp(a) is a potential linkage that connects the lipid-related aspects of restenosis with the coagulation- and thrombus-related aspects of restenosis.

Preventing Restenosis

Given the theoretical background and the epidemiologic evidence to date, what evidence is there that lipid-lowering therapy may affect restenosis? The information available to date is limited, and there is as yet no definitive answer. Although some of the preliminary data can be viewed as cautiously encouraging, there is still no evidence that lipid lowering in and of itself can affect the process of restenosis.

Gellman and coworkers examined the effect of lovastatin (an HMG-CoA reductase inhibitor) on intimal hyperplasia after balloon angioplasty in atherosclerotic hypercholesterolemic rabbits (59). Initial atherosclerotic lesions were created by air desiccation injury followed by a high cholesterol diet. Balloon angioplasty was performed on the atherosclerotic lesions, and the animals were randomized to either lovastatin or control, and killed 39 days after the procedure. The percent decrease in luminal diameter was significantly less in the lovastatin-treated group than in the control group, and intimal thickness in the lovastatin group was also significantly less than in the control group (Figure 11.7). Theoretically, lovastatin could work by inhibiting DNA synthesis and cell growth, by reducing serum cholesterol, by some combination of the two, or by some as yet unknown mechanism. The authors believed that the cholesterol-lowering effect alone was not adequate to explain the beneficial effects of lovastatin in these overtly hypercholesterolemic animals, but that HMG-CoA reductase inhibitors may have a role in preventing restenosis.

Figure 11.7. Quantitative histologic analysis of intima, lumen, and media in rabbits with restenosis following angioplasty treated with lovastatin. (Reprinted with permission of the American College of Cardiology from J Am Coll Cardiol 1991;17:251–259.)

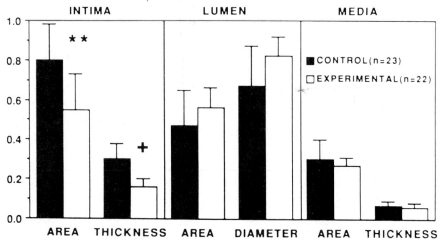

Preliminary results of a randomized, controlled clinical trial of lovastatin for the prevention of restenosis were reported by Sahni and colleagues (60). They found that 4% of the treated vessels and 14% of the PTCA sites developed restenosis in the lovastatin group, in comparison to 38% of the treated vessels and 47% of the PTCA sites in the control group. The authors concluded that lovastatin significantly reduced the incidence of restenosis following successful PTCA.

In contrast, a study by Hollman and coworkers showed that aggressive cholesterol lowering with a combination of diet, colestipol, and lovastatin had no effect on the incidence of restenosis in 55 consecutive patients (61). A study by Zhao and coworkers examined the role of cholesterol-lowering therapy on "late" regression (at 2.5 years post-procedure) of 18 post-PTCA lesions in the patients participating in the Familial Atherosclerosis Treatment Study (FATS; 62). They showed that late regression of post-PTCA lesions was greater in frequency and magnitude than that of non-PTCA lesions, and that regression occurred only in the setting of intense lipid-lowering therapy (lovastatin plus colestipol or niacin plus colestipol).

The Lovastatin Restenosis Trial is a multicenter, randomized, blinded, placebo-controlled study of approximately 400 PTCA patients treated with diet and either lovastatin or placebo. The results of this trial are not currently available, but they will help to better define whether lovastatin may have a significant role in reducing the incidence of restenosis following PTCA.

Fish Oil Studies

Omega-3 fatty acids, such as eicosapentaenoic acid (EPA) and docosahexaenoic acid (DHA) are present in large quantities in cold water fish such as mackerel, herring, bluefish, and salmon (63). Epidemiologic studies have suggested that Greenland Eskimos (who eat large amounts of fish) have a low incidence of coronary thrombosis (64–66). In general, omega-3 fatty acids will favorably affect the lipid profile (decrease plasma triglyceride and total cholesterol, increase HDL) and will inhibit platelet aggregation and alter neutrophil and monocyte function (Table 11.2).

Two of the major classes of polyunsaturated fatty acids are the n-6 (or omega-6) and the n-3 (or omega-3) fatty acids. Because human beings are unable to synthesize fatty acids with double bonds beyond the ninth carbon atom from the carboxyl terminus, linoleic acid (an n-6 fatty acid)

Table 11.2. Antiatherogenic Effects of Fish Oils

1. Competition with arachidonic acid
   a. Decreased levels of platelet arachidonic acid
   b. Decreased production of thromboxane A_2 (a vasoconstrictor) and prevention of platelet aggregation
   c. Little inhibition of PGI_2 (prostacyclin, a vasodilator and inhibitor of platelet aggregation)
   d. Inhibition of LTB_4 production (leukotriene B_4, a potentiator of inflammation and white blood cell recruitment)
2. Decreased blood viscosity
3. Increased endogenous fibrinolytic activity
4. Decreased arterial blood pressure
5. Decreased vasospastic response to catecholamines
6. Increased endothelial-dependent relaxation in coronary arteries
7. Platelet inhibition

and α-linoleic acid (an n-3 fatty acid) must be ingested as part of the diet. Linoleic acid is a precursor for the subsequent synthesis of eicosanoids, including both prostaglandins (synthesized via the cyclooxygenase pathway) and leukotrienes (synthesized via the 5-lipoxygenase pathway; Figure 11.8). α-Linoleic acid, on the other hand, is the precursor for the synthesis of EPA and DHA. When n-3 fatty acids (such as EPA and DHA) are included in the diet, they compete with arachidonic acid and

Figure 11.8. Metabolism of n-6 (arachidonic acid) and n-3 (eicosapentaenoic acid) fatty acids to prostanoids and leukotriene. (Reprinted with permission of The New England Journal of Medicine from N Engl J Med 1988;318:549–557.)

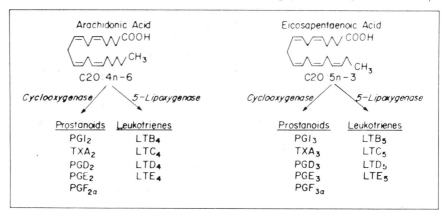

eicosanoic synthesis in three ways: EPA and DHA can inhibit the synthesis of arachidonic acid; they can compete with arachidonic acid for binding sites on phospholipids; and they can inhibit the production of thromboxane A_2 by competing with arachidonic acid as the substrate for cyclooxygenase (63).

The n-3 fatty acids also compete with arachidonic acid as a substrate for conversion (by 5-lipoxygenase) to leukotrienes, which are strong attractants of leukocytes and monocytes, and which participate in allergic, inflammatory, and immune responses and in the vascular response to ischemia. The n-3 fatty acids also have a number of other effects that may inhibit atheroma formation. They decrease arterial pressure (67, 68) and blood viscosity (69; by increasing erythrocyte deformability), thus potentially improving oxygen delivery to distal tissues. They increase endogenous fibrinolytic activity by both decreasing the levels of inhibitors of plasminogen activator and increasing the levels of tissue plasminogen activator itself (70). Administration of n-3 fatty acids also decreases the vasospastic response to catecholamines (67) and increases the endothelial-dependent relaxation in coronary arteries (71). The n-3 fatty acids may also directly inhibit platelets via a direct action on the platelet membrane (72,73).

A number of animal studies strongly suggest that fish oils may retard the development of atherosclerosis. In animal models of atherosclerosis, omega-3 fatty acids inhibit both intimal hyperplasia and coronary atherosclerosis. Landymore and coworkers have shown in dogs that dietary supplementation with cod liver oil prevents intimal hyperplasia in autologous arterial grafts (74,75). Davis and colleagues have shown that fish oil prevents the progression of atherosclerosis in nonhuman primates over a 12-month period, but their results may be confounded somewhat by the simultaneous changes in the dietary content of saturated fats (76). Weiner and coworkers have shown that dietary cod liver oil prevents intimal hyperplasia in coronary arteries in hypercholesterolemic (diet-induced) swine (77). This effect appeared to be independent of any cholesterol-lowering effects.

A number of clinical studies have sought to determine whether dietary therapy with fish oils can prevent restenosis following PTCA. The results of these clinical trials are more contradictory than the initial experimental data might have suggested.

Dehmer and colleagues conducted a randomized, unblinded study in 82 male patients undergoing PTCA who were assigned to either conventional antiplatelet therapy (aspirin 325 mg/day, dipyridamole 225 mg/day) or a similar regimen supplemented with 3.2 g EPA per day, starting 7 days prior to PTCA and continuing for a period of 6 months (78). The incidence of restenosis was significantly decreased in the group receiving fish oils, both per patient (19% versus 46% in the control group) and per lesion (16% versus 36% in the control group; Figure 11.9).

Grigg and coworkers studied 108 patients (89 men, 19 women) randomized either to conventional therapy (aspirin 150 mg/day, verapamil 80 mg tid) plus control capsules (50% olive oil, 50% corn oil) or conventional therapy plus fish oil (1.2 g EPA, 1.2 g DHA), starting the day before angioplasty and continuing for 4 months after the procedure (79). Follow-up angiography (100) or postmortem examination (1) was performed in 101 patients (94%). There was no significant difference in the fish oil versus control restenosis rate, either by patient (34% versus 33%) or by lesion (29% versus 31%). Triglyceride levels were significantly lower in the fish oil–treated group, but no significant differences occurred between groups in cholesterol levels or platelet counts.

Milner and colleagues studied 194 patients who were randomized to receive either conventional therapy (aspirin and a calcium antagonist) or conventional therapy plus high doses of omega-3 fatty acid (Promega, 9 capsules per day = 4.5 g fish oil daily) initiated 24 hours after PTCA

Figure 11.9. The effect of fish oil therapy in 82 male PTCA patients. (Adapted from reference 78.)

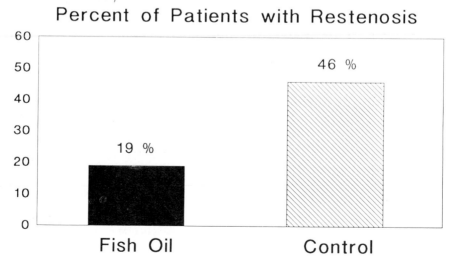

(80). Eighty-four patients continued fish oil therapy for 6 months, 11 patients withdrew from therapy within 1 week, and 99 patients were the control group. The end points were a combination of clinical symptoms (100%), exercise testing (92%), and angiography when clinically indicated (23%). The overall incidence of clinical restenosis was 19% in the fish oil–treated group, 46% in the group who withdrew from therapy within 1 week, and 35% in the control group.

Reis and colleagues conducted a double-blind study in 196 PTCA patients who were randomized to receive either conventional therapy (aspirin 325 mg/day + calcium channel blockers + dipyridamole 50 mg qid) plus olive oil placebo or conventional therapy plus omega-3 fatty acids (6 g/day) given either as ethyl-ester (SuperEPA) or triglyceride (Promega) beginning 5.4 ± 3.2 days before PTCA and continuing for 6 months (81). Follow-up included telephone contact, exercise testing, and coronary angiography if clinically indicated. Angiographic restenosis was present in 42 (34%) of 124 patients on fish oil and 14 (23%) of 62 patients on placebo (Table 11.3). They also noted that 7% of fish oil patients had symptomatic progression of their disease as opposed to 3% of controls, and that 6% of fish oil patients had a myocardial infarction during the 6 months of follow-up, as opposed to no one in the control group. They raised the possibility that fish oils may have had some detrimental effect in the population being tested.

Slack and colleagues reported a study in which patients undergoing PTCA were randomized to conventional therapy (nitrates, aspirin, dipyridamole, calcium channel blockers) or conventional therapy plus fish oils (max EPA, 6 to 9 capsules/day; 82). They found no difference in the clinical restenosis rate in patients undergoing multivessel PTCA (20 of 30 fish oil patients [67%] versus 11 of 19 control patients [58%]).

Table 11.3. Incidence of Restenosis and Clinical Events in 186 PTCA Patients Randomized for Fish Oil or Placebo

	FISH OIL (n = 124)	PLACEBO (n = 62)
Angiographic restenosis	42 (33%)	14 (23%)
Clinical restenosis	44 (35%)	15 (24%)
Progression of other disease	9 (7%)	2 (3%)
Myocardial infarction	7 (6%)	0
Repeat PTCA	36 (30%)	13 (21%)
Late bypass grafting	5 (4%)	3 (5%)
Any major clinical event	47 (38%)	16 (26%)

However, in single vessel disease, 8 of 50 fish oil-treated patients (16%) developed restenosis in comparison to 21 of 63 control patients (33%).

Bowles and coworkers studied 85 PTCA patients randomized to either conventional therapy or conventional therapy plus 2.8 g/day of EPA, started within 24 hours of successful PTCA (83). Patients were followed for 6 months and repeat angiography was performed. They found no significant difference in restenosis rates between groups.

In summary, the fish oil data are not consistent. Fish oils may provide a protective advantage in selected populations (such as single vessel disease or men at high risk for restenosis), but studies will be necessary to more definitively identify those groups that will derive maximum benefit. Other adjunctive therapies (such as calcium blockers or antiplatelet drugs) may also influence the efficacy of fish oil. It may be important to provide pretreatment for up to 1 week prior to PTCA to show a protective effect. It is clear from the data currently available that fish oils are not always protective and that more work is necessary to sort out the other factors contributing to the success or failure of fish oils in preventing restenosis after PTCA. In designing these studies, it will be important to control for the patient population being tested, the time at which fish oil therapy is started, and the adjunctive medications received.

Conclusions and Future Directions

From the currently available data, no inexorable conclusions can be drawn regarding the relationship between lipids and restenosis. The accelerated process of restenosis is different from de novo atherosclerosis, and although lipids clearly play a role in native atherosclerosis, their role in the complex metabolic interactions involved in restenosis is much less clear. Potential areas of overlap between lipids and the coagulation system include the relationship between heparin and lipoprotein lipase and the homology between Lp(a) and plasminogen. However, these remain almost purely theoretical at the present time. Lipids appear to play a role in the progression or regression of native atherosclerosis; they may have a role in the progression or regression of atherosclerotic lesions following PTCA and may also have a role in restenosis following other types of interventional procedures.

Lipid-lowering agents may be of benefit in protecting against restenosis in selected populations, but the potential benefit derived from agents, such as the HMG-CoA reductase inhibitors and fish oils, may not be related solely to their lipid-lowering effects. Lipid-lowering therapy may be of benefit in preventing or modifying restenosis in selected populations and, given some of the initial positive results, certainly deserves further study. The results of the multicenter lovastatin restenosis study are still pending, and hopefully future trials will look at combination therapy such as fish oils plus HMG-CoA reductase inhibitors or even combinations of fish oils or HMG-CoA reduction inhibitors with other agents that may be of benefit in reducing restenosis.

Acknowledgment: The authors would like to acknowledge the invaluable assistance of Angie Ruiz and Jennie Walker in the preparation of the manuscript.

References

1. Sones FM, Shirey EK, Proudfit WL, Westcott RN. Cine coronary arteriography. Circulation 1959;20:773.
2. Favaloro RG. Saphenous vein autograft replacement of severe segmental coronary artery occlusion: operation technique. Ann Thorac Surg 1968; 5:334.
3. Gruentzig AR, Myler RK, Manna EM, Tunha MI. Coronary transluminal angioplasty (abstr). Circulation 1977;55–56:(suppl III):84.
4. American Heart Association. 1990 Heart and Stroke Facts. Dallas: 1990.
5. Bourassa MG, Fisher LD, Campeau L, Gillespie MJ, McConney M, Lesperance J. Long-term rate of bypass grafts. The coronary artery surgery study (CASS) and Montreal Heart Institute experiences. Circulation 1985;72(suppl V):71.
6. Yitzhak B, Antonio MG. Lipoproteins in health and disease: diagnosis and management. Baylor Cardiology Series 1986;9:6–7.
7. Eckel RH. Lipoprotein lipase: a multifunctional enzyme relevant to common metabolic diseases. N Engl J Med 1989;320:1060–1066.
8. Hahn PF. Abolishment of alimentary lipemia following injection of heparin. Science 1943;98:10–20.
9. Ross R, Glonset JA. The pathogenesis of atherosclerosis. N Engl J Med 1976;295:369–377, 420–425.
10. Ross R. The pathogenesis of atherosclerosis—an update. N Engl J Med 1986;314:488–500.
11. Castelli WP. Cholesterol and lipids in the risk of coronary artery disease—The Framingham Heart Study. Can J Cardiol 1988;4:5A–10A.

12. Brown WV. Clinical trials including an update on the Helsinki Heart Study. Am J Cardiol 1990;66:11A–15A.

13. Dayton S, Pearce ML, Hashimoto S, Dixon WJ, Tomiyasu U. A controlled clinical trial of a diet high in unsaturated fat in preventing complications of atherosclerosis. Circulation 1969;40(suppl II):1–63.

14. Leren P. Effect of plasma cholesterol lowering diet in male survivors of myocardial infarction. Bull NY Acad Med 1968;44:1012–1020.

15. Hjermann I, Velve Byre K, Holme I, Leren P. Effect of diet and smoking intervention on the incidence of coronary heart disease. Report from the Oslo Study Group of a randomized trial in healthy men. Lancet 1981; 2:1303–1310.

16. The Lipid Research Clinics Program: the Lipid Research Clinics Coronary Primary Prevention Trial results. Part I. JAMA 1984;251:351–364.

17. Frick MH, Elo O, Hazpa K, et al. Helsinki Heart Study: primary-prevention trial with gemfibrozil in middle-aged men with dyslipidemia: safety in treatment, changes in risk factors, and incidence of coronary heart disease. N Engl J Med 1987;317:1237–1245.

18. Carlson LA, Rosenhamer G. Reduction of mortality in the Stockholm Ischemic Heart Disease Secondary Prevention Study by combined treatment with clofibrate and nicotinic acid. Acta Med Scand 1988;233:405–418.

19. Loscalzo J. Regression of coronary atherosclerosis. N Engl J Med 1990; 323:1337–1339.

20. Anitschkow N. Experimental atherosclerosis in animals. In: Cowdfry EV, ed. Arteriosclerosis: a survey of the problem. New York: Macmillian, 1933:271–322.

21. Friedman M, Byers SO. Observations concerning the evolution of atherosclerosis in the rabbit after cessation of cholesterol feeding. Am J Pathol 1963;43:349–359.

22. Clarkson TB, Bond MG, Bullock BC, Marzetta CA. A study of atherosclerosis regression in *Macaca mulatta*. IV. Changes in coronary arteries from animals with atherosclerosis induced for 19 months and then regressed for 24 or 48 months at plasma cholesterol concentrations of 300 or 200 mg/dl. Rcp Mol Pathol 1981;34:345–368.

23. Van Winkle M, Levy L. Further studies on the reversibility of serum sickness cholesterol-induced atherosclerosis. J Exp Med 1970;132:858–867.

24. Wagner WD, Clarkson TB, Foster J. Contrasting effects of ethane-1-hydroxy-1,1-diphosphonate (EHDP) on the regression of two types of dietary-induced atherosclerosis. Atherosclerosis 1977;27:419–435.

25. Vartiainen I, Kanerva K. Arteriosclerosis and war-time. Ann Med Intern Fenn 1947;36:748–758.

26. Wilens SL. The resorption of arterial atheromatous deposits in wasting disease. Am J Pathol 1947;23:793–804.

27. Ost CR, Stenson S. Regression of peripheral atherosclerosis during therapy with high doses of nicotinic acid. Scan J Clin Lab Invest 1967; 99(suppl):241–245.

28. Brensike JF, Levy RI, Kelsey SF, et al. Effects of therapy with cholestyramine on progression of coronary arteriosclerosis: results of the NHLBI type II coronary intervention study. Circulation 1984; 69:313–324.

29. Levy RI, Brensike JF, Epstein SE, et al. The influence of changes in lipid values induced by cholestyramine and diet on progression of coronary artery disease: results of the NHLBI type II coronary intervention study. Circulation 1984;69:325–337.

30. Blankenhorn DH, Nessim SA, Johnson RL, Sanmarco ME, Azen SP, Cashin-Hemphill L. Beneficial effects of combined colestipol-niacin therapy on coronary atherosclerosis and coronary venous bypass grafts. JAMA 1987;257:3233–3240.

31. Brown G, Albers JJ, Fisher LD, et al. Regression of coronary artery disease as a result of intensive lipid-lowering therapy in men with high levels of apolipoprotein B. N Engl J Med 1990;323:1289–1298.

32. Waller BF, Pinkerton CA, Orr CM, Slack JD, Van Tassel JW, Peters T. Restenosis 1 to 24 months after clinically successful coronary balloon angioplasty: A necropsy study of 20 patients. J Am Coll Cardiol 1991; 17(suppl B):58B–70B.

33. Ross R, Harker L. Hyperlipidemia and atherosclerosis. Science 1976; 193:1094–1100.

34. Garratt KN, Holmes DR Jr, Bell MR, et al. Restenosis after directional coronary atherectomy: differences between primary atheromatous and restenosis lesions and influence of subintimal tissue resection. J Am Coll Cardiol 1990;16:1665–1671.

35. Safian RD, Gelbfish JS, Erny RE, Schnitt SJ, Schmidt DA, Baim DS. Coronary atherectomy: clinical, angiographic, and histological findings and observations regarding potential mechanisms. Circulation 1990;82:69–79.

36. Dick RJ, Haudenschild CC, Popma JJ, Yakubov SJ, Topol EJ. Insights from quantitative histological analysis of excisional atherectomy specimens. Circulation 1990;82(suppl III):311.

37. Myler RK, Topol EJ, Shaw RE, et al. Multiple vessel coronary angioplasty: classification, results, and patterns of restenosis in 494 consecutive patients. Cathet Cardiovasc Diagn 1987;13:1–15.

38. Fleck E, Regitz V, Lehnert A, Dacian S, Dirschinger J, Rudolph W.

Restenosis after balloon dilatation of coronary stenosis: multivariate analysis of potential risk factors. Eur Heart J 1988;9:15–18.

39. Holmes DR Jr, Vlietstra RE, Smith HC, et al. Restenosis after percutaneous transluminal coronary angioplasty: a report from the PTCA Registry of National Heart, Lung and Blood Institute. Am J Cardiol 1984;53:77C–81C.

40. Lambert M, Bonan R, Cote G, et al. Multiple coronary angioplasty: a model to discriminate systemic and procedural factors related to restenosis. J Am Coll Cardiol 1988;12:310–314.

41. Guiteras VP, Bourassa MG, David PR, et al. Restenosis after successful percutaneous transluminal coronary angioplasty: The Montreal Heart Institute experience. Am J Cardiol 1987;60:50B–55B.

42. Leimgruber PP, Roubin GS, Hollman J, et al. Restenosis after successful coronary angioplasty in patients with single-vessel disease. Circulation 1986;73:710–717.

43. Mata LA, Bosch X, David PR, Rapold HJ, Corcos T, Bourassa MG. Clinical and angiographic assessment 6 months after double vessel percutaneous coronary angioplasty. J Am Coll Cardiol 1985;6:1239–1244.

44. Rapold HJ, David PR, Guiteras VP, Mata AL, Crean PA, Bourassa MG. Restenosis and its determinants in first and repeat coronary angioplasty. Eur Heart J 1987;8:575–586.

45. Ellis SG, Roubin GS, King SB III, Douglas JS Jr, Cox WR. Importance of stenosis morphology in the estimation of restenosis risk after elective percutaneous transluminal coronary angioplasty. Am J Cardiol 1989;63:30–34.

46. Austin GE, Lynn M, Hollman J. Laboratory test results as predictors of current coronary artery stenosis following angioplasty. Arch Pathol Lab Med 1987;111:1158–1162.

47. Galan KM, Hollman JL. Recurrence of stenosis after coronary angioplasty. Heart Lung 1986;15:585–587.

48. Schneider W, Vallbracht C, Kadel C, Klepzig H, Kaltenbach M. Plasma lipids and coronary angioplasty (abstr). Eur Heart J 1987;8(suppl 2):250.

49. Jacobs AK, Folan DJ, McSweeney SM, et al. Effect of plasma lipids on restenosis following coronary angioplasty (abstr). J Am Coll Cardiol 1987;9:183A.

50. Califf RM, Fortin DF, Frid DJ, et al. Restenosis after coronary angioplasty: an overview. J Am Coll Cardiol 1991;17(suppl B):2B–13B.

51. Bergelson BA, Jacobs AK, Small DA, et al. Lipoproteins predict restenosis after PTCA (abstr). Circulation 1989;80(suppl II):65.

52. Hearn JA, Donohue BC, King SB III, et al. Does serum LP(a) predict restenosis after PTCA? (abstr). J Am Coll Cardiol 1990;15:204A.

53. Arora RR, Konrad K, Badhwar K, Hollman J. Restenosis after transluminal coronary angioplasty: a risk factor analysis. Cathet Cardiovasc Diagn 1990;19:17–22.

54. Austin GE, Hollman J, Lynn MJ, Meier B. Serum lipoprotein levels fail to predict postangioplasty recurrent coronary artery stenosis. Cleve Clin J Med 1989;56:509–514.

55. Schmidt DA, Kuntz RE, Penny WF, Safian RD, Baim DS. Predictors of angiographic restenosis following coronary atherectomy (abstr). Circulation 1990;82(suppl III):492.

56. Utermann G. The mysteries of lipoprotein (a). Science 1989;246:904–910.

57. Hodenberg EV, Kreuzer J, Hautmann M, Nordt T, Kubler W, Bode C. Effects of lipoprotein (a) on success rate of thrombolytic therapy in acute myocardial infarction. Am J Cardiol 1991;67:1349–1353.

58. Ring ME, Vecchione JJ, Figore LD, et al. Detection of intracoronary fibrin degradation after coronary balloon angioplasty. Am J Cardiol 1991;67:1330–1334.

59. Gellman J, Ezekowitz MD, Sarembock IJ, et al. Effect of lovastatin on intimal hyperplasia after balloon angioplasty: A study in an atherosclerotic hypercholesterolemic rabbit. J Am Coll Cardiol 1991;17:251–259.

60. Sahni R, Maniet AR, Voci G, Banka VS. Prevention of restenosis by lovastatin (abstr). Circulation 1989;80(suppl II):65.

61. Hollman J, Konrad K, Raymond R, Whitlow P, Michalak M, Van Lente F. Lipid lowering for the prevention of recurrent stenosis following coronary angioplasty (abstr). Circulation 1989;80(suppl II):65.

62. Zhao X-Q, Flygenring BP, Stewart DK, et al. Increased potential for regression of post-PTCA restenosis using intensive lipid-altering therapy: comparison with matched non-PTCA lesions (abstr). J Am Coll Cardiol 1991;17:230A.

63. Leaf A, Weber PC. Cardiovascular effects of n-3 fatty acids. N Engl J Med 1988;318:549–557.

64. Bang HO, Dyerbery J, Hjorne N. The composition of food consumed by Greenland Eskimos. Acta Med Scand 1976;200:69–73.

65. Dyerberg J, Bang HO, Hjorne N. Fatty acid composition of the plasma lipids in Greenland Eskimos. Am J Clin Nutr 1975;28:958–966.

66. Kromann N, Green A. Epidemiological studies in the Upernavik district, Greenland: incidence of some chronic diseases 1950–1974. Acta Med Scand 1980;208:401–406.

67. Lorenz R, Spengler U, Fischer S, Duhm J, Weber PC. Platelet function, thromboxane formation and blood pressure control during supplementation of the Western diet with cod liver oil. Circulation 1983;67:504–511.

68. Singer P, Berger I, Luck K, Taube C, Naumann E, Godicke W. Long-term effect of mackerel diet on blood pressure, serum lipids and thromboxane formation in patients with mild essential hypertension. Atherosclerosis 1986;62:259–265.

69. Terano T, Hirai A, Hamazaki T, et al. Effect of oral administration of highly purified eicosapentaenoic acid on platelet function, blood viscosity and red cell deformability in healthy human subjects. Atherosclerosis 1983;46:321–331.

70. Barcelli U, Glas-Greenwalt P, Pollack VE. Enhancing effect of dietary supplement with (ω)-3 fatty acids on plasma fibrinolysis in normal subjects. Thromb Res 1985;39:307–312.

71. Shimokawa H, Lam JYT, Chesebro JH, Bowie EJW, Vanhoutte PM. Effects of dietary supplementation with cod-liver oil on endothelium-dependent response in porcine coronary arteries. Circulation 1987; 76:898–905.

72. von Schacky C, Weber PC. Metabolism and effects on platelet function of the purified eicosapentaenoic and docosahexaenoic acids in humans. J Clin Invest 1985;76:2446–2450.

73. Croset M, Lagarde M. In vitro incorporation and metabolism of eicosapentaenoic and docosahexaenoic acids in human platelets—effect on aggregation. Thromb Haemost 1986;56:57–62.

74. Landymore RW, Kinley CE, Cooper JH, MacAulay M, Sheridan B, Cameron C. Cod-liver oil in the prevention of intimal hyperplasia in autogenous vein grafts used for arterial bypass. J Thorac Cardiovasc Surg 1985; 89:351–357.

75. Landymore RW, MacAulay M, Sheridan B, Cameron C. Comparison of cod-liver oil and aspirin-dipyridamole for the prevention of intimal hyperplasia in autologous vein grafts. Ann Thorac Surg 1986;41:54–57.

76. Davis HR, Bridenstine RT, Vesselinovitch D, Wissler RW. Fish oil inhibits development of atherosclerosis in rhesus monkeys. Arteriosclerosis 1987;7:441–449.

77. Weiner BH, Ockene IS, Levine PH, et al. Inhibition of atherosclerosis by cod-liver oil in a hyperlipidemic swine model. N Engl J Med 1986; 315:841–846.

78. Dehmer GJ, Popma JJ, van den Berg EK, et al. Reduction in the rate of early restenosis after coronary angioplasty by a diet supplemented with n-3 fatty acids. N Engl J Med 1988;319:733–740.

79. Grigg LE, Kay TWH, Valentine PA, et al. Determinants of restenosis and lack of effect of dietary supplementation with eicosapentaenoic acid on the incidence of coronary artery restenosis after angioplasty. J Am Coll Cardiol 1989;13:665–672.

80. Milner MR, Gallino RA, Leffingwell A, et al. Usefulness of fish oil supplements in preventing clinical evidence of restenosis after percutaneous transluminal coronary angioplasty. Am J Cardiol 1989;64:294–299.

81. Reis GJ, Sipperly ME, McCabe CH, et al. Randomized trial of fish oil for prevention of restenosis after coronary angioplasty. Lancet 1989; July:177–181.

82. Slack JD, Pinkerton CA, VanTassel J, et al. Can oral fish oil supplements minimize restenosis after percutaneous transluminal coronary angioplasty? (abstr). J Am Coll Cardiol 1987;9:64A.

83. Bowles MH, Klonis D, Plavac TG, et al. EPA in the prevention of restenosis post PTCA. Angiology 1991;42:187–194.

CHAPTER **12**

. . . .

Gene Therapy
and Restenosis

——

ELIZABETH G. NABEL
GREGORY E. PLAUTZ
GARY J. NABEL

RESTENOSIS after transluminal angioplasty poses a major problem in the long-term management of coronary artery disease. Because it has been refractory to treatment, novel approaches are needed to assist in its management. One potential treatment of restenosis is the introduction of recombinant genes into vascular cells of the coronary lesion that encode for proteins to inhibit cell proliferation. Successful vascular gene therapy requires that sufficient numbers of vascular cells in the restenosis lesion be modified to produce proteins that exert physiologic effects. Gene therapy (1–4) is a novel approach to the treatment of many acquired and inherited disorders, but currently it is an experimental therapy not yet available for cardiovascular diseases. Although in its infancy, gene therapy has considerable promise for the treatment of a variety of cardiovascular disorders, such as restenosis, atherosclerosis, and cardiomyopathy. The goals of this chapter are to define the concepts and methods of cardiovascular gene therapy, to delineate the application of these methods to restenosis, and to discuss current efforts in this field.

Definition and Methods of Gene Transfer

A goal of gene therapy is to insert genes into somatic cells of living subjects to correct inherited or acquired disorders through the synthesis of a missing or defective gene product. Various mechanical, chemical, and viral methods have been used to introduce recombinant genes into host cells of different organ systems. Early efforts at gene therapy were directed toward the bone marrow (5–7), lymphoid system (8,9), and skin fibroblasts (10,11); recent research efforts have developed methods for gene transfer into vascular cells (12–16), cardiac (17,18) and skeletal (19) myocytes, hepatocytes (20,21), and the central nervous system (22).

To develop effective gene transfer, several criteria must be met. First, the defective or missing gene for a particular disease must be identified, isolated, and sequenced. Second, the contribution of the gene product to the pathophysiology of the disease should be well understood. Third, an animal model for the disease should be available for study and a measurable clinical end point for correction of the disease should be defined. Fourth, insertion of the defective or missing gene into host cells of the appropriate organ system should result in correction of the disease, measured by the defined end point.

Traditionally, three methods have been used to correct a defective or missing gene: gene replacement, gene correction, and gene augmentation (reviewed in reference 1). Gene replacement is the removal of the mutant gene and substitution with a normal, functional gene. Removal of a defective gene is technically difficult and not currently practical for human gene therapy, although several approaches have been used successfully in the laboratory. Gene correction alters the defective portion of the mutant gene within the host cell genome to allow the gene to function properly. Even in laboratory studies, this method is possible but technically difficult.

Gene augmentation introduces normal genetic sequences into a host cell genome while leaving the mutant gene unaltered. Normal genetic function is restored by the introduced "correct" gene. Although mutations could arise from the integration of foreign sequences into ectopic sites in the host genome, this complication, fortunately, has not arisen with any notable frequency. Gene augmentation could also be used to replace a missing gene in an inherited disorder, such as factor IX deficiency. At the present time, gene augmentation is the most common approach to gene therapy.

To successfully transfer DNA to cells, a gene transfer system must meet several requirements, including high-efficiency transmission into the host cell; maintenance of foreign DNA in a stable form, either integrated into the host genome or as an extrachromosomal element; expression in the relevant tissue; appropriate and regulated expression in the target tissue; and safety during transfer and the life of the host.

In the laboratory, several mechanical and chemical methods are used to introduce genes into cells in tissue culture, including precipitation with calcium phosphate, electroporation, polycations or polymers to complex with DNA, encapsidation of DNA into liposomes, and delivery with microspheres (Table 12.1). A general characteristic of these transfection methods is the integration of multiple repeated copies of the foreign gene into the host genome in a relatively stable form. These methods are experimental and have not yet been used in clinical protocols.

Clinically, viral vectors have been an efficient delivery system for introducing genes into host cells. The most commonly used viral vectors are retroviruses because they effectively infect cells of many species and are thought to integrate almost entirely into random sites in the host genome (reviewed in reference 23). Several potential problems could arise with the use of viral vectors. First, random integration into host chromosomes could lead to insertional mutagenesis through the interruption of cellular genes or the modulation of cellular gene expression by insertion into the regulatory sequences. Second, wild-type virus could form through recombination between the transfected vector plasmid and endogenous viruses. To minimize the possibility of a viral recombination event, retroviral vectors have been "crippled" (24,25); that is, to render the retroviral vector replication defective, the structural genes required for viral replication are removed from the viral backbone, and the viral vector is packaged in a helper cell line (fibroblasts) that expresses the replication genes, which have been produced from separate plasmids with independent selectable markers (26). This al-

Table 12.1. Methods for Gene Transfer

IN VITRO	IN VIVO
Calcium phosphate	Retroviral vectors
Electroporation	DNA liposome complexes
DNA polymer complexes	Direct injection
DNA liposome complexes	DNA ligand complexes
Viral vectors	Microspheres
Microspheres	

lows an intact viral particle to be produced that is capable of infecting a host cell once but cannot replicate. This feature limits the likelihood that a wild-type virus would be generated.

Given the potential hazard of random integration and expression of specific genes in inappropriate cells, it is important that the expression of such genes be controlled. Several approaches have been taken to regulate the expression of genes in vivo. First, "suicide" vectors, which contain a selectable marker sensitive to a particular drug, would allow elimination of cells containing the recombinant selectable marker gene by the administration of the drug in the event of cell transformation. One example of a suicide vector uses the herpesvirus thymidine kinase (TK) gene (27). Introduction of the herpesvirus TK gene into tumor cells results in elimination of the tumors following administration of the drug, ganciclovir, which is converted by the herpesvirus gene to a form that inhibits DNA replication. Ganciclovir has no effect on cells lacking the recombinant TK gene. A second approach to achieve specificity of expression is through the use of tissue-specific enhancer elements in expression vectors. For these purposes, a variety of cell-specific promoters or enhancers have been defined and will be useful in directing recombinant gene expression to appropriate cells in vivo. Finally, the regulated expression of such genes is important. With increased understanding of cellular transcription factors and regulatory elements, it should soon be possible to design inducible promoters that provide for regulated expression of recombinant genes in vivo. Such promoters could contain different combinations of inducible cis-acting DNA regulatory elements (28).

A second potential method of introducing recombinant genes in vivo is DNA liposome complexes. Liposomes can be prepared from cationic lipid molecules (29,30) that coat the negatively charged DNA and allow incorporation into the cell membrane. Once in the cytoplasm, the liposomes can be degraded by cellular enzymes, and plasmid DNA is transported by an unknown mechanism into the cell nucleus. Plasmid DNA replicates in the nucleus, primarily as an episome. The advantages of transfecting cells in vivo with DNA/liposome complexes are safety, ease of preparation, low cost, and general applicability.

Gene Transfer into the Vasculature

Expression of recombinant genes in the vessel wall achieves several goals. First, the methods are used to study the pathophysiology of various vascular diseases. For example, the function of many gene products has been described in vitro, but their in vivo function is unknown. Direct gene transfer allows the analysis of the activity of a specific gene product in vivo. Second, gene transfer is a therapeutic modality; that is, recombinant genes within a vessel wall or microcirculation can express recombinant gene products with therapeutic effect.

The vasculature is an ideal target tissue for the expression of recombinant genes for cardiovascular disease. The endothelium is a regulatory organ that mediates anticoagulant, vascular contractility, cellular proliferation, and inflammatory mechanisms in the vessel wall. Because endothelial cells play an important role in modulating vascular pathology, they represent important target cells for the transfer of genetic material to diseased vascular sites. Genes expressed in endothelial or vascular smooth muscle cells (SMCs) could exert autocrine or paracrine effects locally and could provide a therapy for focal processes, such as atherosclerosis or malignancy. In addition, because of the proximity to the bloodstream, these cells could also deliver therapeutic factors in the circulation, which would be relevant to the treatment of acquired or inherited systemic diseases, such as hemophilia.

Site-specific gene expression in vivo must be addressed on two levels: the vascular site and the exact cell type where the recombinant gene is expressed. For example, if a gene is expressed in an endothelial cell, its gene products could be secreted into the circulation or released locally on adjacent endothelial cells and SMCs in the intima and media. If gene expression is limited to vascular SMCs, a more restricted effect on the proliferation of surrounding vascular SMCs might be seen.

Cell-Mediated Gene Transfer

Two approaches to the delivery of genes into vessels in vivo have been taken in the laboratory. Cell-mediated gene transfer involves the removal of cells from the host and placement of these cells in tissue culture where they are genetically modified with a vector (Plate XX). Following genetic modification, the cells are reimplanted back onto a vessel wall. This method indirectly transfers the gene into the recipient. In contrast, direct gene transfer can also be used to introduce recombinant genes into the vasculature using retroviral vectors or liposomes. This method, discussed below, eliminates the need for prior cell transfection in vitro (Plate XXI).

In our initial studies, we asked whether endothelial cells could be genetically modified in vitro and reimplanted onto an arterial segment in vivo with expression of the recombinant gene (13). To test this hypothesis, endothelial cells were derived from the Yucatan minipig and grown in tissue culture. The endothelial cells were transfected with a retroviral vector expressing a marker gene (β-galactosidase). This enzyme, derived from *Escherichia coli*, was chosen because it catalyzes the formation of a product that stains blue with standard histochemical techniques. The genetically modified endothelial cells retained endothelial cell character and function, demonstrated by their ability to endocytose acetylated low-density lipoprotein and express mRNA for von Willebrand's factor. The genetically altered endothelial cells were introduced onto the iliofemoral artery of Yucatan minipigs using a catheter. This catheter contained a proximal and distal balloon, which, when inflated, created an inner protected space into which the modified endothelial cells were instilled. A local region of the iliofemoral artery was mechanically denuded of endothelium to allow adherence of genetically modified cells. Examination of arterial segments 2 to 4 weeks later revealed areas of blue coloration, indicating β-galactosidase expression. Microscopically, β-galactosidase-staining endothelial cells were observed in the intima, in contrast to sham-operated control segments. Similar studies have been performed using vascular SMCs, demonstrating that genetically modified SMCs can also be reimplanted onto the vessel wall with expression of the recombinant gene product (31). These studies established a model system for cell-mediated gene transfer of endothelial and vascular SMCs.

Direct Gene Transfer into the Vasculature

Although early studies established the feasibility of altering the genome of endothelial cells in vitro with reimplantation in vivo, this technique would be cumbersome to use clinically. It was therefore advantageous to directly modify vascular cells in vivo, eliminating the need for in vitro transfection. Further experiments demonstrated that vascular cells could be directly transduced in vivo (15). Using the Yucatan minipig model, a retroviral vector or liposomes containing the marker gene was introduced into the iliofemoral artery using a double-balloon catheter. Cells in the intima, media, and adventitia were transduced, and evidence of recombinant gene expression in vivo was observed for up to 5 months. Further immunohistochemical studies revealed that both endothelial and vascular SMCs were transfected. Use of the replication defective retroviral vector appeared safe, because evidence of wild-type virus or reverse transcriptase from replicating retrovirus was not present in serum or lymphocytes from pigs infected with the retroviral vector. These studies then established a model for direct gene transfer into vascular cells. Direct vascular cell gene transfer has been confirmed and extended to the coronary circulation by Swain and colleagues using another reporter gene, leuciferase (32).

From an experimental and practical viewpoint, the ability to directly introduce a recombinant gene in vivo represents a major technical advance, eliminating the time and effort of preparing cells prior to the procedure. By direct infection with retroviral vectors, high levels of expression were observed for over 5 months, although diminution was observed with time. Potential disadvantages are the loss of control over the cell types into which the gene is introduced, and loss of expression over time. However, refinements such as the use of cell-specific transcriptional regulatory elements may overcome the problem of recombinant gene expression in specific cell types. Other experimental approaches are being taken to address the issue of longevity of tissue expression, and these model systems for direct and indirect gene transfer represent advances in the expression of recombinant genes in vivo.

Other methods for the direct introduction of recombinant genes in vivo have also been described. In skeletal muscle, for example, injection of DNA into tissue results in uptake in recombinant genes and expression in vivo (19). This technology may have applications for the treatment of muscle diseases and may also be used for immunization using recombinant genes. This approach was recently proven successful as a means to introduce recombinant genes into the myocardium and will provide another approach to gene therapy for cardiovascular disease (17,18).

Biologic Effects In Vivo

The principle that recombinant genes can be directly introduced in vivo has been demonstrated (14,15,17,19). More recently, it has been possible to document a biologic response to a recombinant gene in the vessel wall (33). To test the hypothesis that recombinant genes could be introduced into the vessel wall, which had potent biologic effect, we constructed a retroviral vector expressing a human class I major histocompatibility complex antigen, HLA-B7. Endothelial cells were infected with the HLA-B7 retroviral vector and tested for the surface expression of HLA-B7 antigen by incubation with a monoclonal antibody directed against HLA-B7. Transduced endothelial cells demonstrated expression of the introduced gene whereas nontransduced cells did not, verifying that the cell surface glycoprotein could be secreted by transfected cells. Porcine iliofemoral arteries infected with the HLA-B7 expressing retrovirus in vivo demonstrated a remarkable mononuclear infiltrate primarily in the adventitial layer of the artery, in contrast to control animals infected with other expression vectors. These studies demonstrate that a specific response to the introduction of particular gene product can be achieved in vivo. This system provides a model for the study of vasculitis and may also have applications to human disease in instances where a significant degree of local immunity may be desirable (i.e., tumor rejection).

Cellular Proliferation

A major interest of our laboratory has been to study mechanisms of cellular proliferation in the vessel wall and the contribution of growth factors to the proliferative process. Direct gene transfer technology allows the selective introduction of specific growth factor genes with subsequent analysis of the effect of the recombinant growth factor gene product on cellular proliferation. Our approach has been to selectively introduce human recombinant growth factors, individually and in combination, into the porcine arterial wall and evaluate their contribution to cellular proliferation several weeks following transfection. The goals are to establish a model of cellular proliferation based on the overexpression of recombinant growth factors and to develop inhibitors of growth factor gene expression that can be tested in this model.

We have begun to examine the function of human platelet-derived growth factor B (PDGF-B) protein in the porcine arterial wall. A major concern in the analysis of recombinant growth factor genes in vivo is the development of a model whereby the surgery and transfection procedures induced minimal or no vascular injury. Such injury can stimulate cellular proliferation, which can obscure the effects of recombinant growth factor genes. To minimize this complication, care is taken to avoid trauma or excessive pressure in the vessel wall. With these precautions, minimal vascular injury and cellular proliferation have occurred following introduction of an irrelevant gene. Preliminary studies suggest that the expression of the recombinant PDGF-B gene is associated with intimal proliferation in porcine iliofemoral arteries compared with control arteries. This process may be a direct effect of the recombinant PDGF-B gene, an indirect effect of the PDGF-B gene initiating a cascade effect, including synthesis and release of other growth factors, or both. These results suggest that this model may be used to develop potential inhibitory factors.

Regulation of Gene Expression In Vivo

The ability to express recombinant genes in vivo offers potential new treatments for human disease provided that questions of safety and toxicity in human use can be addressed. For example, complications of gene transfer could arise from the overexpression of growth or angiogenic factor genes with intended therapeutic effects or by insertional mutagenesis, both of which could cause uncontrolled cell growth. To devise a method to regulate the proliferation of transduced cells, we developed a "suicide" retroviral vector that provides a method to eliminate such cells in vivo (27). A suicide gene renders cells sensitive to a specific drug. The herpesvirus gene, TK, was introduced into cells to render them sensitive to the drug ganciclovir. Administration of ganciclovir to cells containing the TK gene results in cell death. Normal cells without the TK gene, exposed to ganciclovir, continue to proliferate normally. A retroviral vector containing the herpesvirus TK gene was synthesized and its effect was first assessed in vitro by infecting multiple human and porcine cell lines. In particular, NIH 3T3 fibroblasts were infected with the vector containing the herpesvirus TK gene in addition to the reporter β-galactosidase gene, and these cells were then exposed to ganciclovir. Ganciclovir treatment eliminated β-galactosidase expression after 4 days in cells transduced with the herpes virus TK gene (Plate XXII). In contrast, ganciclovir had no effect on control cells infected with the β-galactosidase vector alone. Endothelial, vascular SMC, and various tumor cells were also eliminated by ganciclovir following transfection with the herpesvirus TK gene, implying that this retroviral vector conferred sensitivity to multiple cell types in which it was expressed, including vascular cells.

To study the efficiency of this vector in vivo, a murine adenocarcinoma cell line (CT26) was transduced with this vector in vitro. Transduced cells were injected into the hind limb of a mouse, and tumor growth was monitored in the presence and absence of ganciclovir. Mice in which the tumor was allowed to grow uncontrolled died in 4 to 5 weeks. In contrast, mice transplanted with the transduced tumor cells, who were treated with ganciclovir, experienced no tumor growth (27). In several additional mice, the transfected tumor cells were injected into the hind limb, and the tumor was allowed to grow to a size of 4 to 6 cm^3. Ganciclovir treatment was initiated, and 2 weeks following the cessation of ganciclovir treatment, the tumors had completely regressed (Figure 12.1). This suicide vector eliminated transformed cells, but allowed survival of normal nondividing cells. These studies suggest that a suicide retroviral vector may be useful in regulating cellular proliferation in vivo and provides additional safety measures to gene transfer in living organisms. It was also interesting to note that nondividing cells within the vessel wall were insensitive to ganciclovir, suggesting that recombinant gene expression was selectively affected in vivo.

Figure 12.1. Regression of tumors transduced with a suicide retroviral vector following treatment with ganciclovir in vivo. A mouse was injected subcutaneously in the left posterior flank with adenocarcinoma cells transduced with the suicide retroviral vector. A. Gross appearance of inoculated mouse prior to treatment at day 37 of tumor growth. B. 20 days after a 14-day course of ganciclovir (day 71) showing tumor regression. (Reprinted with permission from Plautz G, Nabel EG, Nabel GJ. Selective elimination of recombinant genes in vivo with a suicide retroviral vector. The New Biologist 1991;3:709–715.)

a   **- Ganciclovir**   b   **+ Ganciclovir**

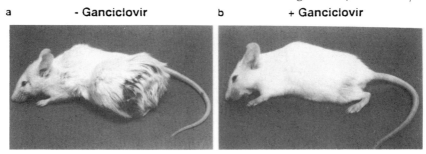

Other approaches can be taken to terminate or regulate gene expression in vivo. For example, the development of tissue-specific promotors will also allow expression only in certain cell types such as endothelium or SMCs. Second, the generation of an inducible promotor will allow regulated expression in vivo by turning on gene expression as opposed to a suicide retroviral vector, which eliminates gene expression.

Endothelial Cell Seeding of Vascular Grafts and Stents

A promising area of research in gene transfer and cardiovascular disease is the use of genetically altered endothelial cells to line implantable biomedical devices to enhance the function of normal endothelial cells. Because many of the implantable devices, including vascular stents and prosthetic grafts, are plagued by thrombosis and cellular proliferation, lining these devices with endothelial cells that have been genetically modified to secrete an antiproliferative agent or an antithrombotic agent would have great clinical utility. Wilson and colleagues first demonstrated that Dacron prosthetic grafts could be lined with canine endothelial cells transduced to express a marker gene (14). These seeded grafts were reimplanted into the carotid artery of the dog, where, 5 weeks after implantation, expression of the recombinant gene was demonstrated. Dichek and colleagues have pioneered endothelial cell seeding of metallic coronary stents as an approach to eliminating in vivo thrombosis (34,35). They demonstrated that sheep endothelial cells can be transduced with retroviral vectors expressing either the marker gene β-galactosidase or the cDNA for human tissue plasminogen activator (tPA). These genetically modified endothelial cells were seeded onto metallic stents in vitro where viability of endothelial cells was demonstrated and secretion of human recombinant tPA into tissue culture supernatant was measured (24). Current limitations to this technology include: a several month time delay between cell harvest, transfection, and seeding of vascular prosthesis; early loss of cells on the luminal surface of the stent following balloon expansion; and viability of endothelial-lined stents following in vivo transplantation. Nonetheless, the ability to augment endothelial cell function through the overexpression of an antithrombotic or antiproliferative agent offers great advances in the utility of gene transfer in vivo and the application to implantable devices.

Conclusions

Considerable progress has been made over the past several years in the field of vascular gene transfer. Recombinant gene expression in both endothelial and vascular SMCs can be performed by indirect or cell-mediated and direct gene transfer. Recombinant genes can be introduced directly into localized vessel segments, where they can induce changes in the biologic function of vessels, as demonstrated in our studies of HLA-B7 antigen. In addition, the overexpression of recombinant growth factors in the vessel wall is associated with cellular proliferation, and this model can be used to study mechanisms of restenosis and atherosclerosis. The ability to regulate gene expression with inducible promoters or suicide vectors is now becoming a reality. Recent progress in the technology of gene transfer in vivo has raised the prospect that it will soon be used for the treatment of a variety of diseases. Although much of the research in gene therapy has focused on the treatment of inherited disorders, it is now increasingly clear that gene therapy will have major benefits in the treatment of acquired diseases. A major challenge is to identify recombinant genes that can serve therapeutic roles and to facilitate their development for in vivo expression. Although several cell-mediated gene transfer protocols have been initiated, it is likely that human clinical trials using direct gene transfer will also become a reality in the foreseeable future. Early human trials are likely to focus on safety and toxicity in vivo and probably will be limited to those clinical diseases with guarded prognosis and limited therapeutic options (36). Subsequent studies will probably deal with improvements in clinical efficacy. The application of gene transfer to cardiovascular disease may take several years because human gene therapy will first treat terminal diseases with limited treatment options. Recent growth of gene transfer methods as well as their application to human diseases would suggest that the application of gene transfer to cardiovascular disease will be evident in the foreseeable future. It is the goal of many investigators that gene therapy fulfill its promise of bringing the power of molecular biology to the treatment of human disease.

References

1. Friedmann T. Progress toward human gene therapy. Science 1989; 244:1275–1280.

2. Miller AD. Progress toward human gene therapy. Blood 1990;76:271–278.

3. Swain JL. Gene therapy: a new approach to the treatment of cardiovascular disease. Circulation 1989;80:1495–1496.

4. Kelley WN. Gene therapy in humans: a new era begins. Ann Intern Med 1991;114:697–698.

5. Joyner A, Keller G, Phillips RA, Bernstein A. Retrovirus transfer of a bacterial gene into mouse haematopoietic progenitor cells. Nature 1983; 305:556–558.

6. Hock RA, Miller AD. Retrovirus-mediated transfer and expression of drug resistance genes in human haematopoietic progenitor cells. Nature 1986;320:275–277.

7. Gruber HE, Finley KD, Hershberg RM, et al. Retroviral vector-mediated gene transfer into human hematopoietic progenitor cells. Science 1985; 230:1057–1060.

8. Kantoff PW, Kohn DB, Mitsuya H, et al. Correction of adenosine deaminase deficiency in cultured human T and B cells by retrovirus-mediated gene transfer. Proc Natl Acad Sci USA 1986;83:6563–6567.

9. Culver K, Cornetta K, Morgan R, et al. Lymphocytes as cellular vehicles for gene therapy in mouse and man. Proc Natl Acad Sci USA 1991; 88:3155–3159.

10. Sorge J, Kuhl W, West C, Beutler E. Complete correction of the enzymatic defect of type I Gaucher disease fibroblasts by retroviral-mediated gene transfer. Proc Natl Acad Sci USA 1987;84:906–909.

11. Palmer TD, Hock RA, Osborne WRA, Miller DA. Efficient retrovirus-mediated transfer and expression of a human adenosine deaminase gene in diploid skin fibroblasts from an adenosine deaminase-deficient human. Proc Natl Acad Sci USA 1987;84:1055–1059.

12. Zwiebel JA, Freeman SM, Kantoff PW, Cornetta K, Ryan US, Anderson WF. High-level recombinant gene expression in rabbit endothelial cells transduced by retroviral vectors. Science 1987;243:220–222.

13. Nabel EG, Plautz G, Boyce FM, Stanley JC, Nabel GJ. Recombinant gene expression in vivo within endothelial cells of the arterial wall. Science 1989;244:1342–1344.

14. Wilson JM, Birinyi LK, Salomon RN, Libby P, Callow AD, Mulligan RC. Implantation of vascular grafts lined with genetically modified endothelial cells. Science 1989;244:1344–1346.

15. Nabel EG, Plautz G, Nabel GJ. Site-specific gene expression in vivo by direct gene transfer into the arterial wall. Science 1990;249:1285–1288.

16. Thompson JA, Anderson KD, DiPietro JM, et al. Site-directed neovessel formation in vivo. Science 1988;241:1349–1352.

17. Lin H, Parmacek MS, Morle G, Bolling S, Leiden JM. Expression of recombinant genes in myocardium in vivo following direct injection of DNA. Circulation 1990;82:2217–2221.

18. Kitsis RN, Buttrick PM, McNally EM, Kaplan ML, Leinwand LA. Hormonal modulation of a gene injected into rat heart in vivo. Proc Natl Acad Sci USA 1991;88:1438–1442.

19. Wolff JA, Malone RW, Williams P, et al. Direct gene transfer into mouse muscle in vivo. Science 1990;247:1465–1468.

20. Wilson JM, Johnston DE, Jefferson DM, Mulligan RC. Correction of the genetic defect in hepatocytes from the Watanabe heritable hyperlipidemic rabbit. Proc Natl Acad Sci USA 1988;85:4421–4425.

21. Wilson JM, Chowdhury NR, Grossman M, et al. Temporary amelioration of hyperlipidemia in low density lipoprotein receptor-deficient rabbits transplanted with genetically modified hepatocytes. Proc Natl Acad Sci USA 1990;87:8437–8441.

22. Palella TD, Hidaka Y, Silverman LJ, Levine M, Glorioso J, Kelley WN. Expression of human HPRT mRNA in brains of mice infected with a recombinant herpes simplex virus-1 vector. Gene 1989;80:137–144.

23. Varmus H. Retroviruses. Science 1988;240:1427–1435.

24. Mann R, Mulligan RC, Baltimore D. Construction of a retrovirus packaging mutant and its use to produce helper-free defective retrovirus. Cell 1983;33:153–159.

25. Cone RD, Mulligan RC. High-efficiency gene transfer into mammalial cells: generation of helper-free recombinant retrovirus with broad mammalian host range. Proc Natl Acad Sci USA 1984;81:6349–6353.

26. Danos O, Mulligan RC. Safe and efficient generation of recombinant retroviruses with amphotropic and ectotropic host ranges. Proc Natl Acad Sci USA 1988;85:6460–6464.

27. Plautz G, Nabel EG, Nabel GJ. Selective elimination of recombinant genes in vivo with a suicide retroviral vector. The New Biologist 1991; 3:709–715.

28. Miller KF, Bolt DJ, Pursel VG, et al. Expression of human or bovine growth hormone gene with a mouse metallothionein-1 promoter in transgenic swine alters the secretion of porcine growth hormone and insulin-like growth factor-I. Endocrinology 1989;120:481–488.

29. Felgner PL. Particulate systems and polymers for in vitro and in vivo delivery of polynucleotides. Advanced Drug Delivery Reviews 1990; 5:163–187.

30. Gao X, Huang L. A novel cationic liposome reagent for efficient transfection of mammalian cells. Biochem Biophys Res Commun 1991;179:280–285.

31. Plautz G, Nabel EG, Nabel GJ. Introduction of vascular smooth muscle cells expressing recombinant genes in vivo. Circulation 1991;83:578–583.

32. Lim CS, Chapman GD, Gammon RS, et al. Direct in vivo gene transfer into the coronary and peripheral vasculatures of the intact dog. Circulation 1991;83:2002–2011.

33. Plautz GE, Nabel EG, Nabel GJ. Expression of a class I MHC antigen in the arterial wall in vivo by direct retroviral infection: an experimental model for vasculitis. Circulation 1990;82(suppl III):697.

34. Dichek DA, Neville RF, Zwiebel JA, et al. Seeding of intravascular stents with genetically engineered endothelial cells. Circulation 1989; 80:1347–1353.

35. Dichek DA, Nussbaum O, Degen SJF, Anderson WF. Enhancement of the fibrinolytic activity of sheep endothelial cells by retroviral vector-mediated gene transfer. Blood 1991;77:533–541.

36. Rosenberg SA, Aebersold P, Cornetta K, et al. Gene transfer into humans—immunotherapy of patients with advanced melanoma, using tumor-infiltrating lymphocytes modified by retroviral gene transduction. N Engl J Med 1990;323:570–578.

· ·

CHAPTER 13

Animal Models of Restenosis

JESSE W. CURRIER
DAVID P. FAXON

Introduction

PERCUTANEOUS transluminal coronary angioplasty (PTCA) has had tremendous impact on the care of patients, yet it is far from a perfect procedure. One of its major imperfections is restenosis, which occurs in 25% to 40% of patients (1). Because of the high cost of clinical studies as well as the risks of using new devices or pharmacologic agents in patients, animal models are necessary to assess the safety and efficacy of new approaches to restenosis. As in any disease model, caution must be exercised in extrapolating the results to patients. One must analyze the strengths and weaknesses of each model and consider the method of delivery, as well as the dose and metabolism of the agent used to determine its potential for clinical use.

There are many models of de novo atherosclerosis, ranging from the pigeon to nonhuman primates (2). Many of these models have also been used to examine restenosis. The ideal model of restenosis would consist of a coronary artery that develops focal, obstructive lesions histologically similar to human atherosclerosis. The arterial diameter would be similar to human coronaries, to facilitate the use of current PTCA equipment and new technologies. The injury used to initiate restenosis would be a standard PTCA balloon inflated to nominal pressures, with acute histologic effects resembling those seen in patients. Development of initial and restenotic lesions would occur in a timely fashion, and restenosis would occur in most animals. The histology of the restenotic lesion would be similar to that seen in human lesions. The animal would be readily obtainable, inexpensive to purchase and maintain, and easy and safe to work with. As in de novo atherosclerosis, however, no ideal model exists. Table 13.1 compares the features of the ideal model with the three animal models most commonly used in the study of restenosis, which will be discussed in the following sections.

Rat Carotid Artery Model

The rat carotid artery injury model was not developed specifically for the study of restenosis. Indeed, it was in use before angioplasty was performed in patients (3) and is a modification of the original aortic bal-

Table 13.1 Models of Restenosis

| | MODEL | | | |
FEATURE	IDEAL	RAT	RABBIT	SWINE
ARTERY	coronary	carotid	iliac	coronary
DIAMETER	2–3 mm	1 mm	2–3 mm	1.5–2.5 mm
UNDERLYING LESION				
Development	brief	0	6 wks	0
Type	obstructive	normal	obstructive	normal
Histology	atherosclerosis	normal	foam cell	normal
INJURY	angioplasty	Fogarty balloon	angioplasty	oversized stent
RESTENOSIS LESION				
Development	brief	2 wks	4 wks	4 wks
Histology	SMC	SMC	SMC and macrophage	SMC
COST*				
Purchase	inexpensive	$11	$32	$144
Board/wk	inexpensive	$4	$10	$39

Current prices at Boston University Medical Center, 1992.
SMC = smooth muscle cells; wks = weeks.

looning technique of Baumgartner, which was used to study the development of de novo atherosclerosis (4). However, the insights provided by researchers using this model have greatly advanced our understanding of the process of restenosis following PTCA.

Technique

Early studies using this model relied on air dessication to create the injury (3,5,6). For this technique, the common carotid artery in 250 to 300-g rats is isolated under systemic anesthesia. A 1.5 cm segment of the artery is ligated at both ends. An exit hole is created with a number 30 needle, and after rinsing with saline, dry compressed air is infused at 50 to 60 cc/min for 3.5 minutes. The ligatures are then removed and flow reestablished. This technique reliably removes the endothelium, as assessed by silver perfusion staining at 24 hours (5,6).

More recently, many researchers have used a Fogarty balloon to accomplish deendothelialization (7–14). For this technique, the common and external carotid arteries of 500-g rats are isolated under systemic anesthesia via a midline incision. A 2F Fogarty balloon catheter is inserted via the external carotid and advanced to the thoracic aorta. It is then withdrawn through the common carotid artery with the balloon inflated sufficiently with saline to generate "slight resistance" (7), usually for a total of three passes. The external carotid artery is then ligated.

With either technique for arterial injury, maximal intimal thickening occurs at 2 weeks, and the animals are killed and perfusion fixed at systemic pressures. The results can be analyzed either as intimal-medial thickness or volume ratios (3). The intimal thickness is measured as the maximal distance from luminal surface to the internal elastic lamina, and the media is measured as the distance from the internal elastic lamina to the most external elastic lamina. Alternatively, intimal cross-sectional area can be measured morphometrically (9).

Histopathology

Air dessication results primarily in endothelial denudation; the use of a Fogarty balloon adds a component of medial smooth muscle cell (SMC) damage (13). The initial response to the injury is platelet deposition over the areas of denudation, but the subsequent cellular response to injury in the normal rat carotid is almost entirely a smooth muscle phenomenon (Figure 13.1). At 2 weeks, the intima is thickened by a factor of 10 or more, from its normal one to two cell layers to twice as thick as the media. Intimal thickening continues to a small degree for several weeks, but the lumen area actually increases over this time because of concurrent relaxation of vasoconstriction seen at the 2-week time point (7).

Advantages and Disadvantages

The rat is easy to work with and inexpensive to procure and maintain. The response to injury is well defined and reproducibly develops over a brief period of time. Most importantly, it consists of the predominant

Figure 13.1. Neointimal proliferation 14 days after air dessication injury; the arrows indicate the internal elastic lamina. Left panel is from a control animal, the right panel is heparin treated. (Reproduced with permission of the American Heart Association from Guyton J et al. Circ Res 1980;46:625–634.)

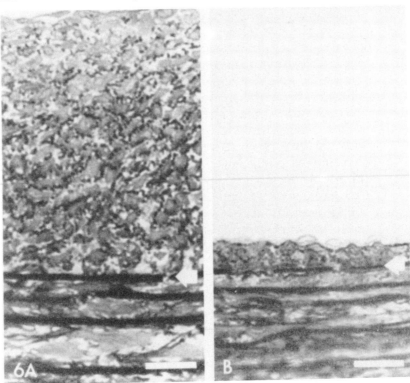

cell type seen in human restenosis after PTCA. An expensive fluoroscopy system is not needed and the investigator is not exposed to radiation using this model. However, the underlying artery is a normal vessel, and the injury does not resemble the degree of vessel trauma induced by PTCA. Because there is no obstructive lesion, flow and shear stress are not altered as in patients (15), although flow is clearly important in this model as well (16). Despite these limitations, a great deal of information about the response of vascular SMCs to injury has been derived from this model.

Results

Clowes and coworkers have used this model extensively to study the response of vascular SMCs to balloon injury (7–12). In a series of experiments they have shown evidence of SMC proliferation 1 to 2 days after injury and that entry of cells into the growth fraction is completed by 3 days after the injury. Further division of SMCs over the next 2 weeks occurs only in those cells previously recruited into the growth fraction; conversion of more quiescent cells to dividing cells does not appear to occur (7,10,12). However, up to 50% of the cells that migrate to the intima do not actually proliferate. In the proliferating fraction, division continues after migration to the intima, but migration alone accounts for a substantial portion of the intimal lesion (8).

Depending on the length of the deendothelialized segment, reendothelialization can occur as soon as 2 weeks (3). Longer segments take longer to reendothelialize because endothelial regrowth occurs from normal endothelium at the ends of the ballooned segment. Other factors such as the stress of administering parenteral medications may also delay reendothelialization (17). Reendothelialization can limit proliferation, but even without an intact endothelium, proliferation ceases at approximately 4 weeks (18).

In patients, Nobuyoshi has described the time course of intimal proliferation after PTCA (19). For the first 10 days after PTCA, no proliferation is present. In lesions dilated from 11 to 30 days previously, 83% of the samples show intimal proliferation. At 1 to 3 months, intimal proliferation is evident in all cases. Intimal SMCs are present for up to 2 years, but the phenotype of these cells reverts to the quiescent type at 6 months. Thus, the temporal sequence of events in patients is similar to that seen in this model, but in a greatly expanded time frame.

Platelet-derived growth factor (PDGF) is one of the factors thought to be important in the pathogenesis of restenosis. This model has been used to study the role of PDGF by inducing thrombocytopenia with a polyclonal antibody. The DNA replication rates after balloon deendothelialization were identical for thrombocytopenic and control animals (9). However, the degree of intimal thickening was less prominent in the thrombocytopenic animals. Thus, platelet products were not essential for proliferation, but appeared to be important in migration of SMC to the intima. This may explain the results of an earlier study, in which standard antiplatelet agents such as aspirin were ineffective in preventing intimal proliferation despite documented inhibition of platelet function (17). The identity of other growth factors that stimulate proliferation is under active investigation.

Most of the work done using this model has concentrated on mechanisms of intimal proliferation, although there has been some investigation of potential means of inhibiting this process. Early studies showed that the continuous administration of heparin could reduce the intimal proliferation by up to 80% (3). In addition to inhibiting proliferation, heparin was also shown to inhibit migration of SMCs into the intima. The inhibition was not due to an anticoagulant effect, since low-molecular weight heparin was also shown to be antiproliferative (5), and the administration of heparin could be delayed for up to 18 hours after the injury without loss of inhibition (11).

More recently, the angiotensin-converting enzyme (ACE) inhibitor cilazapril (10 mg/kg/day) was shown to be effective in limiting intimal proliferation by up to 80% in this model (13). Maximal inhibition required dosing for 6 days before and 14 days after balloon injury. No inhibition was seen with a single dose of cilazapril 1 hour prior to balloon injury or with the continuous use of the calcium channel blocker verapamil dosed to a similar hypotensive effect. The use of nonspecific vasodilators such as hydralazine and minoxidil also were not effective in reducing neointima formation (20). Thus, the mechanism of action was presumably inhibition of the local production of angiotensin II. Alternatively, some other effect of ACE inhibition, such as preventing the normal degradation of bradykinin, may play a role. Interestingly, the effects of cilazapril and heparin appear to be additive in this model, when both drugs were given for 14 days following the balloon injury. Clinical studies based on these data are currently in progress and may help to assess the validity of this model to evaluate therapies to prevent restenosis.

Hypercholesterolemic Rabbit Iliac Artery Model

The hypercholesterolemic rabbit iliac artery model is widely used to study restenosis, and is used most frequently by the authors. It is the only model developed to date that examines the in vivo response of an artery with a focal, obstructive stenosis to the severe damage clinically used in PTCA. It has proven useful to study the mechanisms of angioplasty (21–27), the time course of events following angioplasty (28–32), and potential agents and devices to reduce restenosis (33–48).

Technique

Bilateral iliac atherosclerosis is induced in male New Zealand white rabbits weighing approximately 3 kg by a combination of balloon deendothelialization and a high-cholesterol diet (22–24). After systemic and local anesthesia, the distal femoral arteries are isolated. Via a small arteriotomy, a 3F Fogarty catheter is passed to a distance of 20 cm. The balloon is inflated with saline and deendothelialization is accomplished by gently pulling the catheter down the iliac artery, usually for a total of three to six passes. The catheter is then removed and the distal femoral artery ligated. In our experience, a significant lesion (> 40%) is induced in 80% of arteries by this technique. Other investigators have used air dessication for endothelial injury, in a manner similar to that discussed previously for the rat carotid artery. In an isolated, ligated segment of the femoral artery a number 27 needle is used to create a vent and to infuse dessicated nitrogen gas at 80 cc/min for 8 minutes (29,31,36, 40).

The animals are placed on a diet consisting of rabbit chow supplemented with 1.5% to 2.0% cholesterol and 6% to 7% peanut oil. In prior studies using this model, cholesterol levels have ranged from 1000 to 2000 mg/dL (23,24,40). The animals are maintained on this diet until the time of angioplasty at 6 weeks. Following angioplasty the diet can be maintained or a regular diet resumed; regardless of diet, severe hypercholesterolemia will be maintained for the remainder of the study (Figure 13.2).

Six weeks following endothelial injury, the presence of lesions is documented by angiography. The right carotid artery is isolated and a 4F Swan-Ganz catheter is advanced to the aortic bifurcation. Meglumine diatrizoate is hand injected, and images are obtained either with cut film or with a conventional cineangiographic system with a 6-inch

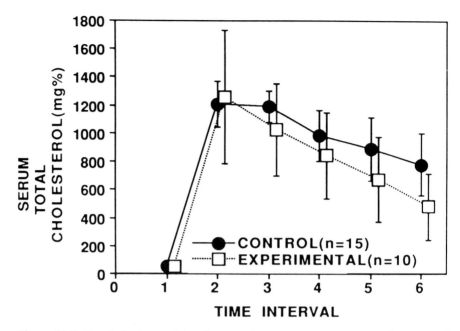

Figure 13.2. Total cholesterol levels over time. Time point 1 is at the time of endothelial injury, point 2 is at the time of angioplasty, points 3, 4, and 5 are 10, 20, and 30 days after angioplasty, and point 6 is at the time of sacrifice. Experimental animals received lovastatin 6 mg/kg daily. A high-cholesterol diet was maintained from time point 1 to time point 2. (Reproduced with permission of the American College of Cardiology from Gellman J et al. J Am Coll Cardiol 1991;17:251–259.)

image intensifier. A 1-cm grid is positioned over the pelvis to allow correction for magnification. Angioplasty is performed under the same anesthesia if a significant iliac stenosis is present.

For angioplasty, the mid femoral artery is isolated. A 2.5 mm Gruentzig intraoperative transluminal angioplasty balloon catheter is passed retrograde to the site of greatest iliac artery stenosis and inflated to a pressure of 5 to 10 atm for 60 seconds for three inflations. The angioplasty catheter is then withdrawn and the result documented by repeat cineangiography using the Swan-Ganz catheter for dye injection. The catheters are then removed and the arteries ligated (22–24).

Alternatively, a 5F sheath can be placed in the carotid artery and advanced to the descending aorta over a 0.014-inch guidewire. Following angiography through the sheath, antegrade angioplasty can be performed with a conventional PTCA balloon (29,31,36,40).

Follow-up angiography is performed at 4 weeks. Using the left carotid artery a Swan-Ganz catheter is introduced for angiography as above. Typical angiographic images before and immediately after angioplasty are shown in Figure 13.3. After the animals are killed with an overdose of pentothal, the iliac arteries are perfused with 10% buffered formalin at systemic pressure for 15 to 30 minutes through a cannula placed in the descending aorta. The entire aortoiliac trunk is removed en bloc, stripped of periadventitial connective tissue, and placed in 10% formalin for at least 72 hours. After review of the angiograms to guide sampling, the appropriate sections of the treated iliac artery are removed and embedded in paraffin, and stained with hematoxylin-eosin, van Gieson-elastin, and modified trichrome-fibrin stains. In addition to morphometric analysis of the histologic sections, the minimal lumen diameter of the iliac arteries can be measured from the angiograms obtained preangioplasty, immediately postangioplasty, and at 4-week follow-up.

Histopathology

The lesions induced by this technique differ from human atherosclerosis. Typically, the lesions are concentric with a thickened neointima consisting of foam cells with an overlying fibrous cap of varying depth (Figure 13.4; 26). Fibrosis, calcification, eccentricity, and necrosis are generally less prominent than in human lesions. A more fibrous type

Figure 13.3. Aortoiliac angiogram of hypercholesterolemic rabbit 4 weeks after balloon deendothelialization. The left panel shows a focal iliac stenosis (arrow), the middle panel shows a 2.5-mm angioplasty balloon inflated to 5 atm, and the right panel shows the immediate result. A small tear is evident at the site of balloon inflation (arrow). (Reproduced with permission of the American Heart Associaton from Faxon DP et al. Arteriosclerosis 1982;2:125–133.)

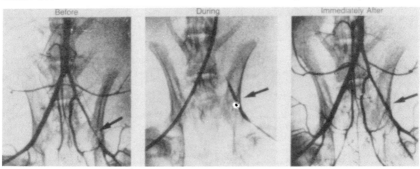

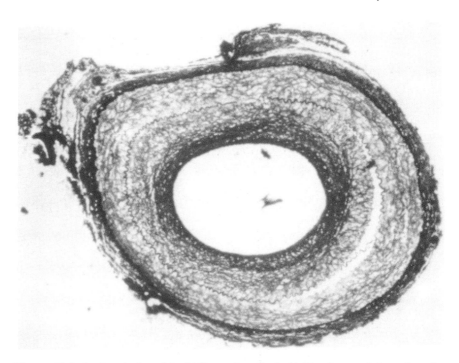

Figure 13.4. Lesion induced by balloon deendothelialization and 4 weeks of a high-cholesterol diet shows neointimal proliferation of foam cells with an overlying fibrous cap. The separation along the internal elastic lamina is an artifact of preparation. (Reproduced with permission of the American Heart Association from Sanborn TA et al. Circulation 1983;68:1136–1140.)

eccentric lesion can be induced by leaving an indwelling catheter across the iliac artery for 8 weeks (Figure 13.5; 22).

The acute effects of angioplasty on these lesions are demonstrated in Figure 13.6 (22,26). These include fracture of the neointimal plaque, dissection between the neointima and media, disruption of the internal elastic lamella, and frequently fracture of the media and stretching of the adventitia.

Prior studies have shown nearly 100% restenosis rates in untreated animals, over a 4-week follow-up period. A typical proliferative restenotic lesion consists of foam cells with abundant extracellular matrix (Figure 13.7; 24). As in the primary lesions, often a fibrous cap overlies the foam cells. Frequently, the original neointimal plaque can be seen, with the fracture induced by the angioplasty evident.

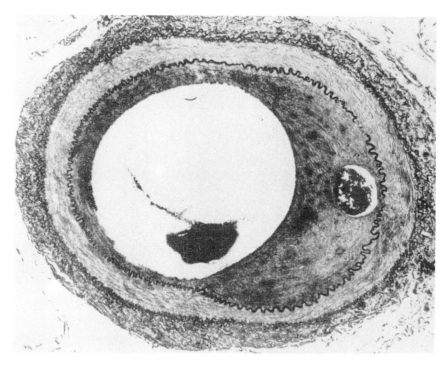

Figure 13.5. Fibrous lesion induced by a chronic indwelling catheter. The circular defect in the thickest portion of the eccentric lesion is due to the catheter. (Reproduced with permission of the American Heart Associaton from Faxon DP et al. Arteriosclerosis 1982;2:125–133.)

Advantages and Disadvantages

This model allows interaction of platelet deposition, thrombus formation, endothelial denudation, and plaque disruption. The effects of flow reduction and deep arterial trauma, with exposure of the inner components of the atherosclerotic plaque to circulating blood, are more similar to PTCA than other models. The use of obstructive primary lesions and the severe degree of stenosis 4 weeks after angioplasty allow the use of angiography, in addition to histology, to assess therapeutic benefit. The rabbit is inexpensive, but the time course of development of lesions and restenosis is longer than other models.

Limitations of this model include the use of iliac as opposed to coronary arteries, the expense and operator risk of radiation exposure, and

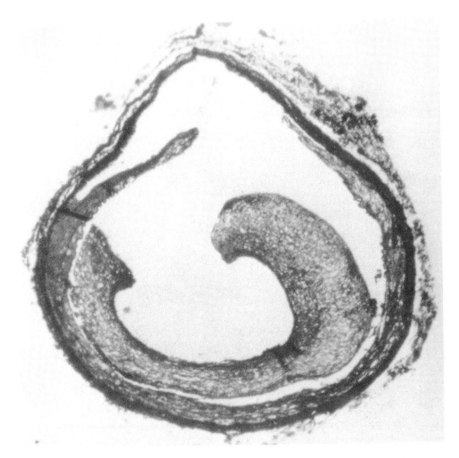

Figure 13.6. The acute result of angioplasty in a lesion such as that shown in Figure 13.4. There is fracture of the neointimal plaque, internal elastic lamina, and media. The adventitia is stretched, resulting in a local aneurysm. (Reproduced with permission of the American Heart Association from Sanborn TA et al. Circulation 1983;68:1136–1140.)

the degree of hyperlipidemia required for the development of lesions. The latter results in a prominent foam cell component to both the primary and restenotic lesion. However, immunocytochemical studies in the hypercholesterolemic rabbit have verified that these lipid-containing cells are of both macrophage and SMC origin (49). Proliferating cells in de novo lesions are approximately 30% macrophages and 45% SMCs (50).

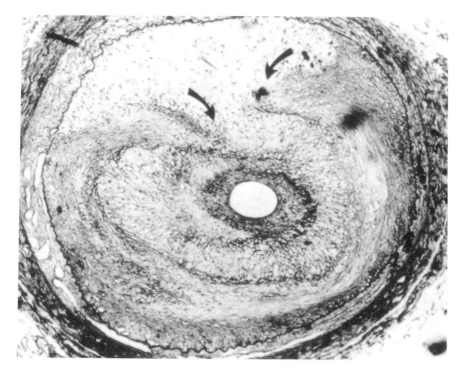

Figure 13.7. Restenosis after angioplasty. The original neointimal plaque was split by angioplasty (arrows), the resultant lumen has been largely filled in by a foam cell proliferative process, with a dense fibrous cap. (Reproduced with permission of the American Heart Association from Faxon DP et al. Arteriosclerosis 1984;4:189–195.)

Results

Our initial studies using this model concentrated on the mechanism of angioplasty and restenosis (22–27). At that time, it was felt that angioplasty increased lumen size by compressing or redistributing the atherosclerotic plaque. When a conventional, appropriately sized angioplasty balloon is inflated to nominal pressure in an artery with a significant focal stenosis, the histopathology in this model suggested a much more traumatic mechanism. These effects have been confirmed in patients by angioscopy (51), intravascular ultrasound (52), and necropsy (53). Later studies showed that, in addition to neointimal plaque fracture and dissection, local aneurysm formation occurred by stretching of the less atherosclerotic portions of the vessel (26). Despite the severe degree of arterial injury, there was no evidence for distal embolization (27).

In addition to allowing the study of mechanisms of angioplasty, it became apparent that, as in patients, angioplasty in this model was frequently followed by restenosis (23–25). Our laboratory and others have attempted to define this process. Removal of the endothelium is essentially unavoidable because pressure must be exerted on the artery wall to dilate the lesion. Deendothelialization and deeper damage to the arterial wall exposes collagen, lipid, and other elements of the extracellular matrix circulating blood, leading to platelet deposition and thrombus formation (Figure 13.8).

In the rabbit iliac artery model, platelet deposition occurs rapidly following balloon injury (28). Using ^{51}Cr-labelled platelets, we showed that large numbers of platelets are present as soon as 30 minutes following injury, and a peak in platelet deposition occurs at 2 hours. Over the subsequent 24 hours a small amount of deposition occurs, and there is little

Figure 13.8. Platelet deposition 30 minutes following angioplasty at the site of neointimal plaque fracture (large arrow) and extending into dissection plane (small arrow). (Reproduced with permission of the American Heart Association from Wilentz JR et al. Circulation 1987;75:636–642.)

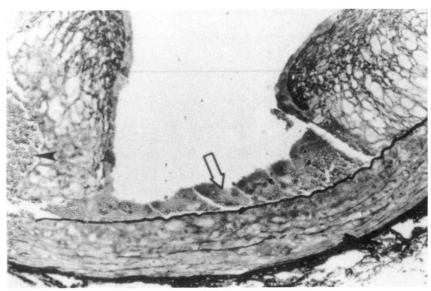

further platelet deposition over the next 4 weeks. Histologically, platelet deposition is most pronounced at sites of plaque fracture and least in areas where there is deendothelialization only.

As soon as 24 hours following injury, large numbers of polymorphonuclear leukocytes are present (22). Over the next 2 days the inflammatory infiltrate involves deeper layers of the artery, and by day 5 it has essentially resolved. Chronic inflammatory cells are present, but not prominent (unpublished data).

Endothelial regrowth after balloon injury occurs by 2 weeks in normal arteries (30). The cells appear structurally abnormal but are identifiable with an immunocytochemical stain for factor VIII-related antigen. Endothelial-dependent relaxation is abnormal up to 2 weeks after moderate injury and 4 weeks after severe injury, whereas endothelial-independent relaxation is not altered. In contrast, after balloon injury in atherosclerotic arteries with induced stenoses, endothelial-independent relaxation is impaired for 2 weeks with an appropriately-sized balloon, and for 4 weeks with an oversized balloon (29).

The SMCs show evidence of pressure necrosis at even low-pressure dilations (26). With higher pressure dilations, evidence of dissection and medial necrosis is increased, and the arteries dilated with higher pressure show increased intimal proliferation at 28 days (31). Other studies have shown that in the rabbit aorta, a stretch of approximately 45% leads to loss of vascular reactivity and that precontraction with a vasoconstrictor increased the degree of damage for any given balloon size (32).

After characterizing the mechanism of angioplasty and subsequent events in this model, many studies have been directed at reducing restenosis. Since one of the earliest events is platelet deposition, antiplatelet agents were among the first examined. High-dose oral sulfinpyrazone (33 mg/kg daily) was effective in limiting the extent of neointima formation (25). The combination of oral aspirin (10 mg/kg daily) and high-dose dipyridamole (8 mg/kg daily) was less effective but still significantly better than control. Subsequently, we showed that intravenous aspirin, but not oral, could significantly reduce early platelet deposition (33). The combination of oral aspirin and dipyridamole was much better than oral aspirin alone, but not as effective as intravenous aspirin at inhibiting platelet deposition. From these results it was concluded that high-dose antiplatelet agents could limit restenosis in this model, whereas oral aspirin alone at an extrapolated human dose was ineffective.

In addition to platelet deposition, thrombosis also occurs early after balloon injury. To inhibit both of these processes, we have used a regimen of aspirin at a dosage sufficient to decrease thromboxane B_2 levels by more than 95% (20 mg/kg daily) with warfarin to maintain the prothrombin time 1.5 times control (0.8–1.6 mg/kg daily), started 1 week prior to angioplasty (34). This regimen was also successful in limiting restenosis, with lumen diameter 1.3 ± 0.3 mm at follow-up, versus 0.6 ± 0.3 mm in controls. Other investigators have used this model to evaluate antiplatelet agents such as trapidil, a PDGF antagonist (35). Subcutaneous trapidil administered twice daily (30 mg/kg) for 4 weeks had a modest but statistically significant effect in reducing intimal proliferation. More recently, the potent thrombin inhibitor desulphatohirudin given intravenously for 2 hours following femoral artery angioplasty reduced intimal proliferation at 4 weeks (36). Treated animal vessels lost only 0.3 ± 0.3 mm diameter from immediately postangioplasty. In the control animals (treated with a 150 U/kg bolus of heparin), the diameter at follow-up was reduced by 0.9 ± 0.6 mm from postangioplasty. The lack of benefit with heparin is not surprising given its inability to prevent platelet deposition; it was not administered long enough to directly inhibit SMC proliferation (33).

Other components of the restenotic process have also been examined. Coronary spasm was a frequent event in the early days of angioplasty, and we hypothesized that spasm may play a role in restenosis in this model. However, nifedipine in doses of 3 mg/kg daily was unsuccessful in reducing the occurrence of restenosis in this model (37), and subsequent human studies with nifedipine and diltiazem also gave negative results (1).

The failure of antiplatelet agents in the usual doses to prevent restenosis in patients led us to examine other aspects of restenosis in this model, and we have focused on the proliferative component of the process. Colchicine was an attractive agent for a number of reasons, including its antiproliferative, anti-inflammatory, and migration inhibiting effects. In the extrapolated human dose, colchicine was ineffective in preventing restenosis (38). However, at high dose (0.2 mg/kg daily), generating serum levels approximately 10 times the usual therapeutic human level, an inhibitory effect was noted. This suggested that therapy directed at later events in restenosis could also be effective.

The inhibitory effects of heparin on SMC proliferation in the rat carotid model have been discussed (3). Low-molecular weight heparin has several advantages over unfractionated heparin, including more favorable pharmocokinetics and less bleeding complications. Several studies in this model showed that, although low-dose (1 mg/kg per day) enoxaparin was not effective, high-dose (10 mg/kg per day) enoxaparin given for either 2 or 4 weeks following the procedure was able to significantly reduce restenosis (39). The magnitude of the effect was similar to colchicine, with mean luminal diameter at follow-up 1.2 ± 0.1 mm for high-dose 4-week enoxaparin, 1.0 ± 0.2 mm for high-dose 2-week enoxaparin, 0.8 ± 0.2 mm for low-dose 4-week enoxaprin, and 0.6 ± 0.1 mm for control vessels. These results formed the basis for a multicenter, randomized, placebo-controlled trial of this agent in patients.

Lovastatin has also been used to inhibit intimal proliferation in this model (40). After femoral angioplasty, 6 mg/kg per day of oral lovastatin significantly reduced intimal area and thickness compared with controls. Although cholesterol levels fell more in the treatment group, both treatment and control animals had severe hypercholesterolemia throughout the study (see Figure 13–2). Thus, the mechanism of action presumably related to a direct effect on proliferation rather than an indirect effect through reducing cholesterol.

As discussed in the previous section, ACE inhibition inhibits myointimal proliferation in the rat carotid model. We showed a similar effect using cilazapril (5 mg/kg daily) in this model (41), and are currently performing studies to investigate the mechanism of this effect.

One of the important sources of SMC activators is the platelet. The role of other cellular elements of the response to injury is less well defined. Proliferating SMCs express class II antigens concurrent with T lymphocyte infiltration, and T cell supression with cyclosporin A limited the proliferative response after balloon injury in the rat carotid artery (42). However, in this model cyclosporin A did not inhibit intimal proliferation as assessed by angiography (43). Histologically, there was an increase in medial thickening in the treatment group. These results may reflect a different degree of inflammatory cell infiltration in the two models.

In addition to the study of restenosis, we and other investigators find this model useful for the continued investigation of new devices such as lasers, microwave catheters, and stents (44–48). Recognizing some of the limitations of this model, other investigators have used various modifications. One modification is to harvest SMCs from the artery at various times after angioplasty and measure the propensity of the cells to migrate and divide in culture (54). We are currently using this technique to examine the difference between in vivo and in vitro effects of ACE inhibitors. Another modification is to use the descending thoracic aorta in nonhypercholesterolemic rabbits (55,56). This technique is essentially a modification of the rat carotid model, and inhibition of myointimal proliferation with somatostatin analogue angiopeptin was significant in both the rabbit aorta and rat carotid (55–57). Angiopeptin was also effective in another model of accelerated atherosclerosis, the cardiac transplant model (58).

Other modifications include the use of heterozygous Watanabe rabbits, resulting in a primary lesion more resembling human atherosclerosis (59). The Flemish giant rabbit has been used as well; this allows the air dessication method of induction to be used in a larger femoral artery (60). Finally, a more calcific lesion can be created by supplementing the diet of hypercholesterolemic rabbits with vitamin D_2 and calcium (61). This results in a less distensible lesion that may respond to dilatation more like human lesions.

Thus, the rabbit model has been widely used, and a variety of therapies have been shown to be effective. When effective, all agents to date have been used in doses much higher than the usual or safe human dose. Attacking platelet deposition and cell proliferation with potent agents limits restenosis, but drugs directed at inflammation or spasm even in high dose do not appear to be effective.

Swine Coronary Stent Model

This model of restenosis is the newest of the three models discussed in this chapter, but the early experience suggests that this may be a useful way to study the events of restenosis. The model consists of normal swine coronary arteries injured by the placement of an oversized stent, or by simple oversized balloon inflation.

Technique

Juvenile pigs weighing 20 to 30 kg are used for study (62). With systemic anesthesia, the right carotid artery is isolated and an 8F sheath is placed via an arteriotomy. Standard PTCA guides are used (JR4 for the left coronary, JL4 for the right coronary). A 0.005-inch tantalum coil stent is mounted on a 3.0-mm PTCA balloon and advanced to the target artery over a 0.014-inch guidewire. The stent is deployed with a single 14-atm inflation. The balloon is deflated and removed, and the stable location of the stent is confirmed by fluoroscopy and angiography. The carotid artery is then repaired or ligated. Initial studies were performed using 5000 U heparin before and after the procedure. Subsequently, the investigators have added a single dose of aspirin (650 mg) and sustained-release nifedipine (30 mg) on the day prior to the procedure (R. S. Schwartz, personal communication).

Balloon overinflation alone can be used to injure the artery as well, without using a stent. However, the induced lesions are less significant than with a stent and less reproducible (62).

After 4 weeks, the animals are sacrificed and the hearts' perfusion fixed at systemic pressure for 24 hours. The stented segments are removed, embedded and stained as described previously for the rabbit iliac arteries. The original native lumen is measured as the area enclosed by the internal elastic lamella (calculated by measuring major and minor axes and assuming an elliptical shape). The restenotic lumen is measured similarly, using the endothelial surface instead of the internal elastic lamina. Results are expressed as percent area stenosis. Alternatively, the mean intimal thickness can be measured as the distance from lumen to internal elastic lamina.

Histopathology

The acute effects of stent deployment include rupture of the internal elastic lamina by the coil wires; occasionally they are even forced through the media to the adventitia. Within the first 6 hours, there is evidence of extensive platelet deposition and thrombus formation, which often significantly obstructs the lumen (63). The subsequent healing of the artery results in a severe restenotic lesion (see Figure 8.2). Histologically, this lesion closely resembles human restenosis (Figure 13.9). The initial trauma of stent deployment is still evident, with stent wire defects present in the adventitia. The neointimal proliferation is impressive and consists of SMCs and abundant extracellular matrix.

Advantages and Disadvantages

The main advantage of this model is the close gross and histologic resemblance between these lesions and human restenosis. The lesions are easily and reproducibly induced (at least with the stent) and develop over a brief period of time. The deep arterial trauma more closely simulates angioplasty than mere deendothelialization, and the muscular pig

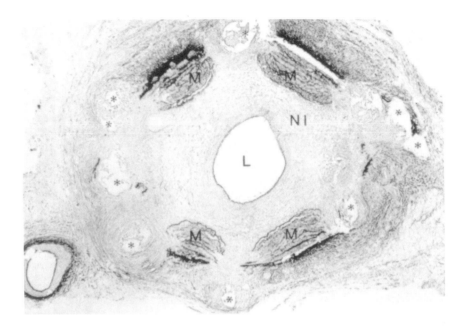

Figure 13.9. Neointimal (NI) proliferation with severe luminal obstruction. * indicates stent coils, and M denotes residual media. (Reproduced with permission of the American Heart Association from Schwartz RS et al. Circulation 1990;82:2190–2200.)

coronary artery is more like human coronaries than the elastic rabbit iliac and rat carotid arteries.

Pigs are more difficult to use and more expensive than either rats or rabbits. The model uses normal arteries and leaves an indwelling foreign body. Given the prominent early thrombotic component to the lesions, the contribution of platelets and thrombus to restenosis may be more pronounced in this model. Although experience with this model is limited, it may represent a useful way to evaluate potential therapies for restenosis in patients.

Results

The concept of severe injury in normal arteries resulting in a marked proliferative lesion has been noted previously. In the normal pig carotid artery, balloon injury with an oversized balloon (8 mm in a 5–6 mm artery) results in intimal tears, SMC necrosis, marked platelet deposition, and thrombus formation (64). The thrombus can significantly reduce the lumen (Figure 13.10), and organization of this mural thrombus can result in a significant obstructive fibrotic plaque. Analogous to the results in the rabbit model, the depth of injury appears to be directly related to the degree of platelet deposition (65), because the presence of a mild or moderate dissection was clearly associated with an increased number of platelets. The importance of platelet deposition in patients was recently emphasized by a necropsy series reported by Nobuyoshi and colleagues (19). In analyzing a group of 20 patients dying at various times after angioplasty, mural thrombus was common in lesions dilated from 11 to 30 days previously. In a limited number of lesions less than 10 days after dilatation, thrombus was present in one third. Organized thrombus was found later than 1 month in a few cases but did not constitute the obstruction in patients with restenosis.

Over the 4 days following stent placement the thrombus begins to orga-

Figure 13.10. Eccentric neointima (NI) formation after oversized balloon injury alone. Lumen (L) is more preserved, and media (M) is less disrupted than in Figure 13.9. (Reproduced with permission of the American Heart Association from Schwartz RS et al. Circulation 1990;82:2190–2200.)

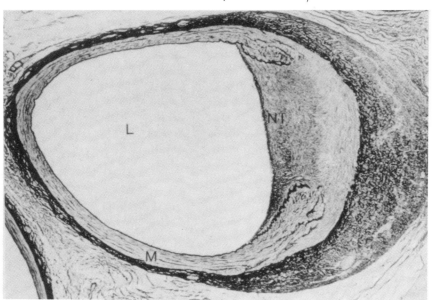

nize and the surface begins to reendothelialize (63). By day 14, inflammatory cells, including lymphocytes and monocytes, are prominent. SMCs begin to grow into the thrombus, growing in from the lateral borders. Over the subsequent 2 weeks the migrating SMCs form a fibrous cap over the luminal aspect of the organizing thrombus and grow down toward the media. The end result is a homogenous lesion with large numbers of SMCs and a prominent extracellular matrix.

From histologic sections in which only a few of the stent wires perforated the internal elastic lamina, it is apparent that the deeper the degree of damage, the more prominent the intimal proliferation (62). In arteries damaged by an oversized balloon alone, a more eccentric pattern of injury and resultant lesion formation is seen (Figure 13.11). Again, the deeper injury reflected by internal elastic lamina disruption results in a more prominent neointimal lesion. Although disruption of the internal elastic lamina may facilitate migration of SMCs (66), it clearly is not necessary because in the rat carotid artery model it is not damaged and extensive migration occurs.

Results of intervention in this model are just becoming available. Methotrexate and azathioprine are unsuccessful in limiting the neointimal lesions in this model (67). Preliminary data show that neither ACE inhibitors nor external irradiation prevent the development of neointimal lesions (R. S. Schwartz, personal communication). Trials of other agents are currently in progress.

In addition to the coronary stent model, some investigators have used a Yucatan microswine model in which lesions are created in iliac arteries by hypercholesterolemia and balloon deendothelialization. The advantage of this model over the rabbit iliac model is that the lesions resemble the human de novo lesion more closely, with fibrosis, calcification, and collagen (68). Additionally, this species attains a body weight of only 20 kg at maturity. The disadvantage is that it requires 20 weeks of atherogenic diet after balloon deendothelialization to develop lesions.

Hanford microswine have also been used as a model of atherosclerosis (69–72). Coronary abrasion followed by 5 months of a high-cholesterol diet results in angiographically visible, although not critical, lesions. Stent deployment in this model is followed by intimal hyperplasia at 1 month even with minimal oversizing (stent-arterial ratio of 1.2:1; 72). Neither aspirin and dypridamole nor warfarin significantly modified this response. Again, the length of time necessary to develop lesions is a distinct disadvantage.

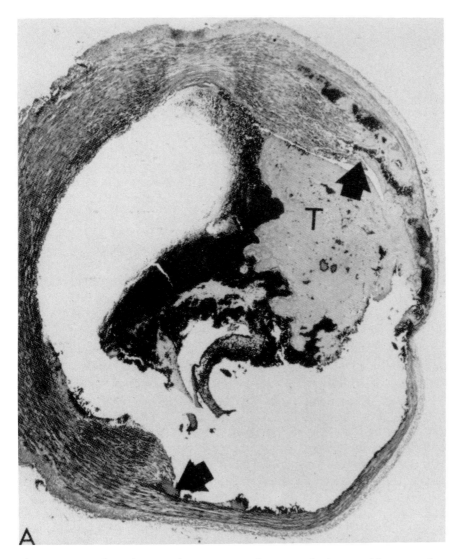

Figure 13.11. Thrombus (T) formation in the normal pig carotid artery after inflation of an oversized balloon. Arrows denote sites of medial dissection. (Reproduced with permission of the American College of Cardiology from Lam JYT, et al. J Am Coll Cardiol 1986;8:1380–1386.)

Conclusions

In summary, there is no ideal animal model for restenosis following PTCA. The process of restenosis is complex, with many components that may be targeted by different strategies (Table 13.2). The importance of any one component may vary from patient to patient, and different animal models emphasize different components of the process. Successful results in any one model may reflect activity against only the predominant mechanism of restenosis in that model.

Thus, the rat carotid artery model is primarily a SMC proliferation model. Although platelet deposition occurs and may lead to increased neointimal thickening, it is not required for proliferation. In the swine coronary stent model, the predominant early histologic feature is thrombus. Certainly the final histologic result resembles human restenosis, but the contribution of thrombosis to its genesis may be more important than occurs in most cases clinically. The hypercholesterolemic rabbit iliac artery model combines several mechanisms of restenosis including recoil, platelet deposition, SMC proliferation, and alterations in shear stress. However, by virtue of the marked elevation in cholesterol it adds another feature (i.e., foam cell development) that is not usually apparent in human restenosis. Although evidence is accumulating that lipids may play a role in restenosis, the histologic features seen in this model are not present clinically (81,82).

Because human restenosis occurs by a number of separate but related mechanisms, therapy directed at any one mechanism may have only a small impact on the overall occurrence of restenosis, despite encouraging results in an animal model. Effective therapy in patients will likely need to target several different mechanisms and may require combined therapeutic modalities. Thus, elimination of recoil may reduce the degree of intimal narrowing by up to 50% in some patients (83), but the successful reduction of clinical restenosis may require the addition of another agent directed at such processes as platelet deposition or SMC proliferation. Many of the different mechanisms are under active investigation (see Table 13.2). Additive effects have been described for the combination of cilazapril and heparin in the rat carotid artery model (20) and warfarin and aspirin in the rabbit iliac model (34).

Another reason to combine different modes of therapy is to minimize side effects. Many of the agents shown to be effective in animal models require the use of high doses, which may be poorly tolerated in patients. Additionally, as more potent inhibitors of platelet deposition or cell pro-

Table 13.2 Mechanisms of Restenosis and Potential Therapies

MECHANISM	POTENTIAL THERAPY
Recoil	stents (46,47,72)
Platelet deposition	antibody to glycoprotein IIB/IIIA (73)
Thrombus formation	thrombin inhibitors (36,74)
	warfarin/aspirin (34)
	heparins (3,39)
Inflammation	steroids (75)
	cyclosporin A (42,43)
	colchicine (38,78)
Growth factors	trapidil (PDGF; 35)
	ketanserin (5-HT; 76)
	ACE inhibitors (A II; 20,41)
	angiopeptin (IGF, PDGF, FGF; 56,77)
	SQ29548 (thromboxane A_2; 76)
	heparins (FGF, EGF, IGF; 3,39)
Smooth muscle cell	
migration	ACE inhibitors (20,41)
	colchicine (38,78)
proliferation	ACE inhibitors (20,41)
	lovastatin (40)
	heparins (3,39)
	antimetabolites (67,78)
	gene transfer (79)
hypertrophy	ACE inhibitors (20,41)
	thrombin inhibitors (36,74)
Matrix production	colchicine (38,78)
	heparins (3,39)
	thrombin inhibitors (36,74)
Delayed reendothelialization	endothelial cell seeding (80)
	gene transfer (79)

ACE = angiotension-converting enzyme; PDGF = platelet-derived growth factor; IGF = insulinlike growth factor; EGF = epidermal growth factor; FGF = fibroblast growth factor; 5-HT = serotonin, A II = antiotension II (Modified from Currier JW, et al. Pathophysiology of restenosis: clinical implications. Submitted for publication.)

liferation are used, the potential for significant "side effects" due to the desired effect occurring in a nontarget tissue increases. Local delivery systems may circumvent some of these problems (14).

A final reason to combine therapies is that the different mechanisms of luminal narrowing occur at different times. For example, therapy directed at platelet deposition need not continue for 6 months, but must be started prior to angioplasty. Conversely, it may not be important to start antiproliferative agents for several days after the procedure, but they must be given over several weeks.

Using agents with known mechanisms of action in the model that emphasizes the appropriate mechanism of restenosis offers the best chance of evaluating therapies that may be effective in patients. These and other lessons learned from animal models will be important in enabling us to combine these therapies in a rational manner for human use that will reduce the incidence of restenosis following PTCA.

References

1. Blackshear JL, O'Callaghan WG, Califf RM. Medical approaches to prevention of restenosis after coronary angioplasty. J Am Coll Cardiol 1987; 9:834–848.
2. Armstrong ML, Heistad DP. Animal models of atherosclerosis. Atherosclerosis 1990;85:15–23.
3. Clowes AW, Karnovsky MJ. Suppression by heparin of smooth muscle cell proliferation in injured arteries. Nature 1977;265:625–626.
4. Baumgartner HR. Eine neue Methode zur Erzeugung der Thromben durch gezeilte Uberdehnung der Gefasswand. Z Ges Exp Med 1963; 137:227–249.
5. Guyton J, Rosenburg R, Clowes A, Karnovsky M. Inhibition of rat arterial smooth muscle cell proliferation by heparin. In vivo studies with anticoagulant and nonanticoagulant heparin. Circ Res 1980;46:625–634.
6. Fishman JA, Ryan GB, Karnovsky MJ. Endothelial regeneration in the rat carotid artery and the significance of endothelial denudation in the pathogenesis of myointimal thickening. Lab Invest 1975;32:339–351.
7. Clowes AW, Reidy MA, Clowes MM. Mechanisms of stenosis after arterial injury. Lab Invest 1983;49:208.
8. Clowes AW, Schwartz SM. Significance of quiescent smooth muscle migration in the injured rat carotid artery. Circ Res 1985;56:139–145.
9. Fingerle J, Johnson R, Clowes AW, Majesky MN, Reidy M. Role of platelets in smooth muscle cell proliferation and migration after vascular injury in rat carotid artery. Proc Natl Acad Sci USA 1989;86:8412–8416.
10. Clowes AW, Clowes MM. Kinetics of cellular proliferation after arterial injury. IV. Heparin inhibits rat smooth muscle mitogenesis and migration. Circ Res 1986;58:839–845.
11. Majesky MW, Schwartz SM, Clowes MM, Clowes AW. Heparin regu-

lates smooth muscle S phase entry in the injured rat carotid artery. Circ Res 1987;61:296–300.

12. Clowes AW, Clowes MM, Fingerle J, Reidy M. Regulation of smooth muscle cell growth in injured artery. J Card Pharm 1989;14:S12–S15.

13. Powell JS, Clozel JP, Muller KM, et al. Inhibitors of angiotensin-converting enzyme prevent myointimal proliferation after vascular injury. Science 1989;245:186–188.

14. Edelman ER, Adams DH, Karnovsky MJ. Effect of controlled adventitial heparin delivery on smooth muscle cell proliferation following endothelial injury. Proc Natl Acad Sci USA 1990;87:3773–3777.

15. Liu MW, Roubin GS, King SB. Restenosis after coronary angioplasty. Potential biologic determinants and role of intimal hyperplasia. Circulation 1989;79:1374–1387.

16. Kohler TR, Jawien A, Clowes AW. Effect of shear on intimal hyperplasia following arterial injury in rats. Circulation 1990;82(suppl III):400.

17. Clowes AW, Karnovsky MJ. Failure of certain antiplatelet drugs to affect myointimal thickening following arterial endothelial injury in the rat. Lab Invest 1977;36:452–464.

18. Reidy MA, Clowes AW, Schwartz SM. Endothelial regeneration: V. Inhibition of endothelial regrowth in arteries of rat and rabbit. Lab Invest 1983;49:569.

19. Nobuyoshi M, Kimura T, Ohishi H, Horiuchi H, et al. Restenosis after percutaneous transluminal coronary angioplasty: Pathologic observations in 20 patients. J Am Coll Cardiol 1991;17:433–439.

20. Powell JS, Muller RK, Baumgartner HR. Suppression of the vascular response to injury: the role of angiotensin converting enzyme inhibitors. J Am Coll Cardiol 1991;17:137B–142B.

21. Block PC, Baughman KL, Pasternak RC, Fallon JT. Transluminal angioplasty: correlation of morphologic and angiographic findings in an experimental model. Circulation 1980;61:778–785.

22. Faxon DP, Weber VJ, Haudenschild C, Bottsman SB, McGovern WA, Ryan TJ. Acute effects of transluminal angioplasty in three experimental models of atherosclerosis. Arteriosclerosis 1982;2:125–133.

23. Faxon DP, Sanborn TA, Haudenschild CC. Mechanism of angioplasty and its relation to restenosis. Am J Cardiol 1987;60:5B–9B.

24. Faxon DP, Sanborn TA, Weber VJ, et al. Restenosis following transluminal angioplasty in experimental atherosclerosis. Arteriosclerosis 1984;4:189–195.

25. Faxon DP, Sanborn TA, Haudenschild CC, Ryan TJ. Effect of antiplatelet therapy on restenosis after experimental angioplasty. Am J Cardiol 1984;53:72C–76C.

26. Sanborn TA, Faxon DP, Haudenschild CC, Gottsman SB, Ryan TJ. The mechanism of transluminal angioplasty: evidence for formation of aneurysms in experimental atherosclerosis. Circulation 1983;69:1136–1140.

27. Sanborn TA, Faxon DP, Waugh D, Small SM, Haudenschild CC, Gottsman SB, Ryan TJ. Transluminal angioplasty in experimental atherosclerosis: analysis for embolization using an in vivo perfusion system. Circulation 1982;66:917–922.

28. Wilentz JR, Sanborn TA, Haudenschild CC, Valeri CR, Ryan TJ, Faxon DP. Platelet accumulation in experimental angioplasty: time course and relation to vascular injury. Circulation 1987;75:636–642.

29. LaVeau PJ, Sarembock IJ, Sigal SL, Yang TL, Ezekowitz MD. Vascular reactivity after balloon angioplasty in an atherosclerotic rabbit. Circulation 1990;82:1790–1801.

30. Weidinger FF, McLenachan JM, Cybulsky MI, et al. Persistent dysfunction of regenerated endothelium after balloon angioplasty of rabbit iliac artery. Circulation 1990;81:1667–1679.

31. Sarembock IJ, LaVeau PJ, Signal SL, et al. Influence of pressure and balloon size on the development of intimal hyperplasia after balloon angioplasty. Circulation 1989;80:1029–1040.

32. Fischell TA, Grant G, Johnson DE. Determinants of smooth muscle cell injury during balloon angioplasty. Circulation 1990;82:2170–2184.

33. Balelli LA, Sanborn TA, Haudenschild CC, Valeri CR, Ryan TJ, Faxon DP. The effect of antiplatelet therapy on platelet accumulation after experimental angioplasty. Submitted for publication.

34. Franklin SM, Currier JW, Cannistra A, et al. Warfarin/aspirin combination reduces restenosis after angioplasty in atherosclerotic rabbits. Circulation 1990;82(suppl):427.

35. Liu MW, Roubin GS, Robinson KA, et al. Trapidil in preventing restenosis after balloon angioplasty in the atherosclerotic rabbit. Circulation 1990;81:1089–1093.

36. Sarembock IJ, Gertz SD, Gimple LW, Owen RM, Powers ER, Roberts WC. Effectiveness of recombinant desulphatohirudin in reducing restenosis after balloon angioplasty of atherosclerotic femoral arteries in rabbits. Circulation 1991;84:232–243.

37. Faxon DP, Sanborn TA, Haudenschild CC, Gottsman SB, Ryan TJ. The effect of nifedipine on restenosis following experimental angioplasty. Circulation 1984;70(suppl II):175.

38. Currier JW, Pow TK, Minihan AC, Haudenschild CC, Faxon DP, Ryan TJ. Colchicine inhibits restenosis after iliac angioplasty in the atherosclerotic rabbit. Circulation 1989;80(suppl II):66.

39. Currier JW, Pow TK, Haudenschild CC, Minihan AC, Faxon DP. Low molecular weight heparin reduces restenosis following angioplasty in the hypercholesterolemic rabbit. J Am Coll Cardiol 1991;17:118B–125B.

40. Gellman J, Ezekowitz MD, Sarembock IJ, et al. Effect of lovastatin on intimal hyperplasia after balloon angioplasty: a study in an atherosclerotic hypercholesterolemic rabbit. J Am Coll Cardiol 1991;17:251–259.

41. Bilazarian SD, Currier JW, Haudenschild CC, et al. Angiotensin converting enzyme inhibition reduces restenosis in experimental angioplasty. J Am Coll Cardiol 1991;17:268A.

42. Jonasson L, Holm J, Hansson GK. Cyclosporin A inhibits smooth muscle cell proliferation in the vascular response to injury. Proc Natl Acad Sci USA 1988;85:2303–2306.

43. McKenney P, Currier JW, Haudenschild CC, Faxon DP. Cyclosporin A does not inhibit restenosis in experimental angioplasty. Abstract submitted to 1991 AHA Scientific Sessions.

44. Sanborn TA, Haudenschild CC, Ryan TJ, Faxon DP. Angiographic and histologic consequences of laser thermal angioplasty: comparison to balloon angioplasty. Circulation 1987;75:1281–1286.

45. Hanke H, Haase KK, Hanke S, et al. Morphological changes and smooth muscle cell proliferation after experimental excimer laser treatment. Circulation 1991;83:1380–1389.

46. Robinson KA, Roubin GS, Siegel RJ, Black AJ, Apkarian RP, King SB. Intra-arterial stenting in the atherosclerotic rabbit. Circulation 1988;78:646–653.

47. Sutton CS, Tominaga R, Harasaki H, et al. Vascular stenting in normal and atherosclerotic rabbits: studies of the intravascular endoprosthesis of titanium-nickel alloy. Circulation 1990;81:667–683.

48. Landau CL, Currier JW, Haudenschild CC, Heymann D, Minihan AC, Faxon DP. Microwave balloon angioplasty to treat arterial dissections in an atherosclerotic rabbit model. J Am Coll Cardiol 1991;17:234A.

49. Tsukada T, Rosenfeld M, Ross R, Gown AM. Immunocytochemical analysis of cellular components in atherosclerotic lesions: use of monoclonal antibodies with the Watanabe and fat-fed rabbit. Arteriosclerosis 1986;6:601–613.

50. Rosenfeld ME, Ross R. Macrophage and smooth muscle cell proliferation in atherosclerotic lesions of WHHL and comparably hypercholesterolemic fat-fed rabbits. Arteriosclerosis 1990;10:680–687.

51. Remee S, White C, Jain A, et al. Percutaneous coronary angioscopy versus intravascular ultrasound in patients undergoing coronary angioplasty. J Am Coll Cardiol 1991;17:125A.

52. Lasardo D, Rosenfield K, Ramaswamy K, et al. How does angioplasty work? Intravascular ultrasound assessment of 30 consecutive patients demonstrating that angiographic evidence of luminal patency is the consistent result of plaque fractures and dissections. Circulation 1990; 82: (suppl III):338.

53. Waller BF, Pinkerton CA, Orr CM, et al. Restenosis 1 to 24 months after balloon angioplasty: a necropsy study of 20 patients. J Am Coll Cardiol 1991;17:58B–70B.

54. Grunwald J, Haudenschild CC. Intimal injury in vivo activates vascular smooth muscle cell migration and outgrowth in vitro. Arteriosclerosis 1984;4:183–188.

55. Conte JV, Foegh ML, Calcagno D, Wallace RB, Ramwell PW. Peptide inhibition of myointimal proliferation following angioplasty in rabbits. Trans Proc 1989;21:3686–3688.

56. Asotra S, Foegh ML, Conte JV, Cori BR, Ramwell PW. Inhibition of ^{3}H-thymidine incorporation by angiopeptin in the aorta of rabbits after balloon angioplasty. Trans Proc 1989;21:3695–3696.

57. Lundergan C, Foegh ML, Vargas R, et al. Inhibition of myointimal proliferation of the rat carotid artery by the peptides angiopeptin and BIM 23034. Atherosclerosis 1989;80:49–55.

58. Foegh ML, Khirabadi BS, Chambers E, Amamoo S, Ramwell PW. Inhibition of coronary artery transplant atherosclerosis in rabbits with angiopeptin, an octapeptide. Atherosclerosis 1989;78:229–236.

59. Atkinson JB, Hoover RL, Berry KK, Swift LL. Cholesterol fed heterozygous Watanabe heritable hyperlipidemic rabbits: a new model for atherosclerosis. Atherosclerosis 1989;78:123–126.

60. LeVeen RF, Wolf GL, Villaneuva TG. New rabbit model for the investigation of transluminal angioplasty. Invest Radiol 1982;17:470–475.

61. Demer LL. Effect of calcification on in vivo mechanical response of rabbit arteries to balloon angioplasty. Circulation 1991;83:2083–2093.

62. Schwartz RS, Murphy JG, Edwards WD, et al. Restenosis after balloon angioplasty: a practical proliferative model in porcine coronary arteries. Circulation 1990;82:2190–2200.

63. Schwartz RS, Edwards WD, Murphy JG, Camrud A, Holmes D. Restenosis develops in four stages: serial histologic studies in a coronary injury model. J Am Coll Cardiol 1991;17:52A.

64. Steele PM, Chesebro JH, Stanson AW, et al. Balloon angioplasty: natural history of the pathophysiological response to injury in a pig model. Circ Res 1985;57:105–112.

65. Lam JY, Chesebro JH, Steele PM, et al. Deep arterial injury during exper-

imental angioplasty: relation to a positive indium-111 labeled platelet scintigram, quantitative platelet deposition and mural thrombus. J Am Coll Cardiol 1986;8:1380–1386.

66. Schwartz RS, Murphy JG, Edwards WD, et al. Coronary artery restenosis and the "virginal membrane": smooth muscle cell proliferation and the intact internal elastic lamina. Invas Cardiol 1991;3:239–244.

67. Murphy JG, Schwartz RS, Edwards WD, et al. Methotrexate and azathioprine fail to inhibit procine coronary restenosis. Circulation 1990; 82(suppl III):429.

68. Gal D, Rongione AJ, Slovenkai GA, et al. Atherosclerotic Yucatan microswine: an animal model with high-grade, fibrocalcific, nonfatty lesions suitable for testing catheter-based interventions. Am Heart J 1990 Feb;119(2 Pt 1):291–300.

69. Scott RF, Kim DN, Schmee J, Thomas WA. Atherosclerotic lesions in coronary arteries of hyperlipidemic swine. Atherosclerosis 1986;62:1–14.

70. Weiner BH, Ockene IS, Jarmolych J, Fritz KE, Daoud AS. Comparison of pathologic and angiographic findings in a porcine preparation of coronary atherosclerosis. Circulation 1986;72:1081–1086.

71. Nam SC, Lee EM, Jarmolych J, Lee KT, Thomas WA. Rapid production of advanced atherosclerosis in swine by a combination of endothelial injury and cholesterol feeding. Exp Mol Pathol 1973;18:369–379.

72. Rodgers GP, Minor ST, Robinson K, et al. Adjuvant therapy for intracoronary stents: investigations in atherosclerotic swine. Circulation 1990;82:560–569.

73. Ellis SG, Bates ER, Schaible T, Weisman HF, Pitt B, Topol EJ. Prospects for the use of antagonists to the platelet glycoprotein IIb/IIIa receptor to prevent post angioplasty restenosis and thrombosis. J Am Coll Cardiol 1991;17:89B–95B.

74. Heras M, Chesebro JH, Penny WJ, Bailey KR, Badimon L, Fuster V. Effects of thrombin inhibition on the development of acute platelet-thrombus deposition during angioplasty in pigs: heparin versus recombinant hirudin, a specific thrombin inhibitor. Circulation 1989;79: 657–665.

75. Berk BC, Gordon JB, Alexander RW. Pharmacologic roles of heparin and glucocorticoids to prevent restenosis after coronary angioplasty. J Am Coll Cardiol 1991;17:111B–117B.

76. Willerson JT, Eidt JF, McNatt J, et al. Role of thromboxane and serotonin as mediators in the development of spontaneous alterations in coronary blood flow and neointimal proliferation in canine models with chronic coronary artery stenosis and endothelial injury. J Am Coll Cardiol 1991; 17:101B–110B.

77. Lundergan CF, Foegh ML, Ramwell PW. Peptide inhibition of myointimal proliferation by angiopeptin, a somatostatin analogue. J Am Coll Cardiol 1991;17:132B–136B.

78. Muller DWM, Ellis SG, Topol EJ. Colchicine and antineoplastic therapy for the prevention of restenosis after percutaneous coronary interventions. J Am Coll Cardiol 1991;17:126B–131B.

79. Nabel EG, Plautz G, Nabel GJ. Gene transfer into vascular cells. J Am Coll Cardiol 1991;17:189B–194B.

80. Dichek DA, Neville RF, Zwiebel JA, et al. Seeding of intravascular stents with genetically engineered endothelial cells. Circulation 1989; 80:1347–1353.

81. Jacobs AK, Folan DJ, McSweeney SM, et al. Effect of plasma lipids on restenosis following coronary angioplasty. J Am Coll Cardiol 1987; 9:183A.

82. Bergelson BA, Jacobs AK, Small DM, et al. Lipoproteins predict restenosis after PTCA. Circulation 1989;80(suppl II):65.

83. Rensing BJ, Hermans WRM, Beatt KJ, Laarman J, et al. Quantitative angiographic assessment of elastic recoil after percutaneous transluminal coronary angioplasty. Am J Cardiol 1990;66:1039–1044.

· ·

CHAPTER 14

Coronary Stents and Restenosis: Potential Solution for a Vexing Problem?

GEORGE I. FRANK
ULRICH SIGWART

Introduction

In the late 1960s a cardiologist in Spokane, Washington treated a few patients who were suffering an acute myocardial infarction with intracoronary thrombolytic therapy. Although his efforts were never published, they helped convince his colleagues that patients suffering an acute myocardial infarction could safely be catheterized. This group aggressively performed angiography on patients presenting with chest pain, with and without evidence of an acute myocardial infarction. Believing that early revascularization could reduce mortality and preserve myocardium, those patients with appropriate anatomy were sent for emergency coronary artery bypass grafting (CABG; 1). This was a major break with standard medical practice. No controlled studies were done, and much of the medical community outside of this small western Washington town decried this new form of medical adventurism. However, some found this therapeutic approach fascinating. Drs. Rentrop, Berg, and Sigwart discussed the potential for aggressive therapy in acute myocardial infarction in Vienna at a coffee house in the mid 1970s. Rentrop followed this new direction a few years later when he reported his attempts to open acutely occluded vessels, initially with a soft guidewire through the clot, and subsequently by instilling intracoronary streptokinase (2). When Gruentzig demonstrated the ability to dilate coronary arteries with a balloon catheter, the floodgates opened for those who wished to change the natural history of coronary disease (3). Of course, basic research in each area preceded these new therapeutic interventions, but the actual basic science detailing their mechanisms of action and subsequent effects are still being investigated more than 12 years after these initial studies were published.

Today cardiologists and the medical–industrial complex, which is so much a part of modern medicine, are vigorously pursuing therapeutic interventions that might alter the course of atherosclerosis. Soft and hard balloons, hot and cold lasers, fast and slow drills, some eccentric, others concentric, as well as stents have been applied to human coronary lesions in the hopes that the therapy will improve coronary blood flow and cause less morbidity than the disease itself. Time has demonstrated that at least some of these approaches are therapeutic, improving on the natural history of the disease. There is no question that thrombolytic therapy reduces mortality and decreases hospitalization for patients suffering an acute myocardial infarction (4,5). Angioplasty has become an accepted alternative to medical therapy for patients suffering from angina, and present investigations may show it to be a reasonable alternative to CABG for selected patient groups. Controlled studies examining the newest advances in interventional therapy to determine their role in the treatment of coronary artery disease are now being initiated.

New problems have arisen from these changing approaches to therapy. We still do not know the best treatment for those whose myocardial infarction was interrupted by thrombolytic therapy. Should they receive long-term anticoagulant therapy? Should further interventions be used in this patient group? Similarly, percutaneous transluminal coronary angioplasty (PTCA) created its own set of problems: abrupt closure and restenosis. Estimates suggest that over 400,000 standard balloon procedures were done worldwide in 1990. If 5% of these procedures were complicated by abrupt closure and 35% recurred due to restenosis, the financial and human costs of these problems are enormous. Attempts to modify the course of abrupt closure and restenosis with medical therapy have been unrewarding thus far. Several investigators have felt that an endoluminal support device, a stent, might be able to tack down flaps, prevent elastic recoil, and provide improved rheology for a diseased vessel segment, promoting healing and preventing restenosis.

The first stent was implanted in a human coronary artery in 1986 (6). Since then more than 1000 stents have been studied under various clinical circumstances.

Some investigators have advised the medical community to be wary of new interventional therapies because we still do not fully understand the process we are attempting to alter or the processes we are stimulating with these new tools (7). Of course these admonitions are wise. Some of the experimental forms of intervention will prove unsuccessful and perhaps more deleterious in the long-term than investigators thought initially. They will be discarded in favor of new tools as our knowledge expands. But for many medical advances, serendipity and a receptive mind have led the way before the basic sciences have studied and explained the phenomenon. Though intravascular endoluminal devices have been described as early as 1912, the primary areas of investigation involved their use in the peripheral circulation. Several different investigators realized their potential for the coronary circulation after the problems of balloon angioplasty became apparent. Stents have become a major focus for clinical and basic science research efforts. In this chapter we describe the current status of stents and their potential role in the future treatment of coronary artery disease.

Geometry and Histology of Stents

Animal research has demonstrated that stents inserted into vascular structures show variable degrees of endothelialization over time. These differences, in part, are related to the species of animal studied. In dogs a stent is likely to be covered with neointima in 4 weeks, whereas in a pig the process may require 12 weeks (8,9). The thickness of the metal wires is also a significant factor. Wright and colleagues demonstrated that stents placed in dogs with 0.46-mm stainless steel struts were only 30% covered with endothelium at the end of 4 weeks (10); others have shown that struts 0.09 mm thick are completely covered in 3 to 4 weeks (6,11). In dogs the neointima can have a "crazy quilt" pattern at 3 weeks, but in 3 months it appears normal under scanning electron microscopy (12). The neointima varies between 150 to 500 μm in thickness. Investigators have not observed pressure necrosis, but thinning and minimal fibrosis of the underlying media have been identified (12). Although growth of the endothelium occurs both from the ends and between pores of the stents, in animal models side branches covered by these prostheses have remained patent (Figure 14.1). The porosity factor also helps determine the early success of endothelialization. Designs with low porosity factors are more likely to induce fibrin deposition with thicker intima and greater luminal narrowing, whereas those with high porosity factors may cause increased turbulence, suboptimal hemodynamics, and decreased structural support.

Once a stent is fully covered with endothelium, the risk of thrombosis becomes negligible. Human studies have shown that acute stent thrombosis occurs most often in the first 48 hours and then becomes progressively less frequent over the ensuing 4 weeks. There may be enormous variability for the time needed to completely endothelialize a stent in a human coronary vessel because of the underlying disease. Potentially the process of fibrointimal proliferation could be affected by the underlying atherosclerosis as well as scarring induced by a prior angioplasty procedure (13).

Figure 14.1. Canine femoral artery 9 months after stent implantation. Scanning electron micrograph shows complete endothelialization with patent side branch. (Reprinted with permission from Sigwart U et al. Intravascular stents to prevent occlusion and restenosis after transluminal angioplasty. N Engl J Med 1987;316:701–706.)

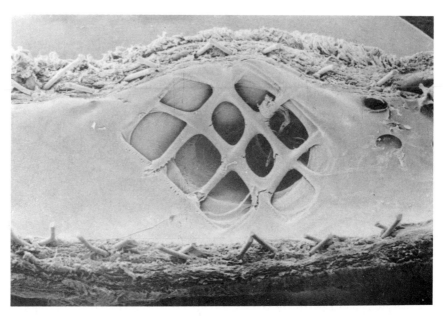

Clinical Results

The self-expanding mesh stent (Figure 14.2) has intrinsic expansile properties and is made from 0.06- to 0.08-mm surgical stainless steel manufactured in lengths of 15 to 30 mm. When the stent is released from the delivery system by removing a doubled-over membrane, it expands along its horizontal axis while it contracts longitudinally until reaching the limits of the vessel wall diameter. Stents are chosen 10% to 20% larger than the vessel luminal diameter to ensure that residual force is exerted against the wall preventing stent migration and vessel wall recoil. The stent has an 80% porosity factor and considerable structural strength while remaining quite flexible. Because of the delivery system design, the device profile is only 1.57 mm but can carry stents varying between 2.5 to 6.0 mm in diameter. In our experience the stent can be maneuvered easily through serpiginous vessels to the point of a stenotic lesion. No cases of stent migration or embolization have been reported with this device.

The other stents presently under clinical investigation are balloon expandable. The devices are delivered to the lesion on a standard angio-

Figure 14.2. Diagrammatic representation of the delivery system and self-expanding mesh stent. **A.** Central shaft. **B.** Guidewire. **C.** Inflation port. **D.** Restraining membrane. **E.** Self-expanding stent. (Reprinted with permission of the publisher from Sigwart U, Urban P. Use of coronary stents following balloon angioplasty. In Braunwald E, ed. Heart disease—update. Philadelphia: WB Saunders, 1989;5:111.)

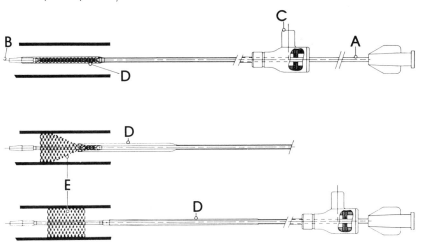

plasty balloon, which is inflated to release the prostheses into the vessel lumen. All but one of the stents under clinical investigation are made from surgical stainless steel, which is nearly radiolucent. The stent is not visualized unless very high-resolution flouroscopy is available. The balloon-expandable design has the advantage that precise placement can be accomplished more easily using the balloon markers. The Medtronic–Wiktor stent is made from tantalum, a relatively soft radiopaque metal. Because of the metal's plastic deformability, the wire elements composing this coiled device require greater thickness to create sufficient radial force (Figure 14.3). This device is the most recent to enter clinical investigation and few results are presently available.

The Palmaz–Schatz prosthesis (Figure 14.4) has been implanted in more patients than any other device (14). Originally Palmaz designed this stent as a tube with rectangular slots that assumed a diamond-shaped configuration when expanded by the balloon. When the stent is stretched, it loses its intrinsic elasticity, preventing significant elastic recoil. Each strut measures 76 by 100 μm. Early studies demonstrated that the device was quite stiff. Schatz modified the original design by adding a straight metal rod that connects two short tubular segments,

Figure 14.3. Picture of a Medtronic–Wiktor stent.

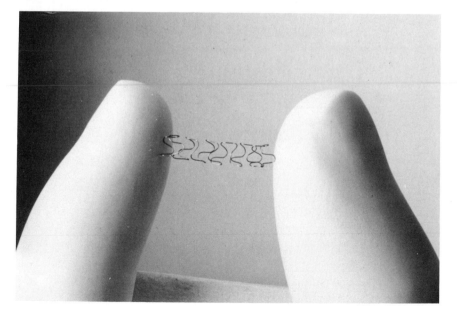

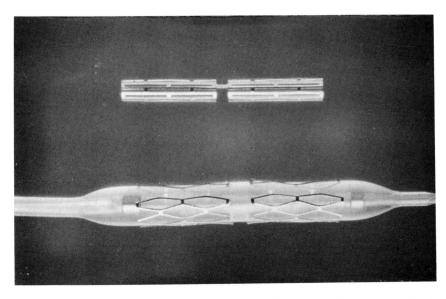

Figure 14.4. Palmaz–Schatz balloon expandable stent. (Courtesy of R. A. Schatz, Scripps Clinic, La Jolla, Calif.)

providing considerably more flexibility (15). However, the stent is still difficult to maneuver beyond major bends in the coronary tree.

More than 1000 patients have received this device during its clinical trials worldwide (14; Schatz RA, personal communication). The stent has been delivered successfully over 95% of the time. The delivery has been improved by the use of a plastic sleeve over the balloon and stent, which is removed only when the device is positioned at the lesion. Before this modification in the delivery system, stent embolization occurred in several situations (16). Since the institution of an ongoing anticoagulation program, approximately 3.5% of patients have experienced stent thrombosis within 30 days of deployment. Emergency CABG occurred in 1.1% of the stented patients, and 1.9% of the patients died within 30 days of stent implantation. Approximately 25% of all patients who came to repeat angiography within 6 months of stenting had evidence of at least 50% luminal narrowing within the stent (Schatz RA, personal communication; Marco J, personal communication). But nearly half these patients had no clinical evidence of ischemia when measured by the presence of angina, positive exercise tests, or thallium tests. A preliminary analysis of the data suggested that the major predictors for restenosis related to the initial angiographic result from stenting, the placement of two or more stents in tandem, a prior history of total occlusion, and perhaps most important, a prior history of restenosis, which increased the likelihood of stent restenosis three-fold (31% versus 10%; 17).

The Gianturco–Roubin stent is made from stainless steel, 150 μm thick and 20 mm long (Figure 14.5). Initially the device was studied only under circumstances of abrupt closure with all stented patients proceeding to CABG (18,19). The second study phase involved using the stent under circumstances of abrupt closure and sending patients for emergency surgery only if clinically necessary. More recently, the device has been used in trials as a potential means of avoiding restenosis. Roubin reported that more than 200 stents have been deployed for abrupt closure in phase I and II of the study protocol (20). The stent was implanted in 95% of this patient group successfully with an acute, or subacute, thrombosis rate of 6%. Two patients died, and 12 patients required emergency CABG among the phase II group. Angiographic

Figure 14.5. Diagrammatic representation of the Gianturco–Roubin coil spring stent. (Courtesy of G. S. Roubin, University of Alabama, Birmingham.)

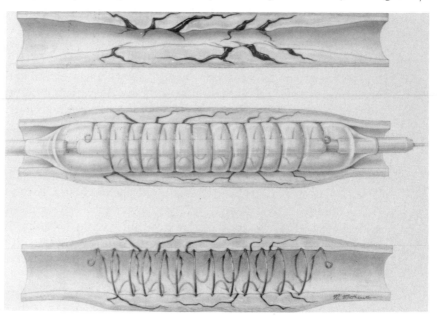

restenosis was seen in 50% of the patients restudied in the first 6 months after implantation for abrupt closure. For patients stented primarily to prevent restenosis, 2% suffered acute or subacute thrombosis, 4% required emergency surgery, and 1% died. In a small follow-up group, 30% demonstrated restenosis.

Our experience with self-expanding mesh stents now comprises 172 stents in 136 patients, including a number of stents placed in tandem. In our series stent thrombosis occurred in 6.4% of patients, 4.4% required emergency CABG, and 3.3% died from cardiac causes (Figure 14.6). We have angiographic follow-up from 71% of our patient group 4 to 6 months after implantation. In this group, 14% of patients demonstrated at least 50% narrowing within the stent. A number of these patients have no measurable evidence of myocardial ischemia and are being followed clinically without further intervention. Like the preliminary analyses from the Palmaz–Schatz device, our data suggest that higher rates of restenosis occurred in patients who were stented for prior restenosis, particularly when the previous procedure occurred within 3 months of the stent deployment.

Discussion

The endoluminal prostheses reviewed have been implanted under variable circumstances in a heterogeneous patient population. Although tempting, it is inappropriate to compare the results from these different devices. These stents have been modified during the course of their clinical trials and the indications for deployment have evolved with clinical experience. In some cases even the mechanisms for insertion have been altered during the course of clinical trials. With these various changes, the success rates for deployment have improved and the potential complications have decreased significantly (21).

These studies demonstrate that emergency surgery for abrupt closure after standard balloon angioplasty can be a rare occurrence with the use of an intracoronary stent. The studies performed until now with these devices are descriptive investigations. They involved the researchers' observations of these prostheses under various clinical circumstances. These investigations achieved the primary goal for a new therapeutic modality, demonstrating that patient morbidity is less with the intervention than without it. Enough time has passed for investigators to observe patients several years after stent insertion. Cases of a significant inflammatory response or of infection because of the stent have not

A

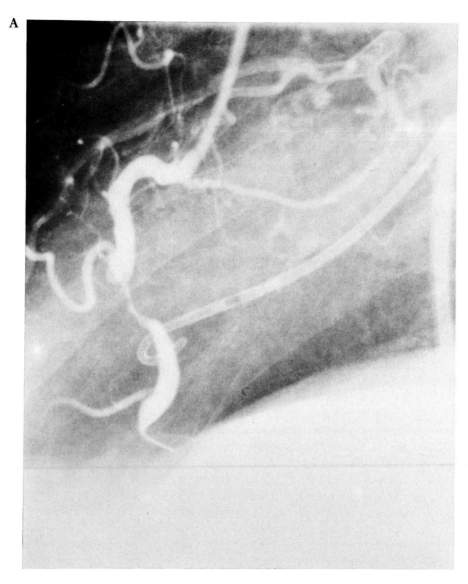

Figure 14.6. Stenting for abrupt closure. (A) Right coronary artery prior to angioplasty. (Courtesy of Dr. Miles Williams. Reproduced with permission from Prog Cardiol 1990;3/2:89.)

B

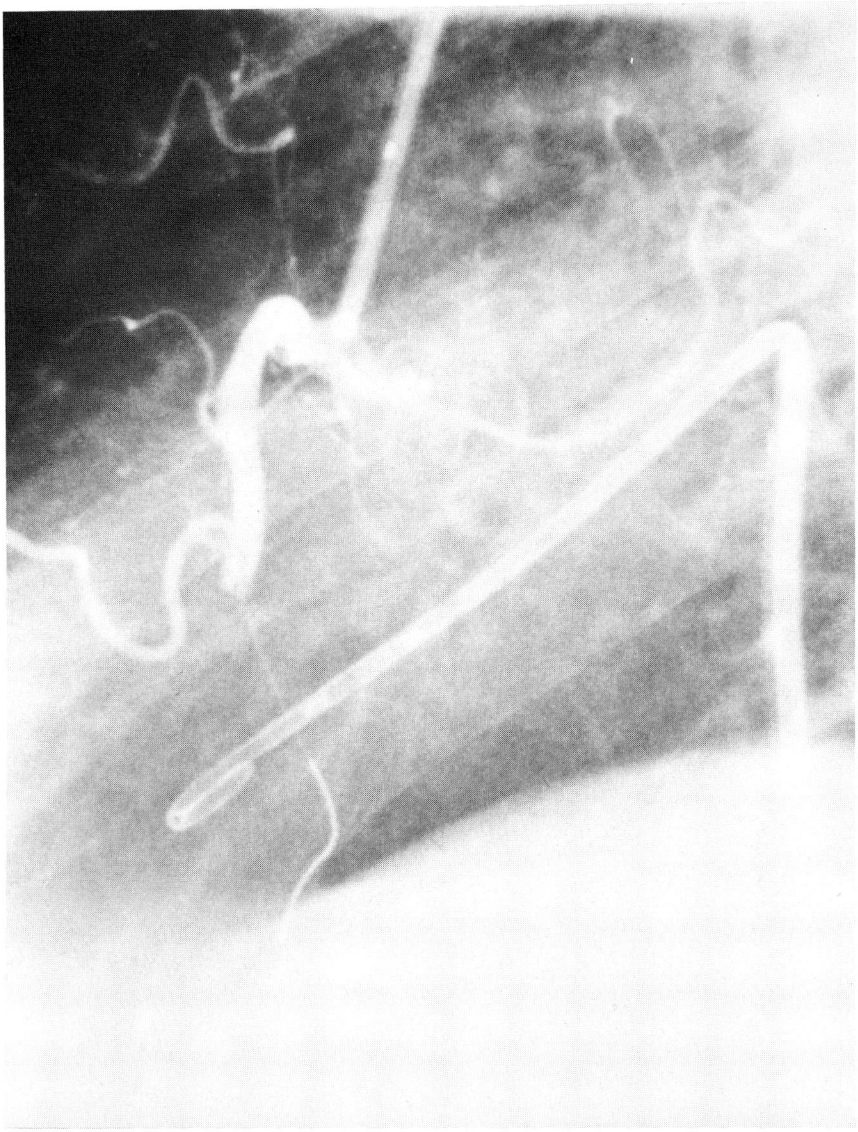

Figure 14.6 *(cont.)* (B) A guidewire is across the lesion, no distal flow is evident.

C

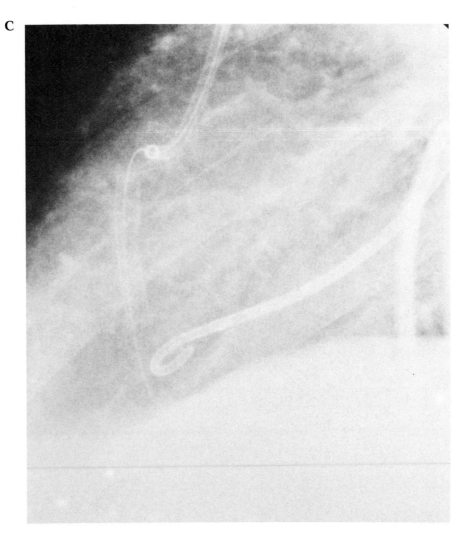

Figure 14.6 *(cont.)* (C) A self-expanding mesh stent is visualized after placement in the vessel.

D

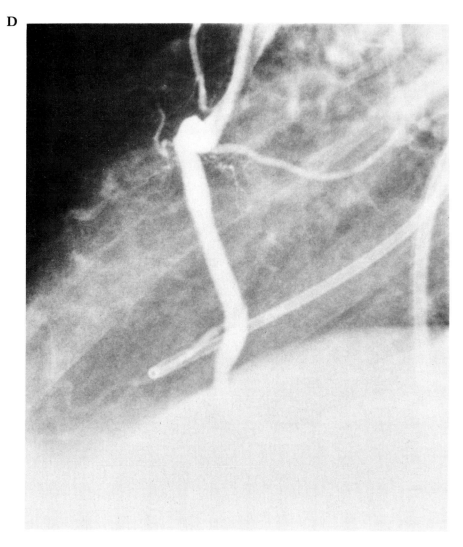

Figure 14.6 *(cont.)* (D) The vessel after stenting demonstrates excellent ante-grade flow and no residual stenosis.

been reported. Several observers have performed serial angiography on patients with coronary stents. At 1 year follow-up the luminal diameter within the prostheses is not significantly different from observations made at 6 months (16).

An unanswered question is the potential role these devices may play in preventing restenosis. This issue cannot be resolved until studies are performed that compare standard balloon angioplasty to intracoronary stenting. The descriptive data published suggest that stents may decrease rates of restenosis, particularly in certain patient subgroups. Patients with bypass graft disease and those patients who receive stents as a primary intervention appear to have lower rates of restenosis than historic controls. However, to properly evaluate this data we must understand that the definitions of acute stent thrombosis and restenosis vary among different investigators and different institutions.

Several chapters in this book are devoted to the subjects of defining and measuring restenosis. We will not attempt to review these discussions here, but some issues are particularly relevant for understanding intracoronary stent data. Moreover, the assessment of intracoronary stent restenosis may require different measurements than those applied to standard balloon angioplasty. Stents become embedded in neointima varying between 150 to 500 μm in diameter. If a stent were circumferentially covered by neointima of 400 μm, a measurement of its luminal diameter at follow-up angiography should be approximately 0.8 mm less than when it was inserted. In a stent of 3.0 mm this would represent a 22% decrease in luminal diameter. If one used a computer-derived measurement of 0.72 mm as the indicator of restenosis (22), this example would be included among the restenosis group. In our opinion, this is an expected finding when dealing with stents and does not represent restenosis. We can pursue this reasoning further by looking at the hypothetical course of a patient with a 4.0 mm stent in a bypass graft. At follow-up angiography, the stent area is decreased by a focal narrowing of 50% and therefore is included statistically as a case of restenosis. However, the luminal opening is still 2.0 mm, and the patient is totally asymptomatic and has no objective evidence of ischemia. If 0.7 to 0.8 mm represents the potential luminal narrowing related to the formation of the neointima, the actual hyperplastic response represents 1.2 mm or 30% of the original luminal diameter. This narrowing may represent a scientific measure of intimal hyperplasia, but is it clinically a case of restenosis? Perhaps almost as important, does this degree of fibrointimal hyperplasia represent the same tissue response as a 50%

narrowing observed after standard balloon angioplasty? We and other investigators have found that many of our patients with "stent restenosis" as defined by 50% luminal narrowing are asymptomatic and can be followed clinically without serious sequelae.

Several other issues affect our understanding of stent restenosis. Some investigators believe a lesion that develops in a stented vessel proximal or distal to the stent should also be considered evidence for restenosis. They argue that the hyperproliferative response related to the stent deployment must play a role in a new, or advanced, lesion that develops in proximity to the stent. Others believe the issue of stent restenosis should be considered in the same fashion as standard balloon angioplasty and only luminal narrowing within the stent represents restenosis. Finally, the issue of stent thrombosis is defined differently by various researchers. We feel that an episode of stent thrombosis that occurs in the hospital after leaving the catheterization laboratory and is treated successfully should not eliminate a patient from further follow-up evaluation as a measure for stent success or failure. Others treat a single episode of thrombosis as an end point. Some investigators believe that any episode of stent occlusion within 30 days of deployment represents stent thrombosis, whereas others analyze any event beyond 2 weeks as a case of stent restenosis. A few researchers believe a sudden, acute event occurring in the distribution of the stented vessel, even at 3 months, probably represents thrombosis and not restenosis. We have had several patients who abruptly discontinued anticoagulant medications and within 10 days suffered an acute myocardial infarction, in one case even 3 months after the stent was inserted. It seems likely that these events were related to stent thrombosis although we have chosen to include these few patients for analyses within the restenosis group.

A common standard is necessary to measure and compare results from different interventions. When we make decisions regarding these standards, we must keep in view the primary goals of therapy. Balloon angioplasty was developed as a noninvasive means to decrease a critical coronary narrowing, relieving symptoms of angina and decreasing the potential for an acute coronary event. The true measure of a coronary intervention must be its therapeutic success or failure. An arbitrary standard created because the human eye can distinguish 50% narrowing or a computer program can reliably reproduce measurements at 0.72 mm should not determine the judgment of the scientific community or the role of an intervention in clinical practice. We feel a better measure should be clinical end points: angina pectoris, objective measures of ischemia, myocardial infarction, or death. As coronary stenting evolves from the descriptive clinical phase to a phase of comparative studies with standard angioplasty or surgery, it will become much easier to apply these types of end points. It would be useful for investigators in the field to decide on a common set of rules and measurements that would allow the scientific community to assess these data more readily. To compare the results from different interventions, we should use a continuous measurement of the degree of luminal narrowing, rather than arbitrarily defining distinct categories of doubtful clinical relevance.

The Future of Coronary Stenting

We should not be surprised that the current generation of endoluminal support devices also stimulate excessive fibroinitimal hyperplasia in some cases. They are composed of metal struts of varying thickness surrounding empty space that allows tissue to protrude into the lumen. This geometry creates potential areas of flow turbulence. The struts, as well as the tissue, may cause local eddy currents affecting laminar flow. Rheology is improved after coronary stenting, but it is still not ideal. The metal struts may serve as a focus for excessive platelet deposition and clot formation or serve as a platform for the development of neointima. Local turbulence as well as local tissue factors may be significant in the development of exuberant smooth muscle cell hyperplasia. Thus far, clinical results suggest that stents with high porosity factors may lead to higher rates of restenosis. Those stents with low porosity factors have greater structural support but are more likely to cause thrombotic events. The optimal material-pore ratio has not yet been defined.

The next generation of intravascular devices should substantially improve local fluid dynamics by improvements in geometric design probably involving the use of finer filaments composed of nonmetallic substances. These filaments should permit the development of neointima but avoid the problems of clot formation, possibly by changing the local hemostatic environment. Some investigators are examining the potential of coating struts with heparin or hirudin, another potent anticoagulant, antiplatelet agent. Others are attempting to modify the local environment by seeding struts with endothelial cells genetically engineered to produce tissue thromboplastin-activating agent. These devices could provide an opportunity to instill agents locally that modify smooth muscle cell migration or proliferation and avoid the potential for systemic toxicity. Finally, the future prostheses may be composed of biodegradable polymers that support the vessel wall for 6 to 9 months then gradually resorb. These second- and third-generation stents are presently under investigation in different laboratories throughout the world and should enter clinical evaluation over the next several years.

Conclusion

Endoluminal support devices have been studied for 80 years, but their importance in clinical medicine has been demonstrated only in the past few years (23). The enormous growth of standard balloon angioplasty created the problems of abrupt closure and restenosis for which this type of device seems uniquely suited. Clinical studies have demonstrated that the problems of abrupt closure can be surmounted by coronary stenting, but the problems of restenosis persist. The present generation of intracoronary stents are about to enter controlled, comparative studies with standard angioplasty that will determine their role in clinical practice. As these clinical events unfold, we are beginning to understand the biochemical controls over smooth muscle cell hyperplasia. It seems probable that the endoluminal prosthesis will eventually be used as a temporary support to permit vessel healing while locally instilling agents that promote this healing process in a controlled manner.

References

1. Berg R Jr, Kendall RW, Duvoisin GE, et al. Acute myocardial infarction: a surgical emergency. J Thorac Cardiovasc Surg 1975;70:432–439.
2. Rentrop P, Blanke H, Krsch KR, et al. Acute myocardial infarction: intracoronary application of nitroglycerin and streptokinase. Clin Cardiol 1979;2:354–363.
3. Gruentzig AR, Senning A, Siegenthaler WE. Nonoperative dilatation of coronary-artery stenosis: percutaneous transluminal coronary angioplasty. N Engl J Med 1979;301:61–68.
4. Gruppo Italiano per lo Studio della Streptochinasi nell'Infarcto Miocardico (GISSI): Effectiveness of intravenous thrombolytic treatment in acute myocardial infarction. Lancet 1986;1:397–401.

5. Kennedy JW, Martin GV, Davis KB, et al. The Western Washington Intravenous Streptokinase in Acute Myocardial Infraction randomized trial. Circulation 1988;77:345–352.

6. Sigwart U, Puel J, Mirkovitch V, et al. Intravascular stents to prevent occlusion and restenosis after transluminal angioplasty. N Engl J Med 1987;316:701–706.

7. Serruys PW, Strauss BH, van Beusekom HM, et al. Stenting of coronary arteries: has a modern Pandora's box been opened? J Am Coll Cardiol 1991;17 (suppl B):143B–154B.

8. Roubin GS, Robinson KA, King SB, Gianturco C, et al. Early and late results of intracoronary arterial stenting after coronary angioplasty in dogs. Circulation 1987;76:891–897.

9. Steele PM, Chesebro JH, Stanson AW, et al. Balloon angioplasty: natural histology of the pathophysiologic response to injury in a pig model. Circ Res 1985;57:105–109.

10. Wright KC, Wallace S, Charnsangavej C, et al. Percutaneous endovascular stents: an experimental evaluation. Radiology 1985;15:69–72.

11. Schatz RA, Palmaz JC, Tio FO, et al. Balloon expandable intracoronary stents in the adult dog. Circulation 1987;76:450–457.

12. Palmaz JC, Windeler SA, Garcia F, Tio FO, Sibbitt RR, Reuter SR. Atherosclerotic rabbit aortas: expandable intraluminal grafting. Radiology 1986;160:723–726.

13. Urban P, Sigwart U, Kaufmann U, Kappenberger L. Restenosis within coronary stents: possible effect of previous angioplasty (abstr). J Am Coll Cardiol 1989;13:107–A.

14. Ellis SG, Savage M, Baim D, et al. Intracoronary stenting to prevent restenosis: preliminary results of a multicenter study using the Palmaz–Schatz stent suggest benefit selected high risk patients. J Am Coll Cardiol 1990;15:118A.

15. Schatz RA. A view of intravascular stents. Circulation 1988;79:445–450.

16. Schatz RA, Palmaz JC. Balloon expandable intravascular stents (BEIS) in human coronary arteries: report of initial experience. Circulation 1988; 78 (suppl II):415.

17. Ellis SG, Savage MS, Fischman D, et al. Restenosis after placement of Palmaz–Schatz stents in native coronary arteries: initial results of a multicenter experience. Hertz 1990;15:307–318.

18. Roubin GS, Douglas JS, Lembo NJ, et al. Intracoronary stenting for acute closure following percutaneous transluminal coronary angioplasty (PTCA). Circulation 1988;78 (suppl II):407.

19. Roubin GS, Hearn JA, Carlin SF, et al. Angiographic and clinical follow-

up in patients receiving a balloon expandable stent for prevention or treatment of acute closure following PTCA. Circulation 1990;82 (suppl III):191.

20. Roubin GS. Balloon expandable coil. Presented at 2nd International Coronary Stenting Symposium, Birmingham, Ala., March 1991.

21. Sigwart U, Urban P, Sadeghi H, Kappenberger L. Implantation of 100 intracoronary stents. Learning curve effect on the occurrence of acute complications (abstr). J Am Coll Cardiol 1989;13:107A.

22. Reiber JHC, Serruys PW, Kooijman CJ. Assessment of short-, medium-, long-term variations in arterial dimensions from computer assisted quantitation of coronary cineangiograms. Circulation 1985;71:280–288.

23. Carrel A. Results of the permanent intubation of the thoracic aorta. Surg Gynecol Obstetr 1912;15:245–248.

CHAPTER **15**

. . . .

Restenosis After PTCA with Coronary Atherectomy and Percutaneous Excimer Laser Coronary Angioplasty

JAMES A. HEARN
SPENCER B. KING III

Introduction

B A L L O O N percutaneous transluminal coronary angioplasty (PTCA) was developed by Dr. Andreas Gruentzig and first used in 1977 (1). A remarkably consistent restenosis rate has persisted for over a decade (2,3). Two major approaches to reduce restenosis have developed. First, numerous pharmacologic agents have been tried in clinical trials without consistent success (4–6). Specific agents are detailed in other sections of this book. Second, several new devices offer alternative ways of removing atheroma instead of displacing the plaque, as occurs in balloon angioplasty. These have yet to be tested in clinical trials against standard PTCA.

Considerations when developing a new device include:

1. Vessel type and anatomy (native coronary artery, vein graft or internal mammary artery)
2. Size of the vessel and distal circulation
3. Length of the plaque
4. Tortuosity present in the proximal vessel and at the plaque
5. Presence of eccentricity

6. Presence of calcium
7. Angiographically visible thrombus
8. Presence of a ruptured atheroma, ulceration, or coronary artery dissection
9. Bifurcations or side branches
10. The number and distribution of lesions to be treated.

Many new devices have obvious limitations (e.g., crossing a tortuous proximal segment before the lesion with directional coronary atherectomy [DCA]). Some may have advantages in the unstable lesion (e.g., extraction–endarterectomy when large amounts of thrombus are present). The overall approach in interventional cardiology is selection of a particular device suited for the anatomy and physiology of the lesion. The ultimate goal is the selection of a device that has both excellent acute success and long-term freedom from restenosis and cardiac events. In trying to optimize acute success, investigators select patients in whom the new device appears appropriate. This makes a comparison of outcomes between devices difficult because baseline clinical and angiographic variables are different due to selection. These clinical and angiographic variables (e.g., angina class, length) influence the potential for restenosis and long-term outcome. The selection of lesions suitable for more than one device illustrates the need for clinical trials from which comparisons can be made.

Although lesion differences could affect selection of cases appropriate for each device, it is increasingly apparent that the response-to-injury hypothesis of coronary atherosclerosis may also be appropriate to the discussion of restenosis following any nonspecific injury to a diseased site. This response to injury may be proportional to the degree of injury. The degree of injury is difficult to discern angiographically, except in cases of large dissections or abrupt closure. The degree of injury may also relate to the production of a satisfactory opening in the artery (e.g., long lesions, eccentric lesions requiring multiple inflations). In an attempt to optimize the acute angiographic appearance, the long-term patency may be reduced. Distinctions between devices may also become blurred when one device is used to improve the results of another.

Recent autopsy evidence suggests that overstretch injury to an arterial wall is directly related to the amount of intimal hyperplasia that follows (7). Animal experiments support this finding (8,9). This extends earlier pathologic studies, which show that disruptions of intima and media, followed by an intense, localized smooth muscle cell hyperplasia, are common in post-PTCA patients (10–18). The alternate approach is minimizing stretch injury by removing the plaque from within rather than displacing it outwardly. This has led to the development of various devices that remove plaque and improve the lumen diameter without the same degree of radial stretching as the balloon. This potential mechanism has been explored with atherectomy and excimer laser angioplasty (19, 20). Also, by removing part of the plaque, its growth-promoting contents (e.g., growth factors, interleukins) are removed. This could theoretically reduce the chance of restenosis. The potential ability of these devices to make a single pass through the artery unaided by balloon PTCA ("stand-alone") may also prove to be an advantage by minimizing repeated stretch injury. However, it may turn out that radial stretching is not the only determinant of restenosis. The disruptions of intima and media may be more important quantitatively and may be caused by any device that is used inside coronary arteries. Repeated stretching may likewise give rise to increased numbers of disruptions. It may be that simple radial stretching, without any histologic evidence of intimal or medial disruptions, also contributes to restenosis. Early data suggest that restenosis is probably not different histologically in response to the various devices used to produce a successful result (21,22).

It is possible that medical therapies postintervention may ultimately reduce the amount of intimal hyperplasia that occurs. Such a therapy would be directed against a process, like arterial healing, that has evolved over many thousands of years and that may be harmful in other situations (e.g., accidents). The combination of a mild but effective medical therapy and an effective interventional technique would be ideal. Attempts to optimize the initial luminal results could then be reassessed among the current devices.

Directional Coronary Atherectomy

Technical and Experimental Aspects

Developed in California by Dr. John Simpson and coworkers, this was the first nonballoon device to receive Food and Drug Administration approval for general use. It is delivered to the coronary circulation through a 9.5F, 10F, or 11F large-lumen catheter. This device consists of a 5F, 6F, or 7F housing with an open side and an internal circular blade (Figure

15.1). It is advanced over a 0.014-inch guidewire. A 2.0-mm balloon opposite the open face of the device is inflated to low pressures (5 to 30 psi) to push the device against the plaque and to minimize the chance of particle embolism. The blade is then rotated at 2000 rpm and advanced the length of the housing. This action results in a cutting of the atheroma protruding into the device. It is directional in that the operator can rotate the entire catheter such that the open face is in the direction of the plaque.

Early results in cadaver coronary artery experiments were promising and the device was submitted for clinical evaluation (23).

Clinical Results

Multiple cuts generally result in a tubular and open appearance of the diseased segment. Initial success rates were approximately 90% in patients selected for this device (24). In a recent study, patients with proximal, eccentric, native artery lesions were treated (25). Lesions in which lower success rates might be expected would be smaller arteries and cal-

Figure 15.1. Simpson Atherocath^{Tm} used in directional coronary atherectomy.

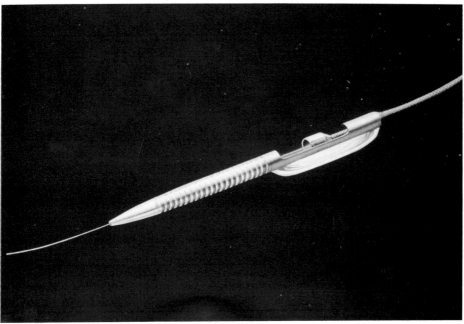

cified lesions or long lesions. This has been recently confirmed by a multicenter, angiographic analysis, with success rates of 93%, 88%, and 75% for ACC/AHA types A, B1 and B2 (too few C lesions to analyze), respectively (26). Complication rates for these lesion types were 3%, 6%, and 13%, respectively.

Restenosis

A recent report on restenosis showed a rate of 36% in patients with follow-up at 3 to 12 months (83% of those eligible; 27; Table 15.1). The restenosis rates have not been as favorable in saphenous venous bypass grafts when restenosis lesions have been treated. In a multicenter report these grafts had a 36% restenosis rate in previously untreated sites and an 81% rate in restenosis lesions (28). In a separate report of 52 vein graft lesions successfully treated, the restenosis rate was 60% with a 46% rate in de novo lesions compared with a 73% rate in restenosis lesions (29). This rate is similar to the restenosis rates seen in older vein grafts treated with balloon PTCA (30).

It can be postulated that restenosis after DCA has been contributed to by the Dottering effect of the catheter (31), the inflation of the balloon on the housing, and need for adjunctive balloon PTCA. In an earlier study with a 50% restenosis rate, a greater depth of tissue removal resulted in a greater chance of restenosis (32). In particular, the presence of media or adventitia (or both) was predictive of restenosis. In previously treated lesions, subintimal resection resulted in a 78% restenosis rate. However, this was not true in primary, previously untreated, coronary artery lesions. In a separate report of 46 lesions with local ectasia after atherectomy (<0% diameter stenosis) the restenosis rate was 63% (33). Some lesions, especially those at the origin of the left anterior descending (LAD) artery have, in the DCA registry, shown a restenosis rate that is comparable to other areas of the coronary tree. This may be a unique advantage for DCA because balloon angioplasty has always shown a higher restenosis rate for that location.

A recent review of atherectomy procedures showed an inverse relation between the size of the artery and restenosis rates, with improved results in vessels greater than 3.0 mm (34). Another study showed a 14% restenosis rate for focal lesions and a 26% rate overall (35). The European experience is similar with a restenosis rate of 36% (36). A multicenter study, CAVEAT, has been started to evaluate whether DCA is associated with an improved restenosis rate compared to balloon angioplasty.

Table 15.1. Directional Coronary Atherectomy

AUTHOR	YEAR	NO.	ANGIO. FOLLOW-UP	DEFINITION	RESTENOSIS RATE		OVERALL RATE
					DE NOVO	RESTENOSIS	
NATIVE ARTERIES							
Hinohara (27)	1991	211	83%	>50% DS	24/82(29%)	52/129(40%)	76/211(36%)
Simpson (35)	1991	117	78%	>50% DS	31/117(26%)	NA	31/117(26%)
Simpson (34)	1990	66	82%	>50% DS	16/66(24%)	NA	16/66(24%)
de Bruyne (36)	1991	22	79%	>50% DS	NA	NA	8/22(36%)
SAPHENOUS VEIN GRAFTS							
Ghazzal (28)	1991	55	80%	≥50% DS	10/28(36%)	22/27(81%)	35/55(58%)
Selmon (29)	1991	52	66%	>50% DS	(46%)	(73%)	31/52(60%)

DS = diameter stenosis; NA = not available.

349

Besides its efficacy in treating coronary stenoses, DCA provides a method of studying coronary histology and its response to various pharmacologic and nonpharmacologic interventions. In addition, it has provided evidence that most of the angiographic luminal obstruction in restenosis lesions is due to intimal hyperplasia (24) instead of elastic recoil alone in a sizable minority (37).

Future modifications of this device include increased flexibility with a lower profile and a shorter housing. Recent changes in technique have been lower pressures in the positioning balloon and decreasing the amount of tissue removal attempted to avoid subintimal resection. This could provide a compromise between maximizing the initial result and reducing restenosis.

Percutaneous Coronary Rotational Ablation

Technical and Experimental Aspects

Developed by Dr. David Auth, this device consists of an olive-shaped, or elliptical, burr attached to a drive shaft that rotates at approximately 175,000 rpm (Figure 15.2; 38–41). This unit is powered by a disposable compressed air turbine. The front half of the burr is coated with diamond microchips and its purpose is to abrade the atheroma. This creates microscopic particles (majority $<10\mu$ in diameter). These are

Figure 15.2. Rotablator^{Tm} used in percutaneous coronary rotational ablation.

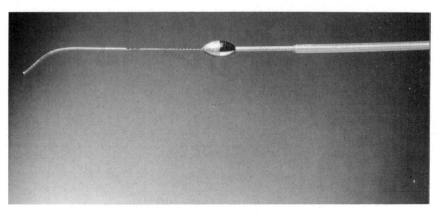

thought to pass through the microcirculation of the heart with little or no harmful effect. However, if enough particles are generated over a brief period of time by rapid advancement through long segments, this device may produce obstruction of the distal circulation resulting in creatine kinase release and transient regional wall motion abnormalities (42). The authors concluded that this was related to the early learning curve and has improved with minor adjustments in technique and patient selection (Auth D, personal communication). In rabbit iliac arteries and coronary arteries this device produced a uniform, smooth lumen with relative sparing of the media (39,43).

This device has been shown in cadaver arteries to achieve a smooth luminal surface and is thought to selectively engage hard tissue as opposed to compliant, normal arterial wall (38). It has a centrally placed 0.009-inch stainless steel guidewire that helps to maintain a coaxial position. Burr sizes range from 1.25 mm to 2.75 mm. The required guide catheter sizes range from 8F to 11F, depending on internal diameter. Burr size is limited by the internal lumen of the guide catheter and the size of the artery.

The technique is to cross the lesion with the guidewire and move the burr through the lesion with a hand-operated advancer while the unit is rotating. Saline is slowly infused through the sheath as a lubricant. One aid to avoiding obstruction of the microcirculation has been to monitor the drop in pitch of the motor as the burr abrades atheromatous plaque. In that case, the burr is withdrawn to allow particle washout and then readvanced. Several slow passes through the lesion are usually required to achieve maximal effect. The strategy has been to start with smaller burrs and work up to an appropriate final size.

Clinical Results

Limited data are available on the initial clinical experiences with this device. O'Neill and colleagues reported data on 30 patients undergoing rotational coronary ablation (44). Primary success, defined as 50% diameter stenosis or less after the procedure, was found in 29 patients (97%). Adjunctive balloon use was not reported. Creatine kinase isoenzymes were elevated in 5 patients (16%). Transient blood flow cessation was seen in 6 patients (20%) but was reversed with intracoronary nitroglycerin and sublingual nifedipine. One patient with multivessel PTCA required emergency coronary artery bypass grafting (CABG). No deaths were reported.

Another series was reported by Ginsburg and members of the Western Collaborative Group on 40 patients (45). All patients were referred for rotational atherectomy because of suboptimal characteristics for balloon PTCA. No adjunctive balloon PTCA was performed in this group. Maximal burr sizes were from 1.5 mm (10 patients) to 2.0 mm (23 patients). Using quantitative angiography the minimum lumen diameter preablation was 0.77 ± 0.10 mm and 1.51 ± 0.09 mm postablation. The reference arterial diameter was 1.57 ± 0.15 mm. Success rates were not reported. However, the complications were similar to the first series: transient spasm in 12 (30%), creatine kinase elevation in 8 (20%), ventricular stunning in 5 (12.5%), and emergency CABG in 1 (2.5%). No flaps, dissections, or Q wave myocardial infarctions occurred. No deaths were reported.

Restenosis

In the first series noted above, 18 patients underwent follow-up angiography at 6 months and restenosis was present in 8 (44%; 44). In a follow-up report on 22 treated patients undergoing quantitative coronary angiography (QCA) assessment at 6 months, the restenosis rate was 50% (46; Table 15.2). In a much larger multicenter follow-up study involving 152 patients, the overall restenosis rate was 32% (47). In another follow-up report on 56 patients, the predictors of restenosis after rotational atherectomy were LAD lesions, ostial and proximal locations, and saphenous vein bypass grafts (48). In addition, there was a trend toward less restenosis in restenosis lesions (see Table 15.2). The European experience with rotational atherectomy was similar with a rate of 39% in 33 patients (49). However, in chronic occlusions this figure jumped to 77% of 13 patients. Further data are needed to properly define the magnitude of restenosis after percutaneous coronary rotational atherectomy.

Transluminal Extraction–Endarterectomy (TEC)

Technical and Experimental Aspects

The initial investigations on this device have been carried out by Dr. Richard Stack and colleagues at Duke University. The device consists of a wire-based, motor-driven, rotating flexible torque tube, 1.8 to 2.5

Table 15.2. Percutaneous Coronary Rotational Ablation

AUTHOR	YEAR	NO.	ANGIO. FOLLOW-UP	DEFINITION	RESTENOSIS RATE		OVERALL RATE
Buchbinder (47)	1991	152	94%	>50% DS			49/152(32%)
Niazi (46)	1990	22	85%	>50% DS			11/22(50%)
Niazi (48)	1991	56	NA	≥50% DS	DE NOVO STENOSES (54%)	RESTENOSIS OCCLUSIONS (29%)	NA
Dietz (49)	1991	46	NA	NA	13/33(39%)	10/13(77%)	23/46(50%)

DS = diameter stenosis
NA = not available

353

mm in diameter (Figure 15.3; 50). It is advanced over a 0.014-inch guidewire through a 10.5F guide catheter. The atheroma is removed by two stainless steel blades at the conical head of the catheter, which rotates at 750 rpm. Five cutter sizes are currently available: 5.5, 6.0, 6.5, 7.0, and 7.5F. Gentle suction is applied by use of small vacuum bottles at the control end of the catheter. As the leading, cutting edge is advanced, luminal contents (atheroma, blood) are evacuated. The cutting blades are positioned inside the limits of the vessel wall to minimize the chance of perforation. The drive unit houses the motor and trigger with terminals for remote battery connection. There is also a connection for a glass reservoir that holds the evacuated debris.

Initial experiments were undertaken in normal and atherosclerotic human cadaver arteries as well as during in vivo canine coronary experiments (50). These studies demonstrated that the TEC device could be easily maneuvered percutaneously in canine peripheral and coronary arteries. It was effective at removing atheroma with the depth of excision

Figure 15.3. Device used for coronary transluminal extraction–endarterectomy.

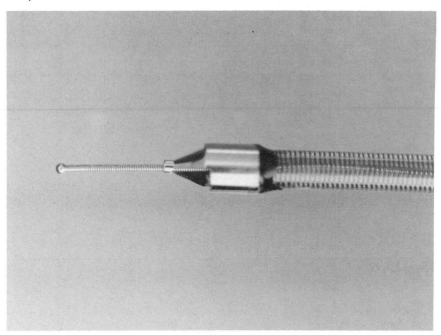

limited to 25% of the medial thickness. There was no evidence of dissection or perforation.

Clinical Results

The primary success rate (final percent stenosis < 50%) using this device has been reported to be 94% in a recent multicenter experience (51). The success rate in 45 vein grafts was 96%; in native coronary arteries it was 92%. In this report it was used without adjunctive devices in 43% of cases. Five percent of patients went for emergency CABG, but no myocardial infarctions, strokes, or deaths occurred.

Restenosis

Angiographic follow-up was obtained in 95 patients of 102 patients eligible (93%) (Table 15.3). The overall restenosis rate was 44% (42 in 95). This was comparable to a balloon PTCA restenosis data base (83% follow-up) in which the restenosis rate was 43%. In a separate report from the William Beaumont Hospital the restenosis rate in 69 patients was 38% at 6 months (52).

Percutaneous Excimer Laser Coronary Angioplasty (PELCA)

Technical and Experimental Aspects

Laser angioplasty developed out of numerous studies in the peripheral arteries with many types of lasers. Some have used the laser to directly ablate plaque, whereas others have used it to heat a metal cap on the end of a catheter. The excimer laser (*excited dimer, light amplification by stimulated emission of radiation*) was developed for use in the coronary circulation by a group of investigators at Cedars–Sinai Medical Center in Los Angeles in close collaboration with a group of scientists working at the NASA Space Program at the California Institute of Technology's Jet Propulsion Laboratory (53,54; Figure 15.4). This system is produced by a pulsed xenon chloride, ultraviolet laser. This particular wavelength (308 nm) was chosen because it ablates calcified plaque, bone, and all tested types of atherosclerotic tissue. In studies on cadaver tissue the microscopic craters created showed little evidence of charring seen

Table 15.3. Coronary Transluminal Extraction–Endarterectomy

AUTHOR	YEAR	NO.	ANGIO. FOLLOW-UP	DEFINITION	RESTENOSIS RATE		OVERALL RATE
					DE NOVO	RESTENOSIS	
NATIVE ARTERIES							
Sketch (51)	1991	95	93%	NA	NA	NA	42/95(44%)
Meany (52)	1991	69	75%	NA	NA	NA	26/69(38%)

NA = not available

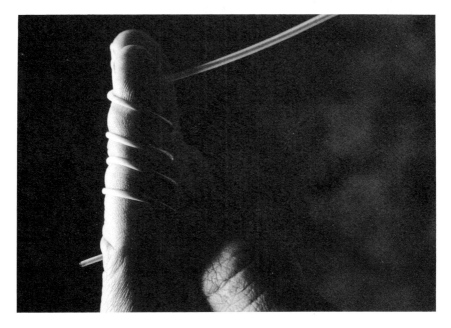

Figure 15.4. Excimer laser catheter used for percutaneous excimer laser coronary angioplasty.

with argon laser. Another reason for using this laser was its excellent transmission through pure silica fibers at energies necessary to ablate tissue. This became feasible when laser scientists reduced the power density by stretching the optical pulse width to greater than 100 ns, avoiding potential fiberoptic damage and providing enough power (30–50 mJ/mm²) to ablate plaque. This also allowed flexibility in the catheter to traverse tortuous segments of artery.

The laser unit weighs 681 kg and measures 32 by 47 by 73 inches; it can be rolled between catheterization laboratories. It requires a 220-volt, 20-ampere current source but no special ventilation. It also requires dedicated personnel for routine on-site maintenance (e.g., gas exchanges). It can be set up in approximately 20 minutes and is relatively simple to operate, with numerous built-in safeguards (e.g., disable switch, gas leakage detection). The unit can deliver 25 to 75 mJ/mm² at up to 30 Hz and is activated by a footswitch.

The laser electromagnetic radiation interacts with living tissue by processes of absorption transmission, reflection, refraction, diffraction, and different types of scattering. The absorption process is the critical aspect for medical applications. With many lasers, this process creates an intense local electric field with breakdown of molecules. Liberation of electrons occurs along with development of gaseous plasma. This sudden expansion of solid to vapor phase products creates a shock wave with localized rupture of tissue. Through experimental research the optimal parameters to ablate tissue and minimize destruction of tissue not directly targeted by the laser have been achieved. When heat is known to be created, the delivery of laser photons is kept below the time and distance normally taken for a given tissue to conduct and diffuse the energy. As long as local heat production is minimized, unwanted damage to normal, nearby tissue can be avoided. For example, protein denaturation and coagulation occur at 50° to 60°C, cell death occurs at 60°C, and melting, boiling, and pyrolysis occur at 90° to 100°C. Calcified tissue ablation may require 500°C. Although thermal damage was hoped to be avoided by using the excimer laser, it is clear that some heat is produced.

Another mechanism for excimer laser ablation is its photochemical effect. The energy of ultraviolet photons exceeds 3.0 electron-volts, which is sufficient to disrupt covalent bonds between atoms and break large organic polymers into smaller, gaseous compounds or particles. The energy absorbed by molecules in rapid expansion away from the original molecule is thought to explain the minimal heat produced. However, kinetic energy usually gives rise to heat as a final form of energy through friction. Thermal energy is more likely to be a problem when high repetition rates are used with insufficient time for thermal relaxation of the tissue (dispersion of heat) or with prolonged irradiation near or below the ablation threshold.

These mechanisms of ablation also represent potential means of inducing arterial injury and restenosis through shock wave energy, thermal energy, or other energy forms. Separation of arterial injury from plaque ablation may be a future research direction.

The delivery catheter used represents a technologic advance in fiberoptic science because of its ability to transmit high-intensity laser light through small (1.3 mm, 1.6 mm, 2.0 mm, 2.2 mm) catheters that have the flexibility to navigate the coronary arteries. Numerous technical publications on the design of the catheter are available (55). It continues to evolve in design (e.g., eccentrically placed laser fibers in the catheter). The 1.3-mm and 1.6-mm catheters require 8F and 2.0-mm catheters require 9F, large lumen, guide catheters.

The lesion to be lased is first crossed with a guidewire. The catheter is then advanced over the guidewire until just proximal to the atheroma. The guidewire is pulled back approximately 2 mm just prior to lasing to cause tissue apposition. Next, the previously calibrated laser catheter is activated for 2 to 3 seconds. Movement of the catheter further than the evolving crater may result in more mechanical expansion effect.

Clinical Results

The clinical success rates reported for PELCA have been high and comparable to conventional balloon PTCA. In a recent, multicenter report laser was successful ($\geq$ 20% reduction of stenosis severity or lumen size $\geq$ catheter size) in 85% of lesions attempted (56). The procedural success rate (final stenosis severity < 50%) was 94%. Interestingly, 41% of lesions were able to be treated with laser alone. The complications were vessel dissection in 12.5%, acute occlusion in 5.4%, spasm in 2%, thrombus in 1.9%, perforation in 1.1%, embolism in 0.8%, aneurysm formation in 0.5%, CABG in 3.5%, myocardial infarction in 1.4%, and death in 0.3%.

Some lesions selected for PELCA would be predicted to have a lower success rate if balloon PTCA were attempted (57). Therefore, the group eligible for restenosis (angiographically successful) may be different from a balloon PTCA group. Long lesions, ostial lesions and, perhaps, saphenous vein grafts are considered appropriate for PELCA because balloon PTCA of these areas suffers from a low success rate or high restenosis rate.

Restenosis

For reasons listed in the introduction, it is difficult if not impossible to compare restenosis rates among different devices due to inherent properties of each device and the different patient populations in which they are first applied. In addition there are differences among operators in skill and experience.

Coronary artery restenosis after PELCA has recently been reported by several groups. Haase and coworkers reported a 43% restenosis rate with 32% restenosis rate seen in stand-alone excimer laser procedures and a 56% rate if adjunctive balloon PTCA were used (Table 15.4; 58). Margolis and colleagues reported on 318 lesions (angiographic follow-up rate of 71%) with a restenosis rate (loss of one half of gain in diameter and a residual > 50% stenosis) of 59% (59). Sanborn and coworkers found a 40% restenosis rate in 74 patients 6 or more months later (60).

Table 15.4. Excimer Laser Coronary Angioplasty

AUTHOR	YEAR	NO.	ANGIO. FOLLOW-UP	DEFINITION	RESTENOSIS RATE STAND ALONE	RESTENOSIS RATE FOLLOW-UP BALLOON	OVERALL RATE
NATIVE ARTERIES							
Haase (58)	1990	107	86%	≥50% DS	18/57(32%)	28/50(56%)	46/107(43%)
Rothbaum (61)	1991	57	90%	>50% DS	15/29(52%)	12/28(43%)	27/57(47%)
Sanborn (60)	1991	74	86%	>50% DS	NA	NA	30/74(40%)
Margolis (59)	1991	318	71%	*	NA	NA	189/318(59%)
SAPHENOUS VEIN GRAFTS							
Unterecker (62)	1991	26	56%	NA	NA	NA	18/26(69%)

*loss of 1/2 gain = >50% DS; DS = diameter stenosis; NA = not available

It was also noted that a post-PELCA stenosis of less than 30% residual was associated with a 25% restenosis rate compared with a 63% rate if this were 30% or greater ($p < 0.05$).

Rothbaum and colleagues reported a 47% restenosis rate in 57 patients overall with a 52% rate in stand-alone procedures and a 43% rate in PELCA combined with balloon (61). An early report of PELCA use in saphenous vein grafts by Unterecker and coworkers showed a restenosis rate of 69% in 26 cases (62).

Conclusion

Data regarding restenosis using these new devices are preliminary. No new device has shown an overall restenosis rate lower than balloon PTCA. Some of these experiences represent restenosis in areas of coronary anatomy and physiology where balloon PTCA is either inappropriate or, when applied, will result in unsuccessful procedures, limiting the investigation of restenosis for a particular indication. Enthusiasm for these devices will depend not only on restenosis rates but perhaps more on the acute outcome. It is anticipated that alterations in patient selection, procedural technique, and device modification will improve the rate of restenosis, but this remains to be proven.

Acknowledgment: Thanks to Ming Wei Liu, M.D. and Sue Mitchell, R.N. for their review of the manuscript and thoughtful recommendations.

References

1. Gruentzig AR, Senning A, Siegenthaler WE. Nonoperative dilatation of coronary artery stenosis: percutaneous transluminal coronary angioplasty. N Engl J Med 1977;301:61–73.
2. Liu MW, Roubin GS, King SB III. Restenosis after coronary angioplasty. Potential biologic determinants and role of intimal hyperplasia. Circulation 1989;79:1374–1387.
3. Block PC. Restenosis after percutaneous transluminal coronary angioplasty—anatomic and pathophysiological mechanisms. Strategies for prevention. Circulation 1990;81:IV2–IV4.
4. Fanelli C, Aronoff R. Restenosis following coronary angioplasty. Am Heart J 1990;119:357–368.

5. McBride W, Lange RA, Hillis LD. Restenosis after successful coronary angioplasty. Pathophysiology and prevention. N Engl J Med 1988; 318:1734–1737.

6. Haudenschild CC. Pathogenesis of restenosis. A correlation of clinical observations with cellular responses. Z Kardiol 1990;79 (suppl 3):17–22.

7. Nobuyoshi M, Kimura T, Ohishi H, et al. Restenosis after percutaneous transluminal coronary angioplasty: pathologic observations in 20 patients. J Am Coll Cardiol 1991;17:433–439.

8. Sarembock IJ, LaVeau PJ, Sigal SL, et al. Influence of inflation pressure and balloon size on the development of intimal hyperplasia after balloon angioplasty. A study in the atherosclerotic rabbit. Circulation 1989; 80:1029–1040.

9. Schwartz RS, Murphy JG, Edwards WD, Camrud AR, Vlietstra RE, Holmes DR. Restenosis after balloon angioplasty. A practical proliferative model in porcine coronary arteries. Circulation 1990;82: 2190–2200.

10. Austin GE, Ratliff NB, Hollman J, Tabei S, Phillips DF. Intimal proliferation of smooth muscle cells as an explanation for recurrent coronary artery stenosis after percutaneous transluminal coronary angioplasty. J Am Coll Cardiol 1985;6:369–375.

11. Block PC, Myler RK, Stertzer S, Fallon JT. Morphology after transluminal angioplasty in human beings. N Engl J Med 1981;305:382–385.

12. Sato T, Takebayashi S, Kohchi K. Increased subendothelial infiltration of the coronary arteries with monocytes/macrophages in patients with unstable angina. Histological data on 14 autopsied patients. Atherosclerosis 1987;68:191–197.

13. Essed CE, van den Brand M, Becker AE. Transluminal coronary angioplasty and early restenosis. Fibrocellular occlusion after wall laceration. Br Heart J 1983;49:393–396.

14. Waller BF, McManus BM, Gorfinkel HJ, et al. Status of the major epicardial coronary arteries 80 to 150 days after percutaneous transluminal coronary angioplasty. Analysis of 3 necropsy patients. Am J Cardiol 1983;51:81–84.

15. Morimoto S, Mizuno Y, Hiramitsu S, et al. Restenosis after percutaneous transluminal coronary angioplasty—a histopathological study using autopsied hearts. Jpn Circ J 1990;54:43–56.

16. Morimoto S, Sekiguchi M, Endo M, et al. Mechanism of luminal enlargement in PTCA and restenosis: a histopathological study of necropsied coronary arteries collected from various centers in Japan. Jpn Circ J 1987;51:1101–1115.

17. Baughman KL, Pasternak RC, Fallon JT, Block PC. Transluminal coro-

nary angioplasty of postmortem human hearts. Am J Cardiol 1981; 48:1044–1047.

18. Waller BF, Pinkerton CA, Orr CM, Slack JD, VanTassel JW, Peters T. Restenosis 1 to 24 months after clinically successful coronary balloon angioplasty: a necropsy study of 20 patients. J Am Coll Cardiol 1991; 17:58B–70B.

19. Hinohara T, Selmon MR, Robertson GC, Braden L, Simpson JS. Directional atherectomy. New approaches for treatment of obstructive coronary and peripheral vascular disease. Circulation 1990;81:IV79–IV91.

20. Litvack F, Forrester JS, Grundfest WS, Mohr FW, Papaioannou T. The excimer laser: from basic science to clinical application. In: Vogel JHK, King III SB, eds. Interventional cardiology: future directions. St. Louis: CV Mosby, 1989:170–181.

21. Waller BF, Pinkerton CA, Rothbaum DA, et al. Restenosis tissue following hot tip laser, excimer laser, primary atherectomy and balloon angioplasty procedures: histologically similar intimal proliferation in 33 atherectomy patients (abstr). Circulation 1990;82(suppl III):312.

22. Forrester JS, Fishbein M, Helfant R, Fagin J. A paradigm for restenosis based on cell biology: clues for the development of new preventive therapies. J Am Coll Cardiol 1991;17:758–769.

23. Simpson JB, Johnson DE, Braden LJ, Gifford HS, Thapliyal HV, Selmon MR. Transluminal coronary atherectomy (TCA): Results in 21 human cadaver vascular segments (abstr). Circulation 1986;74(suppl II):202.

24. Safian RD, Gelbfish JS, Erny RE, Schnitt SJ, Schmidt DA, Baim DS. Coronary atherectomy. Clinical, angiographic, and histological findings and observations regarding potential mechanisms. Circulation 1990;82:69–79.

25. Hinohara T, Vetter JW, Rowe MH, et al. The effect of angiographic risk factors on the outcome of directional coronary atherectomy (abstr). J Am Coll Cardiol 1991;17:23A.

26. Ellis SG, de Cesare NB, Pinkerton CA, et al. Relation of stenosis morphology and clinical presentation to the procedural results of directional coronary atherectomy. Circulation 1991;84:644–653.

27. Hinohara T, Selmon MR, Robertson GC, et al. Angiographic predictors of restenosis following directional coronary atherectomy (abstr). J Am Coll Cardiol 1991;17:385A.

28. Ghazzal ZMB, Douglas JS, Holmes DR Jr., et al. Directional coronary atherectomy of saphenous vein grafts: recent multicenter experience (abstr). J Am Coll Cardiol 1991;17:219A.

29. Selmon M, Hinohara T, Robertson GC, Rowe MH, et al. Directional coronary atherectomy for saphenous vein graft stenoses (abstr). J Am Coll Cardiol 1991;17:23A.

30. Platko WP, Hollman J, Whitlow PL, Franco I. Percutaneous transluminal angioplasty of saphenous vein graft stenosis: long-term follow-up. J Am Coll Cardiol 1989;14:1645–1650.

31. Haine E, Materne P, Renkin J, Boland J, Wijns W. Contribution of a "Dotter effect" in directional coronary atherectomy: a quantitative angiography analysis (abstr). Eur Heart J 1991;12:395.

32. Garratt KN, Holmes DR Jr., Bell MR, et al. Restenosis after directional coronary atherectomy: differences between primary atheromatous and restenosis lesions and influence of subintimal tissue resection. J Am Coll Cardiol 1990;16:1665–1671.

33. de Cesare NB, Popma JJ, Whitlow PL, et al. Excision beyond the "normal" arterial wall with directional coronary atherectomy—acute and long-term outcome (abstr). J Am Coll Cardiol 1991;17:384A.

34. Simpson JB, Rowe MH, Selmon MR, et al. Restenosis following directional coronary atherectomy in de novo lesions of native coronary arteries. Circulation 1990;82(suppl III):313.

35. Simpson JB, Baim DS, Hinohara T, Cowley MJ, Smucker ML, Williams DO. Restenosis of de novo lesions in native coronary arteries following directional coronary atherectomy: multicenter experience (abstr). J Am Coll Cardiol 1991;17:346A.

36. de Bruyne B, Wijns W, Materne P, et al. Directional coronary atherectomy: results of the Belgian Multicenter Registry (abstr). Eur Heart J 1991;12:292.

37. Waller BF, Pinkerton CA, Orr CM, Slack JD, VanTassel JW. Two distinct types of restenosis lesions after coronary balloon angioplasty: intimal proliferation and atherosclerotic plaques only. An analysis of 20 necropsy patients (abstr). Circulation 1990;82(suppl III):314.

38. Ritchie JL, Hansen DD, Intlekofer MJ, Hall M, Auth DC. Rotational approaches to atherectomy and thrombectomy. Z Kardiol 1987;76(suppl 6):59–65.

39. Hansen DD, Auth DC, Vracko R, Ritchie JL. Rotational atherectomy in atherosclerotic rabbit iliac arteries. Am Heart J 1988;115:160–165.

40. Ahn SS, Auth D, Marcus DR, Moore WS. Removal of focal atheromatous lesions by angioscopically guided high-speed rotary atherectomy. Preliminary experimental observations. J Vasc Surg 1988;7:292–300.

41. Erbel R, O'Neill W, Auth D, et al. High-frequency rotablation of occluded coronary artery during heart catheterization. Cathet Cardiovasc Diagn 1989;17:56–58.

42. Teirstein PS, Ginsburg R, Warth DC, Hoq N, Jenkins NS, McCowan L. Complications of human coronary rotablation (abstr). J Am Coll Cardiol 1990;15:57A.

43. Hansen DD, Auth DC, Hall M, et al. Rotational endarterectomy in normal canine coronary arteries: preliminary report. J Am Coll Cardiol 1988;11:1073–1077.
44. O'Neill WW, Friedman HZ, Cragg D, et al. Initial clinical experience and early follow-up of patients undergoing mechanical rotary endarterectomy (abstr). Circulation 1989;80(suppl II):584.
45. Ginsburg R, Teirstein PS, Warth DC, Haq N, Jenkins NS, McCowan LC. Percutaneous transluminal coronary rotational atheroblation: clinical experience in 40 patients (abstr). Circulation 1989;80(suppl II):584.
46. Niazi KA, Brodsky M, Friedman HZ, Gangadharan V, Choksi N, O'Neill WW. Restenosis after successful mechanical rotary atherectomy with the Auth rotablator (abstr). J Am Coll Cardiol 1990;15:57A.
47. Buchbinder M, Warth D, O'Neill W, et al. Multi-center registry of percutaneous coronary rotational ablation using the rotablator (abstr). J Am Coll Cardiol 1991;17:31A.
48. Niazi K, Cragg DR, Strzelecki RN, Friedman HZ, Gangadharan V, O'Neill WW. Angiographic risk factors for coronary restenosis following mechanical rotational atherectomy (abstr). J Am Coll Cardiol 1991; 17:218A.
49. Dietz U, Erbel R, Rupprecht HJ, et al. Acute and longterm results after percutaneous transluminal coronary rotational angioplasty (PTCR) (abstr). Eur Heart J 1991;12:291.
50. Sketch MH Jr, Phillips HR, Lee MM, Stack RS. Coronary transluminal extraction–endarterectomy. J Invas Cardiol 1991;3:13–18.
51. Sketch MH Jr, O'Neill WW, Galichia JP, et al. The Duke Multicenter Coronary Transluminal Extraction–Endarterectomy Registry: acute and chronic results (abstr). J Am Coll Cardiol 1991;17:31A.
52. Meany TB, Grines CL, Choksi N, O'Neill WW. Early and late outcome following coronary transluminal extraction atherectomy: the Beaumont experience. Eur Heart J 1991;12:290.
53. Grundfest WS, Litvack F, Goldenberg T, et al. Pulsed ultraviolet lasers and the potential for safe laser angioplasty. Am J Surg 1985;150:220–226.
54. Litvack F, Grundfest WS, Goldenberg T, et al. Pulsed laser angioplasty: wavelength power and energy dependencies relevant to clinical application. Lasers Surg Med 1988;8:60–65.
55. Goldenberg T, Anderson WB, Kupfer S. Laser delivery systems. In: White RA, Grundfest WS, eds. Lasers in cardiovascular diseases: lasers, alternative angioplasty devices, and guidance systems. 2nd ed. Chicago: Year Book Medical Publishers, 1989:42–55.
56. Bresnahan JF, Litvack F, Margolis J, et al. Excimer laser coronary an-

gioplasty: initial results of a multicenter investigation in 958 patients (abstr). J Am Coll Cardiol 1991;17:30A.

57. Cook SL, Eigler NL, Shefer A, Goldenberg T, Forrester JS, Litvack F. Percutaneous excimer laser coronary angioplasty of lesions not ideal for balloon angioplasty. Circulation 1991;84:632–643.

58. Haase KK, Mauser M, Baumbach A, Voelker W, Karsch KR. Restenosis after excimer laser coronary atherectomy (abstr). Circulation 1990; 82(suppl III):672.

59. Margolis JR, Krauthamer D, Litvack F, et al. Six month follow-up of excimer laser coronary angioplasty registry patients (abstr). J Am Coll Cardiol 1991;17:218A.

60. Sanborn TA, Bittl JA, Torre SR. Procedural success, in-hospital events, and follow-up clinical and angiographic results of percutaneous coronary excimer laser-assisted angioplasty (abstr). J Am Coll Cardiol 1991; 17:206A.

61. Rothbaum D, Linnemeier T, Landin R. Excimer laser coronary angioplasty: angiographic restenosis rate at six month follow-up (abstr). J Am Coll Cardiol 1991;17:205A.

62. Unterecker W, Roubin G, Margolis J, et al. Excimer laser coronary angioplasty of saphenous vein grafts (abstr). J Am Coll Cardiol 1991; 17:23A.

· ·

CHAPTER 16

Restenosis: Recent Advances and Future Prospects

JAMES S. FORRESTER
PETER BARATH
BOJAN CERCEK
JAMES FAGIN

VIEWED from the perspective of patient outcome, preventive therapy of restenosis has been an abysmal failure over the 15 years since coronary angioplasty first began. Nonetheless, in the past 2 years new insights about the pathogenesis of restenosis have emerged. These new insights are helping us understand the cause of our previous failures to influence the restenosis rate. We will first describe these new ideas, then show how they illuminate our previous failures, and finally describe innovative approaches that hold promise for the ultimate prevention of restenosis following successful angioplasty.

New Ideas About Restenosis

Restenosis Rate Is No Longer 30%: Perhaps the most telling insight of the last 2 years has been the recognition that the problem of restenosis is considerably greater than the 30% rate originally reported. There is compelling evidence that the restenosis rate following balloon angioplasty is in the range of 40% to 55% (Table 16.1). The recognition of this

Table 16.1. Restenosis Rate as Determined by Coronary Angiography Before and After Angioplasty

	NO.	%
Nobuyoshi (1)	229	49
Pepine (2)	250	42
Vandormael (3)	129	52

increase in restenosis rate can most reasonably be traced to the remarkable serial angiographic study of Nobuyoshi and colleagues (1) in which patients were restudied at monthly intervals following successful percutaneous transluminal coronary angioplasty (PTCA). The angiographic restenosis rate at 6 months was 49%. Furthermore, the most comprehensive single angiographic study, comprising 520 patients treated by the M-HEART group (2) placed the angiographic restenosis rate at 42%, while Vandormael and coworkers placed the restenosis rate at 46% in a smaller angiographic follow-up study (3).

Is it possible that the restenosis rate has worsened as both the equipment and the techniques of angioplasty have dramatically improved? Remarkably, this is the most reasonable explanation for these results. Early in the history of balloon angioplasty, only the least complex lesions were treated. At the beginning of the 1980s, for instance, only 5% of patients were considered candidates for interventional therapy. Now the number of eligible patients is approximately 50% (4). Inclusion of more complex lesions carriers a higher risk for acute complications and apparently also a higher risk for restenosis. Concomitant with the inclusion of higher risk lesions has been the emergence of more rigorous angiographic criteria for the diagnosis of restenosis. Thus, whereas the 30% restenosis rate was based on clinical criteria of recurrent symptoms, the angiographic restenosis rate is independent of symptoms and includes patients who have no clinical evidence of recurrence. Given these data, in our view the best estimate of the restenosis rate following balloon angioplasty is 45%.

Restenosis Rate Is Independent of Method of Angioplasty: The past year has brought the first reports of restenosis rates using alternative methods of recanalization. These multicenter registries involve several thousand patients. Table 16.2 compares the restenosis rate following directional atherectomy (5), rotational atherectomy (6), excimer laser angioplasty (7), and laser balloon angioplasty (8) to conventional balloon

Table 16.2. Angiographic Restenosis After Different Methods
of Angioplasty

Balloon angioplasty (1)	49%
Directional atherectomy (5)	50%
Rotational atherectomy (6)	50%
Excimer laser (7)	46%
Laser balloon (8)	51%

angioplasty. Remarkably, although the angioplasty procedures involve different patients at different medical centers using different devices, obviously the restenosis rates cluster in the range of 45% to 50%. Thus, in addition to the conclusion that the restenosis rate following balloon angioplasty is no longer 30%, we can add a second remarkable insight from the past 2 years: the restenosis rate is independent of the method of angioplasty.

As we will see, this insight may be crucial to our understanding of the pathogenesis of restenosis. If the restenosis rate is independent of the method of angioplasty, then a logical speculation is that restenosis is a fundamental biologic process, that is, the general wound healing response. Expressed specifically within the blood vessel, the wound healing response is termed intimal hyperplasia. There is now powerful evidence that intimal hyperplasia is the anatomic substrate of the clinical and angiographic syndrome of restenosis (9–15).

Restenosis Rate Is Determined by Lesion Morphology: Late in 1990, Ellis and coworkers reported remarkable differences in the acute success rate for balloon angioplasty for lesions stratified by the AHA/ACC Task Force classification for degree of complexity (16). The complication rate for type A (short, noncomplex) lesions was 2%, whereas the acute complication rate for type C (long, complex) lesions was 21%. This insight confirmed the widely held belief of experienced interventionalists; it also catalyzed analogous subset analyses for restenosis. Whereas the 45% restenosis rate describes the patient population, it is totally inadequate for an individual lesion in a single patient. For different types of lesions, restenosis rates range from 10% to 65% (17).

At least four crucial anatomic variables determine restenosis rate: vessel type, length, residual stenosis, and lesion complexity. Lesions in vein grafts have a higher restenosis rate than coronary arterial locations. Lesions greater than 20 mm are at much greater risk for restenosis than short lesions (17). As shown by the study of Vandormael and colleagues (3; Figure 16.1), the restenosis rate progressively increases with lesion length, reaching levels severalfold higher when the subsets of longest and shortest lesions are compared. Several studies have shown that the lumen diameter following angioplasty is a potent determinant of restenosis rate (18,19). When the posttreatment coronary artery diameter is greater than 3 mm, for instance, the restenosis rate may be as low as 10% to 25% (Table 16.3). Finally, lesion complexity is a catchall term that includes factors such as the presence of intimal disruption and thrombosis, the curvature of the vessel segment treated, and the composition of the lesion. This understanding that lesion anatomy markedly influences restenosis rate is crucial, because analyses of future therapies for restenosis must necessarily include a description of the frequency of each lesion type. For instance, imagine that we find that the restenosis rate following placement of stents is less than 20%. Stents are placed in large-diameter vessels, however, so the appropriate risk–benefit comparison must be to nonstented vessels of similar residual diameter, not to the angioplasty population as a whole.

Definition of Restenosis and Hidden Pitfalls: The histopathology of the restenotic lesion was first established by autopsy in patients who died

Figure 16.1. The restenosis rate in 313 lesions according to initial lesion length at the time of coronary angioplasty. The restenosis rate increases approximately threefold between lesions less than 5 mm and those greater than 20 mm. (Reproduced with permission of the American College of Cardiology, from J Am Coll Cardiol 1987;10:250.)

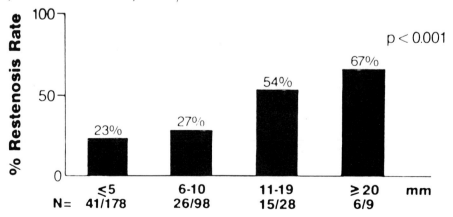

Table 16.3. Angiographic Restenosis Rate for Arteries Greater than 3 mm

Atherectomy (18)	23%
Intracoronary stents (19)	16%

several months after angioplasty, and later by tissue removed by atherectomy from living patients (9–15). The histologic appearance of restenotic tissue is independent of both the type and location of vascular injury. Thus balloon inflation, atherectomy, lasers, and even Gortex grafts produce the same response in peripheral and coronary arteries. The restenotic lesion consists of proliferating smooth muscle cells (SMCs) in a loose connective tissue matrix of proteoglycans and collagen. In this tissue mass, there is also an abundance of new capillaries, representing vigorous endothelial cell proliferation. The histologic pattern is termed intimal hyperplasia.

Intimal hyperplasia always follows significant vascular injury in animals (20). Assuming this same response occurs in man, then we must recognize an important semantic distinction. If we consider restenosis to be the angiographic representation of intimal hyperplasia, it probably occurs in every patient following angioplasty. Serruys and colleagues performed quantitative coronary arteriography in 342 patients at 1, 2, 3, or 4 months following balloon angioplasty. They observed that almost all lesions deteriorate to some extent by 120 days after coronary angioplasty (21). The important inference from these data is that the angiographic restenosis rate is entirely dependent on the measurement cut point selected by the investigator. Given the inherent inaccuracy in the quantitative measurement of small vessel contours by x-ray, the use of a single angiographic cut point to define the frequency of restenosis is a major limitation. Thus, the hidden pitfall is that angiographic cut points suggest that restenosis is present or absent, whereas histologic analysis clearly demonstrates hyperplasia "always" occurs but differs in magnitude.

The Pathogenesis of Restenosis: A Basis for Preventive Therapy

The pathogenesis of intimal hyperplasia following vascular injury is now being defined at cellular and molecular levels (22–24). Most methods of angioplasty cause circumferential removal of endothelial cells from the blood vessel surface. The dilating force causes fissures in the atheroma and stretches or tears the normal wall. When the dilating force exceeds the limit of the normal segment to stretch, the intima is torn and dissected. Platelets aggregate at injury site, releasing biologically active substances, the most important of which are growth factors. These growth factors induce both endothelial cells and SMCs to proliferate. Depending on the area of injury, endothelial cells cover the surface by about 1 week. Concomitant with coverage of the wound surface, the proliferating SMCs begin to produce increased cellular matrix, filling the tissue gap created by the original injury. As the healing response evolves over a period of several months, the typical histologic appearance of SMCs in a mass of extracellular matrix evolves. Typically this mass of intimal hyperplasia encroaches on the vascular lumen. When the mass of intimal hyperplasia is sufficiently large the angiographic and clinical syndromes of restenosis result.

Given our new understanding of the pathogenesis of hyperplasia, we can test pharmacologic interventions at each of the rate-limiting steps in the process (Table 16.4). In broad concept these therapies might interfere with platelet functions, growth factor release or action, SMC migration or replication, or extracellular matrix production. As described by O'Keefe in Chapter 4, however, clinical trials for pharmacologic prevention of restenosis have universally failed.

Why Have Clinical Trials Failed?

We can speculate as to the reasons why attempts to prevent restenosis over the past 15 years have failed (Table 16.5). First, the dose of the agent delivered to the injury site may have been inadequate. For instance, although thrombocytopenia substantially inhibits intimal hyperplasia in animals, antiplatelet agents have been entirely ineffective in humans. It is likely that the dose of antiplatelet agent at the injury site is inadequate to completely prevent platelet adhesion. Second, the timing of the drug administration may have been inappropriate. For instance, if a drug that inhibits proteoglycan synthesis is administered in the first week following injury, it would be much less likely to have an important effect on the mass of intimal hyperplasia than if it were administered in the period 2 weeks to 2 months following injury. Third, if the magnitude of the intimal hyperplasia response is relatively

Table 16.4. Potential Therapies in Restenosis

TARGET	ACTION	EXAMPLES
Platelets	Inhibit adhesion and aggregation	Aspirin, dipyridamole
	Block thromboxane receptor	Sulotroban
	Block IIa/IIIb fibrinogen receptor	Monoclonal antibodies
	Block thrombus formation	Hirudin
Inflammatory cells	Inhibit accumulation and activation	Steroids
	Inhibit activation	Fish oil
	Inhibit T lymphocytes	Cyclosporin A
SMC	Destroy SMCs	Vincristine/actinomycin
SMC receptor	Inhibit SMC growth	Heparin
	Antagonize PDGF action	Trapidil*
Synthetic SMC	Reduce secretory organelles	Colchicine, DMSO
Mesenchymal cells	Inhibit matrix synthesis	Retinoids
	Inhibit matrix synthesis	ACE inhibitor*

*The mechanism of action is not clearly established.
SMC = smooth muscle cells; PDGF = platelet-derived growth factor; DMSO = dimethyl sulfoxide; ACE = angiotensin-converting enzyme.

fixed, for example, a thickness of 0.75 mm, then the size of the residual lumen at the time of injury will be critical to subsequent development of restenosis. It follows that the removal of atheroma mass may be a necessary, although not sufficient, step for the prevention of restenosis. Finally, because intimal hyperplasia is the vascular response to injury, reducing the magnitude of injury might reduce the restenosis rate. These potential sources of failure are also the genesis of promising but untested solutions. The methodologies we will discuss aim for local delivery of therapies and reduction of balloon-induced vascular injury.

**Table 16.5. Reasons for Failure
of Clinical Trials**

Inadequate local drug concentration
Timing of therapy inappropriate
Inadequate residual lumen
Extensive injury area/depth

*One reasonable speculation is that
elimination of several of the above factors could substantially reduce the
restenosis rate.*

Preventing Restenosis: Three Innovative Solutions

Local Delivery of Drugs to Vessel Surface: The infusion–perfusion catheter is designed to increase the concentration of a therapeutic agent at
the injury site and to isolate the site while simultaneously measuring
blood flow. This can be achieved by the catheter shown in Figure 16.2.
Its essential components are a distal balloon for occluding the blood vessel, a central inflow–outflow lumen for perfusion of the vessel distal to
the balloon, a port just proximal to the balloon that allows delivery of
drugs, and a port just proximal to the balloon that allows sampling from
the treatment area.

The advantage of this system is that it allows continuous delivery of
oxygenated blood to the heart through the autoperfusion system, while
maintaining high concentration of an agent (e.g., an antithrombin such
as hirudin) in a specific area. While the local concentration can be made

Figure 16.2. The infusion–perfusion catheter. The catheter has a distal balloon
that occludes flow. The catheter has an autoperfusion construction in which
oxygenated blood enters a proximal lumen and exits a distal one, maintaining
distal perfusion. An additional lumen allows for local delivery of drugs and
sampling of the concentration of drugs and metabolites. (Photo produced with
permission of the patentor, Dr. T. A. DonMichael, Bakersfield, Calif.)

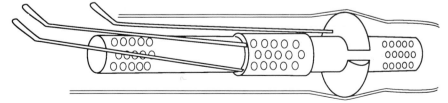

very high, the systemic concentration remains quite low. Finally, the sampling system allows the operator to measure the level of both drug concentration and important metabolites in the local treatment area.

Local Delivery to Vessel Wall—Injection Balloon: In principle it is also possible to deliver therapeutic substances into the vessel wall by high pressure local injection at the local angioplasty site. Figure 16.3 shows such a device developed by Barath in our laboratory. The balloon catheter has nipples on its external surface. As the balloon is inflated the nipples come into direct physical contact with the vessel wall. Drugs are injected directly into the vessel wall through these nipples. Plate XXIII shows an example of heparin delivery into the vessel wall. The current limitation of this technology is that the therapeutic solution rapidly disappears from the vessel wall following delivery. If this technique is to be successful, a method of retaining the drug within the vessel wall must be developed.

Reduction of Stretching and Tearing Injury—Cutting Balloon: An approach to reducing the tearing and stretching injury produced by balloon angioplasty has been developed by Barath and colleagues in our laboratory (25). The device consists of a balloon with tiny blades imbedded in its surface (Figure 16.4). The blades make radial incisions in the vessel surface. The magnitude of intimal hyperplasia induced by this type of radial cutting injury appears to be substantially less than that induced by stretching to a similar lumen diameter. Further, the residual lumen at 2 weeks is substantially larger than that obtained with conventional angioplasty, possibly because elastic recoil is limited.

Figure 16.3. The local drug delivery system. The catheter has nipples on its external surface that allow high-pressure injection of therapeutic solutions into the blood vessel wall.

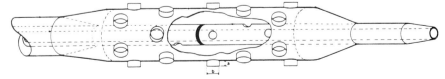

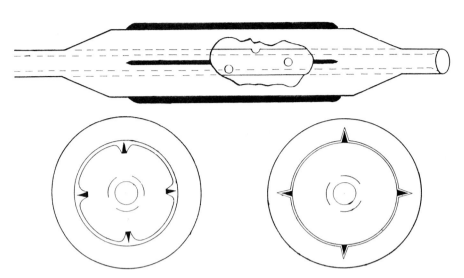

Figure 16.4. The cutting balloon. The catheter has small blades embedded in the balloon surface, which allow the operator to produce clean incisions in the vessel wall. The magnitude of intimal hyperplasia following these incisions is substantially less than that observed following conventional angioplasty.

Summary

In the past several years, research in the field of restenosis underwent dynamic and dramatic change. There are a series of new clinical insights: the restenosis rate is 45% (not 30%), is independent of the method of angioplasty, and is determined by anatomic features of the lesions treated. We also now understand that intimal hyperplasia, the biologic process responsible for restenosis, occurs in every treated vessel. Thus, the angiographic definition of restenosis rate using a measured cut point must be understood as entirely arbitrary. Combined with these new clinical insights is the first complete description of the temporal histologic sequence of restenotic lesion development. The lesion develops in definable phases, each of which presents the opportunity for pharmacologic interruption. Even with this new understanding of its pathogenesis, however, no pharmacologic intervention has yet had an impact on restenosis rate. We can speculate about the reasons for this failure. They include inadequate local concentration of the drug at the injury site, failure to remove atheroma mass, and excessive angioplasty-induced vascular trauma. These limitations can be reduced by development of new devices for local delivery with pharmacologic agents and reducing the magnitude of vascular injury induced by angioplasty. Thus, although our past attempts to prevent restenosis have been a dismal failure, the future is quite promising: one may reasonably speculate that major advances in prevention of restenosis will occur within this decade.

Acknowledgments: The authors wish to express their appreciation to the Medallions, United Hostesses and Grand Foundations for financial support, and to Ms. Dwana Williams for her managerial support, Ms. Ann Cummings for her word processing assistance, and Ms. Susan Schauer for her assistance in gathering the legend information.

References

1. Nobuyoshi M, Kimura T, Noksaka H, et al. Restenosis after successful coronary angioplasty: serial angiographic follow-up of 229 patients. J Am Coll Cardiol 1988;12:616–623.
2. Pepine C, Hirshfeld J, Macdonald R, et al. A controlled trial of corticosteroids to prevent restenosis after coronary angioplasty. Circulation 1990; 81:1753–1761.
3. Vandormael M, Deligonul U, Kern M, et al. Multilesion coronary angioplasty: clinical and angiographic follow-up. J Am Coll Cardiol 1987; 10:246–252.
4. Brown PW. The outlook for the coronary angioplasty industry. Report from Hambrecht and Quist Inc., December 1986.
5. Roger W, Potkin B, Solus D, Reddy S. Mode of death, frequency of healed and acute myocardial infarction, number of major epicardial coronary arteries severely narrowed by atherosclerotic plaque and heart weight in fatal atherosclerotic coronary artery disease: analysis of 889 patients studied at necropsy. J Am Coll Cardiol 1990;15:196–203.
6. Fourrier JL, Bertrand ME, Auth DC, Lablanche JM, Gommeaux A, Bertrand JM. Percutaneous coronary rotational angioplasty in humans: preliminary report. J Am Coll Cardiol 1989;14:1278–1282.
7. Rothbaum D, Linnemeier T, Landin R, Morgan S. Excimer laser coronary angioplasty: angiographic restenosis rate at 6 month follow-up. J Am Coll Cardiol 1991;17:205A.
8. Spears JR, Reyes VP, Wynne J, et al. Percutaneous coronary laser balloon angioplasty: initial results of a multicenter experience. J Am Coll Cardiol 1990;16:293–303.

9. Austin GE, Ratliff NB, Hollman J, Tabeil S, Phillips D. Intimal proliferation of smooth muscle cells as an explanation for recurrent coronary artery stenosis after coronary angioplasty. J Am Coll Cardiol 1985;6:369–375.

10. Block P, Myler R, Stertzer S, Fallon J. Morphology after transluminal angioplasty in human beings. N Engl J Med 1981;305:382–385.

11. Giraldo AA, Esposo OM, Meis JM. Intimal hyperplasia as a cause of restenosis after coronary angioplasty. Arch Pathol Lab Med 1985;109:173–175.

12. Gravanis MB, Roubin GS. Histopathologic phenomena at the site of coronary angioplasty. Human Pathol 1989;20:477–485.

13. Waller BF. Morphologic correlates of coronary angiographic patterns at the site of coronary angioplasty. Clin Cardiol 1988;11:817–822.

14. Potkin BN, Roberts WC. Effects of coronary angioplasty on atherosclerotic plaques and relation of plaque composition and arterial size to outcome. Am J Cardiol 1988;62:41–50.

15. Johnson DE, Hinohara T, Selmon MR, Braden LJ, Simpson JB. Primary peripheral arterial stenoses and restenoses excised by transluminal atherectomy: histopathologic study. J Am Coll Cardiol 1990;15:419–425.

16. Ellis SG, Vandormael MG, Cowley MJ, et al., and the Multivessel Angioplasty Prognosis Study Group. Coronary morphologic and clinical determinants of procedural outcome with angioplasty in multivessel coronary disease. Circulation 1990;82:1193–1202.

17. Webb J, Myler R, Shaw R, et al. Coronary angioplasty after coronary bypass surgery: initial results and late outcome in 422 patients. J Am Coll Cardiol 1991;16:812–820.

18. Hinohara T, Rowe M, Sipperly ME, et al. Restenosis following directional coronary atherectomy of native coronary arteries. J Am Coll Cardiol 1990;15:196A.

19. Ellis SG, Savage M, Baim D, et al. Intracoronary stenting to prevent restenosis: preliminary results of a multicenter study using the Palmaz–Schatz stent suggests benefit in selected high risk patients. J Am Coll Cardiol 1990;15:118A.

20. Schwartz RS, Murphy JG, Edwards WD, Camrud AR, Vlietstra RE, Holmes DR. Restenosis after balloon angioplasty: a practical proliferative model in porcine coronary arteries. Circulation 1990;82:2190–2200.

21. Serruys PW, Luijten HE, Beatt KJ, et al. Incidence of restenosis after successful coronary angioplasty: a time related phenomenon. A quantitative angiographic study in 342 consecutive patients at 1, 2, and 3 months. Circulation 1988;77:361–372.

22. Forrester JS, Fishbein MC, Helfant RH, Fagin J. A paradigm for restenosis based on cell biology: clues for the development of new preventive therapies. J Am Coll Cardiol 1991;17:758–769.

23. Cercek B, Fishbein MC, Forrester JS, Helfant RH, Fagin JA. Induction of insulin-like growth factor-1 m-RNA in rat aorta after balloon denudation. Circ Res 1990;66:1755–1760.

24. Cercek B, Sharifi B, Bailey EL, Forrester JS. Growth factors in pathogenesis of restenosis: Am J Cardiol 1991;68:24C–33C.

25. Barath P, Fishbein M, Sandor V, Yao F, Forrester J. Endovascular incisions with a novel device: a new approach to angioplasty. J Am Coll Cardiol 1991;17:235A.

Index